Praise for *Happy-People-Pills for All*

"A fascinating and provocative argument, beautifully made. This book challenges everything you believe about who deserves to be happy, and why."

—Daniel Gilbert, Harvard University, author of the bestseller
Stumbling on Happiness

"A game-changing contribution to philosophical debates about happiness. Its arguments are ambitious, novel, and philosophically focused and its discussion wide-ranging."

—Nicholas Agar, Victoria University of Wellington, author of
Humanity's End: Why We Should Reject Radical Enhancement

"*Happy-People-Pills* is a great examination of the increasingly contentious issue of modifying our bodies and our moods through pharmacology. Laying out in precise detail the arguments for and against, Walker explains the importance of happiness for health, life, and love and gives a powerful case for using chemical technology to make more of it."

—Patrick Hopkins, Millsaps College, author of *Sex/Machine:
Readings in Culture, Gender, and Technology*

Happy-People-Pills For All

Mark Walker

WILEY Blackwell

This edition first published 2013
© John Wiley & Sons Inc

Wiley-Blackwell is an imprint of John Wiley & Sons, formed by the merger of Wiley's global
Scientific, Technical and Medical business with Blackwell Publishing.

Registered Office
John Wiley & Sons Ltd, The Atrium, Southern Gate, Chichester, West Sussex, PO19 8SQ, UK

Editorial Offices
350 Main Street, Malden, MA 02148-5020, USA
9600 Garsington Road, Oxford, OX4 2DQ, UK
The Atrium, Southern Gate, Chichester, West Sussex, PO19 8SQ, UK

For details of our global editorial offices, for customer services, and for information about how to
apply for permission to reuse the copyright material in this book please see our website at
www.wiley.com/wiley-blackwell.

The right of Mark Walker to be identified as the author of this work has been asserted in
accordance with the UK Copyright, Designs and Patents Act 1988.

Library of Congress Cataloging-in-Publication Data
Walker, Mark (Mark Alan)
   Happy-people-pills for all / Mark Walker.
        pages cm
   Includes bibliographical references and index.
   ISBN 978-1-118-35738-5 (cloth : alk. paper) – ISBN 978-1-118-35747-7
(pbk. : alk. paper) 1. Medication abuse. 2. Pharmaceutical ethics. 3. Happiness.
I. Title. II. Title: Happy people pills for all.
   RM146.W35 2013
   362.29′9 – dc23
                                                        2012050383

A catalogue record for this book is available from the British Library.

Cover image: © pepifoto / iStockphoto
Cover design by E&P

Typeset in 10.5/13pt Minion by Laserwords Private Limited, Chennai, India
Printed in Malaysia by Ho Printing (M) Sdn Bhd

1   2013

To Mardi and Alan
(to whom I owe a great measure of my happiness)

Contents

Acknowledgments

Looking back I realize that I don't even know when exactly I decided to write a book on happy-people-pills. The idea percolated for some time; I'm just not sure when it metamorphosed into a "project." Still, it is clear to me that the many debts I accumulated precede the actual writing of this book.

Long before I turned to normative issues, I had two wonderful PhD supervisors at the Australian National University. Huw Price provided some wonderful mentoring when I first arrived. Price eventually took a job in Sydney, citing the experience as my supervisor as his reason for leaving. Peter Menzies was next on the chopping block. Although they worked with me on metaphysical and epistemological issues, Huw and Peter left an indelible mark on how I think about and write philosophy. I am very grateful for their guidance and patience. Any errors in this manuscript are directly attributable to their mentoring and they should be blamed equally.

The dissertation that I submitted, "Becoming Gods," argued that if we are to complete the grand project of philosophy, the unity of thought and being, we would need to attempt to enhance human beings to make them more godlike. It is a professional secret, because it is such a professional embarrassment, that philosophers have long compared favorably their cognitive abilities to that of gods. (Plato tells us that we must avoid the siren calls of the city and obey the imperative to realize the godlike part of ourselves. Hegel describes all of human history as a process whereby the first god-man is created at the end of history. The first god-man is Hegel himself – what are the chances? It is as incredible as Lou Gehrig getting Lou Gehrig's disease. This embarrassment is not just old-school: Donald Davidson says our cognitive abilities compare favorably with an omniscient interpreter. Who knew?) My dissertation was written in the conditional, because it seemed to me an unanswered question whether we ought to enhance humans.

I left academic philosophy for a time but I continued to think about the issue of human enhancement, and so my interests turned from "real" philosophy (as we used to say as graduate students) – epistemology and metaphysics – to ethics. My first thought was that the issue of human enhancement could be framed within perfectionist ethics. I soon ran into two problems. The first was that perfectionism is often (but not always) couched in terms of the perfection of human nature. To ask about enhancing human nature is to ask something that cannot even be asked within this version of perfectionism. I soon discovered the problem is endemic: one of the touchstones of most ethical theorizing in the history of philosophy is that ethical theory must be in accordance with human nature. Unfortunately, this means that most of the history of ethics can't help us with the most important question of this century: Should we enhance human nature? The second problem is that perfectionism seems to have little to say about happiness. The problem is not so much that perfectionism downplays happiness, although this too is a problem, but it doesn't tell us why happiness is not as important as the development of physical, moral, and intellectual excellence. The usual perfectionist answer to why physical, moral, and intellectual attributes ought to be perfected – because they are part of human nature – seems to me to apply equally well to happiness. In the end the only reason I could see for perfectionists ignoring the psychological state of happiness is that they have always done so.

It was about this time that I entered into email correspondence with David Pearce, probably the world's leading expert on the enhancement of hedonistic states. David was always generous with his time, answering questions about the pharmacology of happiness. His websites are a treasure trove of information for those thinking about the enhancement of happiness: www.hedweb.com. David is part of an academic underclass: an independent scholar. Those of us who are lucky enough to be paid for our scholarly activity don't do enough to acknowledge their work. So, let me go on record: thank you, David!

Nick Agar commented upon Chapters 3 and 4. I have also benefited from a number of conversations with Nick about issues of human enhancement. I owe debts of gratitude to a couple of colleagues in my department. Professor Jean-Paul Vessel was kind enough to provide detailed comments on Chapters 3 and 4. (Professor Vessel, incidentally, may be one of the hyperthymic that I discuss extensively in this work. I say "may" because I am assuming his exalted hedonic states are au naturel.) Professor Danny Scoccia was kind enough to provide detailed comments on Chapters 3, 4, and 5. Professor Jamie Bronstein, one floor down in the history department, generously commented on a first draft of the manuscript. The style and substance are much improved as a result of her efforts. Thanks, Nick, JP, Danny and Jamie!

The folks at Wiley-Blackwell are wonderful. Lindsay Bourgeois and Jennifer Bray are great to work with. Glynis Baguley did heroic work as copy-editor. (If paid by the correction, she should be fabulously wealthy.) Jeff Dean is a great editor: he is quick to respond to emails and offers great advice. Thanks, Jeff!

Last but not least is my debt to my family. I owe my children, Chantal and Danielle, for making me realize the urgent need in this world for happy-people-pills. (I can hear them already: "Ha, ha, very funny dad.") I would be terribly remiss if I did not thank my wife, Dawn Rafferty, who has helped with every facet and stage of this book. (Helping me with this book has made her realize the urgent need in this world for happy-people-pills.) Finally, as for my parents, Mardi and Alan, I dedicate this book to them as a small token of my debt.

1

Introductory

The title of this book, *Happy-People-Pills for All*, is not offered as some bait and switch tactic. So, yes, to put it bluntly, I am arguing for a future where there is a cheap and readily available supply of happiness-boosting pills for everyone. Having spoken and written on this subject for a few years now, I know all too well that many readers, at least initially, will be skeptical. Indeed, some will even recoil in horror at the idea. However, I hope to show in this introductory chapter that the idea is at least worthy of consideration. By the end of the book I hope you will be asking where you can obtain your dose of happy-people-pills.

1.1 The Ends: Greater Happiness

The happy-people-pills for all project has both a means and an end. The means is to use pharmacology; the end is to increase our happiness. Surely the end or goal is innocent enough. The desire for happiness seems unquestionable; we are all accustomed to hearing testimony as to the importance of happiness in our lives. The refrains "I just want you to be happy," "I just want my children to be happy," "I'm not looking to be rich or famous, just happy" are common. There seems to be no reason to doubt the sincerity of such sentiments, and they seem to attest to the utmost importance of happiness in our lives.

Colloquially we might refer to our slightly tipsy colleagues at the staff party as getting 'happy,' but I am not proposing intoxication for all (at least

Happy-People-Pills For All, First Edition. Mark Walker.
© 2013 John Wiley & Sons, Inc. Published 2013 by John Wiley & Sons, Inc.

not in this work). Rather, by 'happy' I mean what I take people to mean when they make the remarks we just noted, e.g., "I just want my children to be happy." To be sure, I'm not suggesting that the nature of happiness is transparent – far from it. The meaning of happiness figures prominently in this work; indeed, there is an entire chapter devoted to the subject. But even at this preliminary stage it may help to say something on the topic.

The term 'happiness,' I argue in Chapter 3, has both an affective and a cognitive component. The primary affective component is that of positive moods and emotions. In this sense, you are happy if your moods tend to be described by such terms as 'joy' or 'contentment.' A person who experiences frequent positive moods and emotions we would say is a happy person. The cognitive aspect is related to being pleased. So, for example, if walking my dog pleases me, then I may be said to be happy. Happiness in this sense is cognitive because it says something about my view about walking my dog: I find it pleasing. Of course there are many things that we may find pleasing; there are a huge number of ways to fill in the blank in "I am pleased that _____." The cognitive component of happiness is that the fact that I have a certain mental state – "being pleased," happiness – is not the object that fills in the blank. If one enjoys a cold beer on a hot day, it would be wrong to say that happiness *is* a cold beer. Happiness is to be understood as being pleased *by* the cold beer. The beer is the cause of the pleasure, not the pleasure itself. Thus, the happiest amongst us are those most often in a positive mood and who are frequently pleased with the things they are thinking about. The unhappiest are those who experience sadness and other negative emotions, and who take little pleasure in what they are thinking about. As noted, we will discuss happiness in more detail below; the hope here is to have sketched it sufficiently to see that I am attempting to capture what we mean by 'happy' in claims such as, "I just want my children to be happy." It is the wish for them that they generally be in a positive mood and take pleasure in their lives. The wish for happiness for our loved ones is not for a life of intoxication.

With this understanding of happiness in hand, it may seem that we should revisit the wish "just to be happy." Positive moods and being pleased about what we are thinking about may not seem enough. We will consider the question of the role of happiness in the good life in Chapter 4, and I will argue that there are good reasons to think there is more to the good life than happiness. The upshot is that I will recommend that we should hope for more than "only to be happy." Still, I believe that happiness is a very important component of the good life. In any event, whether we think there is more to the good life than happiness (as I do), or we think there is nothing more to the good life than happiness, we should recognize the value of the goal of happy-people-pills, making people happier. As noted, the wish translates into hoping for more frequent positive moods and being more pleased. And this is precisely what happy-people-pills promise: more positive moods, and as a consequence, to be more pleased about things.

1.2 The Means: Pharmacology

No doubt it is the means, that is, popping pills, rather than the end, happiness, of the happy-people-pills-for-all project that most people object to. The idea of taking pills to increase happiness is one that we are familiar with: it is a common practice (at least in many Western nations) of health care practitioners to prescribe various mood-altering pharmacological agents. We have seen a veritable army of antidepressants enter the psychiatrist's medicine chest: drugs like Sertraline, Escitalopram, Fluoxetine, and Bupropion go by trade names that are household words: 'Zoloft,' 'Lexapro,' 'Prozac,' and 'Wellbutrin,' to mention but a few. One would have had to be living in a very deep cave for many years to be unaware of the scientific and philosophical controversies that have swirled around the practice of prescribing antidepressants. A large number of academic and popular works have repeatedly asked: Do the drugs work? Are they over-prescribed? Are they under-prescribed? Do people become dependent? Do antidepressants simply mask the underlying psychological or social causes of depression? While these questions are important, they are not our main concern. We are after bigger game: the use of pharmacological agents to boost the moods of both those diagnosed as depressed and those in the so-called "normal" or "healthy" range of happiness

Invariably, talk of enhancing the happiness of those not clinically depressed invokes images or vague memories of Huxley's *Brave New World*, where citizens regularly take the fictional happy-pill 'soma' as a matter of course. The stereotype suggests taking mood enhancers is not like being intoxicated but equivalent to becoming an emotional zombie. Again, this is not the sort of happiness I am advocating, and combating this stereotype is a going concern of this work.

At least some reason for thinking that taking pharmacological agents will not result in a society of zombies can be derived from a real-world study conducted by Dr. David Healy. Healy had healthy volunteers – mostly medical professionals – take antidepressants in a "cross-over" study. One of two antidepressants, Zoloft and Reboxetine, were randomly (and blindly) given to participants for two weeks, followed by two weeks off where subjects took nothing – a clean-out period – then the study concluded with participants taking the other antidepressant for two weeks. Healy describes one of the surprising findings:

> Our focus group met two weeks after the study ended. We already knew that almost everyone preferred one of the two drugs. But two-thirds rated themselves as "better than well" on one of the two drugs. Although this was a study of wellbeing, antidepressants weren't supposed to make people who were normal feel "better than well." Not even Peter Kramer had said this. The argument of his famous *Listening to Prozac* was that people who were mildly depressed became better than well. Here, people who had never been depressed were claiming to be in some way better than normal.*

The fact that two thirds of these "normal and healthy" volunteers felt "better than well" is, as Healy intimates, quite startling: "antidepressants weren't supposed to make people who were normal feel "better than well." "

That Healy found the result of this study surprising is perhaps surprising in itself. After all, it seems a fair question to ask: why shouldn't antidepressants make persons in the normal range of happiness, that is, showing no signs of clinical depression, get a mood boost from antidepressants as well? It is hard to be sure but I suspect there is a tendency to think of psychopharmacological agents as falling into one of two categories: repairing mood and other psychological disorders, or cognitively distorting. The latter category would include such substances as alcohol, marijuana, heroin, etc. Antidepressants are in the former category. They treat an ailment just as aspirin treats pain. Aspirin relieves pain but does not boost pleasure: you can't use aspirin to get an enhanced feeling of pleasure. Similarly, according to this line of thought, antidepressants relieve depression but they do not promote positive moods.

However, there is another model we might consider. Rather than think of pharmacological interventions as "relieving" we might think that some interventions "boost," just as giving children injections of growth hormone is thought to boost their height. Typically such injections are provided for children who are projected to be in the "below average" height range,

---

* Healy, *Let Them Eat Prozac*, 180. A word on the conventions of this book: Substantive notes are at the bottom of the page. Further references and purely scholarly points are marked as endnotes.

and so might be thought of as "relieving" children of the (mostly) social challenges of being far below average height. Of course, injections "relieve" short stature by boosting height. There is no reason to suppose that the same shots might not be given to a child projected to be in the average range to boost them into the above average range. (I'm making a purely theoretical point here; I'm certainly not recommending this.)

So, in thinking about the efficacy of antidepressants there are at least two models we should consider: we might think that antidepressants work by "relieving" patients of depressed states in the way that aspirin relieves pain, or that they boost moods in the way that growth hormone boosts height. Very little work has gone into sorting out which of these is the best model, so it is perhaps not surprising that we should have fallen more or less uncritically into the "relief only" model. I can only conjecture that we may be misled by the name: 'antidepressant.' If 'antidepressants' were more commonly referred to as 'mood boosters,' then I suspect we would be less surprised. Mood boosters could in theory boost the moods of both those diagnosed as clinically depressed and those who are normally happy.

In any event, the point here is to provide some preliminary indication that the suggestion that we ought to boost the moods of the normally happy is not equivalent to the idea that we ought to become wasted zombies. Most of the nineteen participants in the study functioned quite normally. Indeed, one of the primary purposes of the study was to investigate the question of whether the antidepressant Zoloft caused "emotional blunting." Healy summarized the results thus:

> Chasing the question of whether Zoloft caused emotional blunting, half the group said it had given them a "nothing bothers me" feeling. Reactions were split about this: Some liked the effect; others found it made them emotionally dead. Reboxetine, in contrast, didn't seem to make anyone feel indifferent – calm, perhaps, but not indifferent. Its effects were better described as energizing – again, good for some but not for others.[1]

We will discuss the study some more below – as we shall see, the study is certainly not all glad tidings for happy-people-pills. For the moment the take-home message is this: two antidepressants were used in the study, and only one had any "zombie" effect, and only on half the participants. So, the effect is not a necessary consequence of mood boosters. As will be argued, this is not to suggest that we ought to be satisfied with the current stable of antidepressants. Far from it. In Chapter 7 we will outline a research program for creating better, more advanced pharmacological agents.

1.3   The Biological Basis of Happiness

The happy-people-pills-for-all project depends critically on a scientific insight: happiness is rooted in our neurophysiology and neurochemistry, and indeed, to a large degree, in our genes. It is worth thinking a little about what science tells us about the nature of happiness.

First, an admission: we are just now making serious scientific headway in understanding the neurochemistry, neurophysiology, and genetics of happiness. Yet, even at this early stage, this much seems clear: there are significant neurochemical differences between people who are chronically happy and people who are chronically unhappy. Some of these differences are to be explained in terms of neurochemicals such as serotonin: happier people tend to have more serotonin than those who are unhappy.[2] This is by no means the only difference, and, again, science is still in its infancy in this department, but serotonin appears to be important. A point that will loom large in our subsequent discussion is that not simply are there such neurophysiological differences, but these differences are due, to a significant degree, to individual genetic differences. As we shall see, this has disturbing consequences for the view that we are responsible for our own happiness. After all, we are not responsible for our genes, so to the extent that our happiness is rooted in our genes, we are not responsible for this large influence on our happiness.

Let me hasten to point out that I am not advocating some sort of genetic determinism, specifically, that our individual levels of happiness are due entirely to our genes. To say that genes have a significant influence is not to say that our happiness is solely caused by our genes, any more than saying that since there are genetic influences that determine our height is to claim that genes are solely responsible for our height. Non-genetic influences on height are evident in cases of malnutrition or serious childhood diseases that may inhibit a child's growth. But even while acknowledging non-genetic influences, genetic influences on an individual's height are undeniable: in Western nations where most children grow up under favorable environmental conditions, their height compared to the societal norm is determined to a large extent by genes. Similarly, how happy we are compared with others in society is determined to a large extent by the genes we inherit from our parents. The idea that there is a genetic component to happiness is generally acknowledged, at least with respect to those diagnosed with depression. Again, this is not to say that a person's environment has nothing to do with whether they are depressed or not, but it is to say that some of the explanation for susceptibility to depression is genetically based. However, the fact that genetics affect the happiness of those in the normal range is not widely appreciated beyond specialist circles.

The analogy with height is instructive: it is generally accepted that some forms of dwarfism have a genetic component. But of course genes influence the whole range of observed human heights. Similarly, genes do not simply influence those who are clinically depressed, but also contribute to a range of happiness in the so-called 'normally happy' population as well.

Consider Figure 1.1. This graph tells us what we all know: there are very few extremely short people and very few extremely tall people. Most of us fall somewhere in the middle, so human height fits the classic bell curve model. In North America, for example, the average height of adults is approximately 5ft 7in,[†] with very few people under 4 feet or over 7 feet. The same bell graph can be used to describe human happiness (Figure 1.2).

One point of the graphs is to break the tendency to think of human mood propensity as falling into just two categories: those who are depressed, and those who are not depressed. Of course these two categories are perfectly legitimate, just as we can divide human stature into two categories: dwarves and not dwarves. But in both cases there are further distinctions of interest. The 'not dwarves' category includes persons of average height and

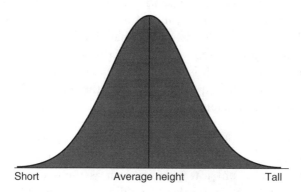

Figure 1.1 Human stature.

[†] There are of course differences in average height when other factors are considered: sex, ethnic background, year of birth, and so on. None of this affects the main point here: human height falls on a normal curve.

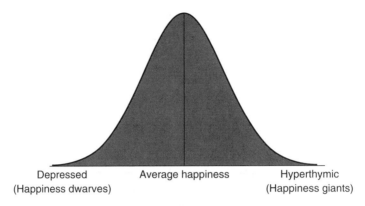

Figure 1.2   Human happiness "stature."

"giants" – extremely tall individuals. A similar point holds with happiness: there are subdivisions within the 'not depressed' range. Some people are just above the cut-off from depression. At the far end are the hyperthymic. The hyperthymic are the "giants" among the normally happy: the happiest 5 to 10 percent. If we could convert their happiness into stature, they would be over about 6ft 1.[3]

A word about the term 'hyperthymia' is perhaps in order. Although it does not have any agreed-upon clinical definition, sometimes the term is used to indicate a pathology, in particular, sometimes it is associated with 'manic'-type personalities and with other characteristics such as risky behaviors, pathological rashness, and insomnia. I'm using 'hyperthymic' in a non-pathological sense to identify the happiest part of the population. Most of us know people who we might describe as 'unusually happy' who don't exhibit pathologies. It is these individuals of whom we shall use the term 'hyperthymia.' It is true that amongst the top 5 to 10 percent of the happiest people we should expect to find some who exhibit pathologies. Of course there is no suggestion that their pathologies are desirable or part of the happy-people-pills-for-all project. Again the analogy with height is instructive: amongst the tallest 5 to 10 percent of the population we will find those with physical maladies such as tumors on the pituitary gland. We would not look to those so afflicted as a model for increasing human height.

The same point about a variety of gradations within the normal range can be made using the grade point idiom (Table 1.1). To convert the happiness of the hyperthymic to a letter grade, they are as rare as the A+ student.

Table 1.1 Happiness grades

Binary classification	Depressed	Normal or healthy range of happiness			
Preponderance of positive moods	Very low	Below average	Average	Above average	Highest (the hyperthymic)
Percentage of the total population	10	20	40	20	10
Happiness "grade"	F–D	C	B	A	A+

Most non-clinically depressed persons will fall into the C and B range of happiness.

As with most analogies, it is possible to misconstrue this one: it makes it sound as if more happiness is always better in the way that one might think a higher grade is always better. We will give a reasonable amount of attention to the idea that it is possible to be "too happy" in Chapter 6. It is worth noting too that it is not obvious that an A+ is always better, all considered. An A+ student who achieves his remarkable grade point average at the expense of alienating his friends and family may not be better off, all considered.

It is the happy giants that are of particular interest to us. As a group, they have not been extensively studied. Indeed, the existence of the hyperthymic surprises even mental health care professionals: Dr. Friedman, a psychiatrist, relates the case of a woman that came to him seeking advice in connection with the loss of her husband. Within the last year the woman's husband had died of cancer and she had lost her job. Despite the terrible circumstances, the woman had not sought out Friedman as a patient herself but for advice about her son who was having a difficult time coping with the loss of his father. Friedman says that he was intrigued by the woman's ability to cope with her circumstances:

> Despite crushing loss and stress, she was not at all depressed – sad, yes, but still upbeat. I found myself stunned by her resilience. What accounted for her ability to weather such sorrow with buoyant optimism? So I asked her directly.
>
> "All my life . . . I've been happy for no good reason. It's just my nature, I guess." But it was more than that. She was a happy extrovert, full of energy and enthusiasm who was indefatigably sociable. And she could get by with five or six hours of sleep each night.[4]

The bottom line for us: there are winners and losers in the genetic lottery for happiness. The woman who piqued Dr. Friedman's curiosity had won the genetic lottery for happiness: it is, as she says, just her nature to be happy.

It will be helpful at this point to draw a distinction between 'happy pills' and 'happy-people-pills.' The former is a slang term for a variety of pharmacological agents, such as Valium, presently on the market. 'Happy-people-pills' refers exclusively to pharmacological agents that will re-create for the rest of us what the hyperthymic have through the stochastic or random process of natural selection. That is, the hope is to put in pill form what the happiest amongst us have received genetically: a pill to allow the rest of us to become happy giants.

What I will propose in Chapter 7 is that we "reverse-engineer" the happy giants: look to see what it is about the biology of the hyperthymic that makes them so happy and put this in pill form for the rest of us. I provide reasons in this same chapter for thinking that the process of reverse-engineering the hyperthymic could take approximately ten years and ten billion dollars. We may not have to wait that long for a pharmacological boost: I will also argue that there is reason to hope that at least some may benefit from experimenting with our current stable of antidepressants. But, and this is an important qualification, there are well-known deficiencies with our current stable of antidepressants, so using them would only be a stopgap measure.

1.4 Therapy versus Enhancement

Happy-people-pills for all seeks to boost the happiness of all – at least those who desire to boost their happiness. As noted, this includes those in the lowest range of happiness – the clinically depressed – and persons in the "normal range" of happiness. I have indicated too that genes play a causal role in the moods of all of us, not just the depressed. This suggests (but hardly necessitates) that there is no significant technical or scientific challenge to boosting the happiness of those in the normal range as compared with the challenge of boosting the depressed into the normal range with pharmacological agents. It should be obvious that the fact that the scientific and technological challenges are similar is in itself no reason for pursuing the use of happy-people-pills for those in the normal range. After all, this would ignore the question of whether there are other non-scientific and non-technological dissimilarities.

One often cited difference is that there is a clear moral difference between therapeutic and enhancement uses of happy-people-pills. Certainly public perception acknowledges a large difference: most citizens in Western democracies agree that, at least in some cases, pharmacology is an appropriate means to treat depression, but often recoil in horror at the prospect of the normally happy availing themselves of happy-people-pills. Thus, the therapy versus enhancement distinction is important because it is often cited as justification for using pharmacology for the depressed, but not for the normally happy. For instance, even Leon Kass, one of the most prominent critics of pharmacological enhancement of happiness, thinks that it is appropriate, at least in some cases, to use the family of antidepressants known collectively as SSRIs (selective serotonin reuptake inhibitors) to treat some forms of depression.[5] At least part of his reasoning seems to be that treating depression is a matter of therapy, rather than enhancement. Therapy here is understood as restoring "normal functioning," but Kass will have no truck with the idea that we should use pharmacology for enhancement purposes, to boost within the normal range, or, more radically, beyond what is possible given human nature. In contrast, happy-people-pills for all says that everyone – every consenting adult, that is – should have access to happy-people-pills. And while Kass and I are at loggerheads, there is also a third possibility: pharmacology should not be available to anyone, including the depressed. To keep these straight, it will help to provide some names to these positions.

'Bioconservatives' endorse the view that the use of pharmacology for therapeutic purposes is permissible, but the use of pharmacology for enhancement purposes is not permissible. Thus, Kass is a 'bioconservative.' We will consider some of his criticisms below, most of which revolve around the idea that happy-people-pills are "dehumanizing." In any event, bioconservatives can consistently maintain that pharmacology is underutilized presently, that is, we should be doing more to deploy happy-people-pills in therapeutic cases.[‡] For example, the World Health Organization predicts that depression will become the second leading cause of death by the year 2020, so one can easily imagine bioconservatives calling for increased use of pharmacology as a means to combat depression.[6] On the other hand, we may think of 'bioabolitionists' as those who believe that

---

[‡] Kass thinks that antidepressants are overprescribed. I am simply making a theoretical point that it would not be inconsistent for a bioconservative to call for greater therapeutic use of pharmacology.

pharmacology is always inappropriate, even as a therapeutic intervention. Amongst mainstream mental health care professionals there is pretty near consensus that bioabolitionism is wrong: at least some pharmacological interventions are appropriate at least some of the time. Naturally, this still leaves lots of room for disagreement in the quest to answer the questions: which pharmacological agents should be used on which patients and for how long?

'Bioprogressivism,' the view advocated here, stands in agreement with bioconservatives in endorsing the therapeutic uses of pharmacology. So, bioconservatives and bioprogressives are united against abolitionists on this point. Where bioprogressives and bioconservatives part company is on the question of whether happy-people-pills should be used for enhancement purposes, to make people feel "better than well," to invoke Peter Kramer's famous phrase.[7] Our primary focus is on the dispute between happy-people-pills progressives and conservatives: the prospect of enhancing the happiness of "normally happy" people. This is not to say that the happiness of those diagnosed with depression is irrelevant or merely a 'side-issue.' Rather, the argument is that if we accept happy-people-pills for the enhancement of happiness of persons in the normal range of happiness, then it seems we have at least as strong a reason to accept it for therapeutic treatment of the depressed.

Our distinction between happy-people-pills conservatives and happy-people-pills progressives is made in terms of a therapy/enhancement distinction which itself has come under extensive scrutiny and criticism. One reason for skepticism is the fact that there looks to be no sharp demarcation between those who are classified as depressed and those in the normal or healthy range. To make the point, let us think again about human height. Figure 1.3 indicates what we all know: people come in a wide range of heights.

Using these data we might define, for example, three categories: 162cm to 194cm in height is 'normal height,' while 'short' refers to persons under 162cm and 'tall' to persons over 194cm. But we can see that there is a real worry that these categories are somewhat arbitrary. After all, it is not as if we find some natural break in human height that separates people into three height categories: under 150cm, 170–80cm, and over 200cm. If people fell naturally into one of these three height categories with no overlap, then we would have some reason to think that our definitions of 'short,' 'normal,' and 'tall' cut nature at its joints, for in this hypothetical scenario there are no persons in the in-between areas, that is, in the 151–179cm range and in the

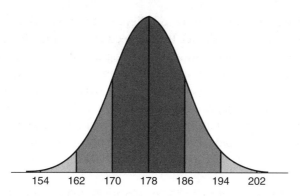

Figure 1.3 Population versus height in cm.

181–199cm range. Given that human height is better represented by our graph with a continuous normal curve, we can see the arbitrary nature of our definitions. It seems we could just as easily have defined 'short' as being under 150cm in height or under 130cm in height, or under 138.3cm in height. In other words, we could take any particular height as a possible cut-off point for one of these categories. The fact that the curve is continuous means that there will be some people who lie just on one side of the distinction or the other. So, for each proposed cut-off point it seems we can ask: why not just a little bit one way or the other on the normal curve? The point here is not that we cannot rigorously define any particular cut-off point: we might say that 'short' means one standard deviation from the mean, and have a well-defined measure of one standard deviation. But this does not solve the problem of *justifying* the cut-off point of one standard deviation: why not one and a half or two standard deviations as the cut-off point for 'short'?

A similar point seems to apply to our happiness curve (Figure 1.3). Just as there are no discontinuities in the populations that might underwrite the categories of short, normal, and tall persons, so too it is the case that there are non-continuous populations of 'depressed,' 'normal,' and 'hyperthymic' persons. Anywhere we happen to draw a line between short and normal, and between depressed and normal, it seems we will have some element of arbitrariness.

At least some bioconservatives are happy to admit that there is some arbitrariness to the line drawing in such cases. Francis Fukuyama, for example, notes that as a matter of policy we must sometimes stipulate rigid divisions where it is implausible to think that such rigid divisions cut nature at its joints.[8] Consider that in some jurisdictions 18 is the legal drinking age. Are we really to believe that persons who are 17 years, 11 months, and 29 days old lack the intellectual and moral development of someone a day older that justifies permitting the latter but not the former to partake of alcohol? Obviously there are many people younger than 18 who are more responsible than many people over 18, but our policy does not recognize this. Policy is a blunt instrument. Still, we seem to have little choice here. We could hardly leave it to the individuals in question to decide. Most 13-year-olds will attest to their nearly infinite maturity. Nor would we want to leave the drinking age to the discretion of sales clerks at liquor stores.

Part of the reason that some bioconservatives do not find it troubling to admit that such distinctions are *somewhat* arbitrary is that clearly it does not follow that the distinction is *entirely* arbitrary. It is not arbitrary to say that five-year-olds are too young to be permitted to drink alcohol and 40-year-olds are old enough. So, some people are clearly too young to drink, and some clearly old enough to drink, and then there is the grey area in between. As a practical matter we cannot always allow grey areas in policy, and so sometimes we are forced to draw precise lines where none exist in nature. By a similar token, the bioconservative can admit that the line between depressed and not-depressed is grey, but as a matter of policy we may have to draw a hard and fast distinction. They might agree that policy will require that some who are at the very low end of the healthy range but not clinically diagnosed with depression may be refused treatment, while those who barely qualify as depressed may be treated.

To illustrate, psychiatrists and other mental health care professionals use the Hamilton Depression Scale as one means to assess a patient's level of depression. The initial version of the test consisted of 17 question items to be put to prospective patients. Questions dealing with suicide, feelings of guilt, depressed moods, etc. are ranked on a 0−4 scale where 0 indicates absence and 4 is the strongest indicator. Other items, such as level of agitation, are ranked on a 0−2 basis, meaning that they will weigh less in the final tally. The highest possible score is 52. Patients who score 30 or above are generally classified as severely depressed while a score of 7 or under is taken to be a sign that the patient is 'normal,' or lacking clinical signs of depression. So, consider Alexandra who scores a 7 on the Hamilton Depression Scale and is barely in the normal range, while Brian scores 8 and so is classified as among the depressed. The bioconservative must say that Alexandra is not a candidate for pharmacological treatment but Brian is. Critics, then, will ask, How can such a small difference – only one point on the Hamilton scale – justify such radically different responses on our part?

For my part I do not think that bioprogressivists ought to make too much of the fact that a line is drawn somewhere between normal and depressed. Again, the fact that there may not be any sharp, non-arbitrary means to draw a sharp distinction does not show that there is no distinction. Anyone who thinks it does should contemplate the standard philosophical question of how many hairs one must lose before one is bald. It is difficult to say exactly how many hairs must vanish before a person is bald, but surely there is a clear difference between the bald and the hirsute. Anyone looking for a reasoned defense of happy-people-pill bioprogressivism will have to do much better than simply pointing out that the line between therapy and enhancement may be fuzzy.[9]

So we will grant the happy-people-pills conservative the therapy/enhancement distinction.[10] I say 'grant' here because it is clearly necessary for the bioconservative position, but it is not necessary for the bioprogressivist. The bioprogressivist could accept, indeed welcome, an argument that showed that there is no viable distinction between therapy and enhancement, since the bioprogressivist wants to enhance the happiness of all those who want to use happy-people-pills. So, happy-people-pills progressivists may object that I grant too much in accepting a therapy/enhancement distinction, but bioconservatives can hardly complain.

Much of this work is an argument to the effect that there are morally compelling reasons to permit or encourage the use of pharmacology for enhancement purposes. The reasoning, in a nutshell, is that the happiest amongst us have enviable lives. As we shall see, not only are they happier than the rest of the population, they tend to have the most success in their love lives, at work, in making friends, in being prosocial, etc. There is a natural tendency to think: "well of course those who are successful in their marriages, at work, making friends, being active in their communities, etc. are happy; after all, they have so much success." As we shall see, however, while success does cause happiness, happiness also causes success. This means that those born with a genetic tendency to be amongst the happiest are doubly blessed: not only are they likely to be happier, but they are also likely to have more success in their love lives, at work, making friends, and so on. Putting in pill form what they have through the genetic lottery will mean more of us can enjoy greater happiness and success.

1.5   Signposts

It may be helpful to conclude this chapter by briefly summarizing what lies ahead. The next chapter is the obligatory excursion into Huxley's *Brave New World*. I argue that as a technological prophecy *Brave New World* offers very little in the way of philosophical elucidation of the issue of pharmacological enhancement of happiness. In part the problem is that *Brave New World* casts a net so wide that it makes it near impossible to gain a clear focus on the issue at hand. True, *soma*, the great happy pill of the *Brave New World*, features prominently in the work, but so too do many other technologies. For example, there is the use of alcohol to stunt the intellectual capacities of the lower classes, ectogenesis (babies in a bottle), the widespread practice of indoctrination rather than education of its denizens, and so on. Even *soma* itself, as we shall see, introduces elements that are not relevant for the present purposes; specifically, it is not just a mood enhancer, but also a tranquilizer and a hallucinogenic. It is not without merit: *Brave New World* offers a useful foil for integrating the question of the relationship and nature of happiness and the good life.

Chapters 3, 4, and 5 examine the question of the good life and engage with millennia-old debates on this subject. The conclusion reached is that the good life comprises happiness and a variety of other goods including knowledge, friendship, and virtue, among others. Chapter 3 attempts to illuminate ordinary-language, social-science, and philosophical uses of the word 'happiness.' As noted above, it is argued there is both a cognitive and an affective component to happiness. Chapter 4 argues, contrary to hedonists and desire satisfactionists, that the best lives contain as many and as much of a long list of goods: positive moods, life satisfaction, friendship, love, autonomy, knowledge, health, virtue, desire satisfaction, and so on. This conclusion, as we shall see, is probably not too far from the "common sense" conception of wellbeing. Chapter 5 argues that moral virtue should also be included in the long list of items that make up the good life.

Chapters 6 and 7 deal with the science of happiness. Chapter 6 shows that contemporary social science research supports the view that happiness (understood as positive moods and emotions) promotes achievement: the "higher" aspects of humanity including work, love, and virtue. Chapter 7 reviews the idea that there is a considerable genetic component to happiness as well as current happiness technology. The best extant possibilities are antidepressants, but there is a lack of scientific studies of their effects on the moods of those in the normal range. A stopgap measure to promote happy-people-pills is to test the efficacy of existing antidepressants on normally happy persons. For the longer term, a research program is proposed for "reverse-engineering" the hyperthymic to garner insights for creating happy-people-pills.

Chapters 8 to 10 deal with the ethical and policy questions that arise on the assumption that we can create happy-people-pills. Chapter 8 looks at the arguments for using happy-people-pills. The arguments in support turn on the claim that happy-people-pills will promote the good life for those taking happy-people-pills *and* for wider society. In particular, it is argued that happy-people-pills will raise the likelihood of people being happier, more productive at work, better in their personal lives with friends and family, and also more virtuous. Chapter 9 seeks to rebut various criticisms of using happy-people-pills, including the ideas that happy-people-pills will lead to false happiness and emotional inappropriateness. Chapter 10 looks at policy implications. It is argued that, at minimum, governments should permit the development of happy-people-pills. Merely permitting the use of happy-people-pills would probably provide plenty of financial incentive for private companies to develop happy-people-pills. On the other hand, if governments have a moral duty to promote the wellbeing of their citizens, then governments have a moral duty to develop happy-people-pills.

Some readers may wish to take a short-cut through the book: Chapters 3, 4, and 5 are the most philosophically dense, and some may wish to skip them initially and head straight to chapter 6. Chapter 6 begins with a very brief summary of the conclusions of these chapters for those readers who wish to follow this route. These chapters are essential for the main argument of this work, but they may be postponed for those who first want to get a sense of the broad contours of the overall argument.

Notes

1. Healy, *Let Them Eat Prozac*, 182.
2. Peirson and Heuchert, "Correlations for Serotonin Levels and Measures of Mood in a Nonclinical Sample"; Williams et al., "Associations Between Whole-Blood Serotonin and Subjective Mood in Healthy Male Volunteers."
3. I have used the vague "over about 6ft 1in" locution because it is surprisingly hard to measure and compare human height. Schilling, Watkins, and Watkins, "Is Human Height Bimodal?"
4. Friedman, "Born to Be Happy, Through a Twist of Human Hard Wire."

5. Kass, "Ageless Bodies, Happy Souls."
6. Patel, "Is Depression a Disease of Poverty?"
7. Kramer, *Listening to Prozac.*
8. Fukuyama, *Our Posthuman Future.*
9. Fukuyama (ibid.) does a nice job of showing that this is not the most promising line of argument for the bioprogressive to take.
10. For more on the therapy/enhancement distinction see Daniels, "Normal Functioning and the Treatment–Enhancement Distinction," and Resnik, "The Moral Significance of the Therapy–Enhancement Distinction in Human Genetics."

References

Daniels, N. "Normal Functioning and the Treatment–Enhancement Distinction." *Cambridge Quarterly of Healthcare Ethics* 9, no. 3 (2000): 309–22.

Friedman, R. "Born to Be Happy, Through a Twist of Human Hard Wire." *New York Times*, December 31, 2002, section F.

Fukuyama, F. *Our Posthuman Future: Consequences of the Biotechnology Revolution.* London: Profile, 2003.

Healy, D. *Let Them Eat Prozac: The Unhealthy Relationship Between the Pharmaceutical Companies and Depression.* New York: New York University Press, 2004.

Kass, L. R. "Ageless Bodies, Happy Souls." *New Atlantis* 1 (2003): 9–28.

Kramer, P. *Listening to Prozac.* New York: Penguin Books, 1993.

Patel, V. "Is Depression a Disease of Poverty?" *Regional Health Forum WHO South-East Asia Region* 5, no. 1 (2001): 14–23.

Peirson, A. R. and J. W. Heuchert. "Correlations for Serotonin Levels and Measures of Mood in a Nonclinical Sample." *Psychological Reports* 87, no. 3 (2000): 707–16.

Resnik, D. B. "The Moral Significance of the Therapy–Enhancement Distinction in Human Genetics." *Cambridge Quarterly of Healthcare Ethics* 9, no. 3 (2000): 365–77.

Schilling, M. F., A. E. Watkins, and W. Watkins. "Is Human Height Bimodal?" *American Statistician* 56, no. 3 (2002): 223–9.

Williams, E., B. Stewart-Knox, A. Helander, C. McConville, I. Bradbury, and I. Rowland. "Associations Between Whole-Blood Serotonin and Subjective Mood in Healthy Male Volunteers." *Biological Psychology* 71, no. 2 (2006): 171–4.

2

What is Living and What is Dead in *Brave New World*

2.1 Introductory

At an early stage of writing this book, I toyed with the idea of not mentioning Huxley's fictional dystopia *Brave New World*. In part it is because I felt (and still feel) slightly annoyed that the book is so technologically unrealistic. As we shall see, much of the technology invoked in the novel is of little relevance to any realistic proposal concerning happy-people-pills. To my mind it is a little like thinking that Jules Verne's *From the Earth to the Moon* should be used to guide current space policy. Verne, writing in the nineteenth century, imagined astronauts being shot from a large cannon to the moon. Imagine telling NASA that their current plans to return to the moon are unrealistic because Verne's cannon is too dangerous. Surely NASA would be right to laugh off this criticism as technologically irrelevant (unless they are planning on sending clowns). As a technological prophecy, *Brave New World* is no better. And yet, I can't think of any sustained philosophical treatment of happy-people-pills that doesn't at least mention Huxley's novel. Some, like Francis Fukuyama, go so far as to maintain that "Huxley was right."[1]

As you can see, I stowed the idea of not mentioning *Brave New World*, but it may be thought that the pendulum has swung back too far in the other direction, given there is an entire chapter devoted to it. Indeed, several readers of an earlier draft of this book asked: "Why put so much emphasis on an eighty-year-old work of fiction in a philosophical work?"

Happy-People-Pills For All, First Edition. Mark Walker.
© 2013 John Wiley & Sons, Inc. Published 2013 by John Wiley & Sons, Inc.

In part my answer is that, as just noted, bioconservatives put a lot of stock in the novel as an objection to happy-people-pills. Secondly, once stripped of its technological irrelevancies, Huxley's novel does provide a useful foil for laying out some of the philosophical issues of happy-people-pills. This will become evident in subsequent chapters as we probe the connection between happiness and what it means for our lives to go well. So, Huxley's work is relevant in terms of its philosophical treatment of the issues and irrelevant in terms of a technological prophecy. Unfortunately, these two strands of his thought are not always sufficiently disentangled.

2.2 Brief Summary of *Brave New World*

It will help to start with a brief summary of the work. Even for those who have read the novel, this may prove useful. Certainly this was so in my case: I read the novel as an undergraduate, but when I reread it recently I was quite surprised at just how much I had forgotten, and how much I had overlooked.

Brave New World is set six hundred years in the future. Most of the events of the novel revolve around two main characters: Bernard Marx and John the Savage. Bernard lives in the highly "civilized" part of the world, which comprises the vast majority of the future world's population and geography. We aren't provided with any hard figures, but it is probably a safe bet to assume that more than 95 percent of the world's population inhabits the civilized portions. A world government has taken on the task of promoting and maintaining the sovereign good: happiness. Interestingly, while it is invariably described as a dystopia, and ultimately it is difficult to disagree with this description, in many ways the world government in *Brave New World* has wrought many desirable aspects by any standard. Food scarcity and other material wants have been eliminated, and wars are a thing of the past. It is easy to forget or overlook these features of *Brave New World* when focusing on its less pleasant aspects, but surely, at least in these areas, we have reason to envy.

The stability and peace of *Brave New World* is credited to careful management by an oligarchy of ten 'Controllers' who run the World State. As noted, the Controllers' primary mission is to make people happy. This is achieved by carefully managing the creation and conditioning of its citizenry. In effect, the Controllers are charged with what Aristotle terms 'soul crafting.' But Aristotle would be horrified at the end the Controllers set for the citizens of *Brave New World*. The book opens with a description of a huge factory devoted to human reproduction: the first step in the citizen-creation process. Embryos are raised in ectogenesis tanks – artificial wombs, or 'bottles' as they are called. Maternity is a thing of the past. Natural birth is seen as primitive and repulsive. Huxley drives home the point by telling us that the very term 'mother' is considered "pornographic" while the word 'father' is not quite so bad, it is merely "scatological." After a nine-month maturation cycle, children are removed from the ectogenesis chamber and raised in state-run nurseries. Families have been dispensed with entirely. The state is the sole agent for socializing and nurturing children. Of course there is one, and only one, goal in socializing children: to maximize happiness.

Hypnopaedia is frequently mentioned throughout the novel as the preferred method for conditioning children. It consists of repeating simple phrases to children as they slumber. A recorded voice echoes a slogan or phrase to condition each generation into the norms of society. For example, part of the conditioning instructs the citizenry on how they are to treat "*soma*," the happy pill of *Brave New World*. The conditioning prescribes the exact dosage of *soma* to take to deal with annoyances and gloom. Thus, as children sleep, they learn phrases such as "A gramme is better than a damn," "A gramme in time saves nine," and "One cubic centimeter cures ten gloomy sentiments."

Hypnopaedia is used for inculcating any number of "civilized behaviors." The norm of happiness is actively promulgated by hypnopaedia phrases such as: "Everybody's happy nowadays." Negative emotions are strongly discouraged as well: "When the individual feels, the community reels." Sexual promiscuity is strongly encouraged by the thousands of repetitions of phrases such as: "Every one belongs to every one else." Sexual license is encouraged even in children. Monogamy, and indeed any exclusive relationships, are strongly discouraged. We are told that sexual relations are a source of pleasure and happiness, but strong emotional attachments, which inevitably develop in exclusive relationships, are a source of much unhappiness.

For most readers one of the most disturbing aspects of the novel is how intelligence is purposely suppressed: alcohol is added to the bottles of some gestating embryos destined for the lower classes in order to keep them "small and backwards."[2] According to its architects, crucial to the happiness of society is social stability, which is maintained in part by the strict caste system. The Alpha and Beta classes are charged with leadership and other more cerebral occupations in society while the Deltas and the Gammas perform the more simple-minded jobs. The Epsilon class is described as having a level of intelligence more akin to that of chimps, so they are assigned tasks like elevator operator. Every level of intelligence is carefully designed to make sure workers are fit for their station and their duties. We are told that the caste system is necessary, for if everyone were bright no one would be happy performing the more menial tasks in society. And so this makes for a perfect fit: the castes with lower intelligence have no ability and no desire to perform the more intellectual tasks. Each caste is conditioned to see its place in society as an enviable one. So the Betas, for example, are told as part of their hypnopaedia conditioning that the lower castes are inferior, while they are lucky not to be Alphas because the Alphas work too hard. So, in effect the argument of the novel is that a stunted intelligence is not a big deal since even the lowest classes, the Deltas and the Epsilons, are happy.

Most relevant for our purposes is the aforementioned *soma*, a technically advanced pharmaceutical agent. Huxley introduces *soma* as having "All the advantages of Christianity and alcohol; none of their defects."[3] With *soma* you can "Take a holiday from reality whenever you like, and come back without so much as a headache or a mythology."[4] The psychological effects of *soma* appear to be very quantity-sensitive. In small amounts, it seems to lift one's mood, and excise negative emotions. Thus, Bernard Marx, in reference to one of his frequent glum moods, is told, "What you need is a gramme of *soma*." In small doses it also seems to increase feelings and propensities for benevolence, and reduce social anxiety. In larger doses, it seems to have psycho-reactive properties similar to those of hallucinogenics such as mushrooms and LSD. So we are told " . . . there is always *soma*, delicious *soma*, half a gramme for a half-holiday, a gramme for a week-end, two grammes for a trip to the gorgeous East, three for a dark eternity on the moon . . . " The ethereal feeling of large doses is underscored towards the end of the work with an inquiry to a physician about the medical safety of consuming large doses of *soma* and whether it will shorten the life of the patient.

> "In one sense, yes," Dr. Shaw admitted. "But in another we're actually lengthening it." The young man stared, uncomprehending. "*Soma* may make you lose a few years in time," the doctor went on. "But think of the enormous, immeasurable durations it can give you out of time. Every *soma*-holiday is a bit of what our ancestors used to call eternity"[5]

The overwhelming majority of the population is said to be – and claims to be – very happy. Bernard Marx is one of the few exceptions. In part,

Bernard's unhappiness is explained by the fact that he is physically different; he is much shorter than the typical Alpha. This leads to him being ridiculed by his own caste and he has trouble commanding the respect he thinks is his due from the lower castes. Several times in the novel we hear of the rumor that his short stature was the result of an accident during gestation: "They say somebody made a mistake when he was still in the bottle – thought he was a Gamma and put alcohol into his blood-surrogate. That's why he's so stunted."[6]

Not only is he physically different, Bernard is also socially awkward. Bernard often prefers solitude to the company of others. Such solitude is strongly discouraged in favor of consumerist social activities, such as sports and entertainment. Bernard's unhappiness is apparent to many of his colleagues, which further alienates him since he is considered strange for being so out of sync with everyone else – unhappy in a world of happiness. The problem, according to his colleagues, is only exacerbated by the fact that he often refuses the socially prescribed solution to unhappiness: *soma*. Sexually too, Bernard is ill matched for *Brave New World*. Ostensibly sex is very egalitarian: "every one belongs to every one else." Yet, it seems that some are more successful in obtaining sexual partners than others; Bernard's physical appearance and social awkwardness mean that he is much less successful in obtaining partners. This fact plays a part in Bernard's pursuit of his love interest Lenina.

Lenina is not quite Bernard's caste equal: she is a Beta. Lenina, as is typical of those in *Brave New World*, has had multiple sexual partners, but is slightly unconventional in having a preference for serial monogamy – a practice that is generally frowned upon. Her interest in Bernard appears to be, in part, to fulfill her duty to refrain from monogamy. Near the beginning of the novel we are told that she had been seeing Henry Foster exclusively for some time and this was cause for some concern among her circle of acquaintances. Henry Foster is the prototypical Alpha-class male: successful at work as assistant to the Director of Hatcheries, happy and completely at ease in *Brave New World*.

The central event in terms of plot development occurs when Lenina acquiesces to Bernard's invitation to visit the "Savage Reservation" in New Mexico. Such reservations constitute relatively autonomous socio-political units. An electric fence separates the reservations from the civilized world and the communities run, for the most part, without interference from the World State. This means that in such 'backwards' communities *soma* and hypnopaedia are absent and people procreate through the disgusting process of pregnancy. As a psychologist specializing in hypnopaedia, Bernard is one of the few civilized persons permitted to visit the uncivilized world. On the reservation, Bernard meets Linda and John. In a critical plot twist, we find that Linda was formerly a resident in the civilized part of the world. She had come to the reservation about two decades ago for a similar 'cultural tourism' trip with Director Tomakin, Bernard's boss. During a storm Tomakin and Linda became separated, and Linda went missing after taking a blow to the head. Tomakin returned to the civilized world leaving Linda for dead. Upon recovery from her injuries, Linda found herself pregnant with John. Too embarrassed to return to the civilized world with a child, and all the ignominy of being a mother, Linda raised John on the Reservation.

Like Bernard, John is out of sync with his world. John is socially isolated in part because he looks different from the indigenous people, and because the locals ostracize John's mother for her promiscuity. Naturally, Linda continued the civilized practice of having multiple sexual partners; after all, as a good civilized citizen she knows that "every one belongs to every one." Such civilized behavior angered the local women, in particular because it led to her "taking their men." Unfortunately for her, Linda found the idea of monogamy absurd. This was not the only aspect of the civilized world she sought to re-create: Linda often used mescal as a substitute for *soma*, but she found that it gave her a headache afterwards and she tended to feel embarrassment for the things that she did under its influence. While Linda's maladaptation to the customs of the savages made childhood difficult for John, the fact that Linda was from the civilized world meant she could read, and she passed on this skill to John. The situation on the reservation meant that books were virtually non-existent, although John managed to get his hands on the collected works of Shakespeare.

Bernard is able to piece together the events of Linda's presence at the reservation and the circumstances of John's birth, and schemes to turn this to his advantage. He persuades Linda and John to return with him to civilization, where Bernard's troubles with his boss, Director Tomakin, stemming from Bernard's unconventional behavior, are solved by Linda and John's presence. Bernard reveals, in front of a large audience at work, the scandalous bit of information that the Director is John's father. Mortified, the Director disappears for good, as does the Director's threat to Bernard of banishment to Iceland. Almost no one has met a savage before, and so there is immense curiosity about the newcomer. As gatekeeper to John, Bernard's social status quickly skyrockets. As toast of London's social scene,

Bernard is happy for the first time in his life. Where Bernard formerly struggled for female companionship in a world of "free love," now he is able to bed at will. However, the Savage soon tires of being paraded before London's social elite, and refuses Bernard's requests to attend any further social functions. Predictably, Bernard's social stock plummets, as does his happiness.

The final events of the book are precipitated by John the Savage's attempt to initiate a revolution through an attack on the *soma* industry: he attempts to demolish a shipment of *soma* destined for a group of Delta workers. A serious riot ensues that has to be quelled by a riot squad, who subdue the crowd with an aerosol version of *soma*. Bernard and his good friend Helmholtz attempt to no avail to rescue John from the center of the uprising. News of the riot makes its way to Mustapha Mond, one of the world Controllers. Mustapha has the police escort the three to his quarters. After some conversation Mustapha decides Bernard and Helmholtz are to be sent to one of the islands for dissidents, the third socio-political unit in *Brave New World*. The islands are necessary since it seems that a certain small percentage of persons in the civilized part of *Brave New World* are not content with their lives. These freethinkers are not imprisoned or tortured for their heretical ideas, but are merely exiled to islands with other freethinkers. Bernard is devastated by the news of his impending banishment, but Helmholtz seems to quite like the idea of pursuing art in a way that is not possible in the civilized world.

With Bernard and Helmholtz out of the way, the story reaches its climax in a philosophical discussion between John and Mustapha. Mustapha offers an eloquent apology for *Brave New World* while John offers a spirited critique. The depth of the conversation – which we will examine more below – is aided by the fact that Mustapha is one of the few persons in *Brave New World* who has access to great works of literature and philosophy, having, like John, read Shakespeare. Mustapha keeps Shakespeare and other heretical authors locked in a safe: to allow the general population access to such works would risk the stability of the civilized world. John is not sent back to the Savage Reservation, nor exiled to one of the islands for misfits with Bernard and Helmholtz; rather, Mustapha keeps him in the civilized part, as he wants to continue the 'experiment.' Disillusioned with the vapidity of the civilized world, John seeks to seclude himself in an abandoned lighthouse. His solitude is short-lived as reporters and the curious hound him. John succumbs to the sins of *Brave New World* one fatal night: he takes *soma* and engages in an orgy. Guilt-ridden, he takes his own life.

2.3   *Brave New World* and Bioconservatives

I mentioned that I toyed with the idea of bypassing Huxley's novel. In part this is because the mere invocation of the title of the book often provokes an almost reflexive action. Mary Winkler describes the reaction thus:

> When the nightly television newscaster invokes the name *Brave New World* to trigger audience response to the latest story of scientific or technological discovery, he is probably not expecting his audience to even have read *Brave New World*. The phrase has entered our cultural vocabulary. Everyone is expected to understand the shorthand. *Brave New World* means science run wild, social control through technology – babies in bottles, mad scientists playing God.[7]

If the novel were simply invoked by critics in this fashion – as a stopper to thought, rather than a prompt to thought – then it would hardly be worth considering. However, there are more thoughtful interpretations.

One line of thought is suggested by Leon Kass. In *Towards a More Natural Science* he asks:

> What kinds of creatures will we become if we obtain our pleasure by drug or electrode stimulation without the usual kind of human efforts and frustrations? What kind of society will we have?
>
> We need only consult Aldous Huxley's . . . *Brave New World* for a likely answer to these questions. There we encounter a society dedicated to homo-geneity and stability, administered by means of instant gratifications, and peopled by creatures of human shape but stunted humanity. They consume, fornicate, take "soma," and operate the machinery that makes it all possible. They do not read, write, think, love, or govern themselves. Creativity and curiosity, reason and passion, exist only in rudimentary and mutilated form. In short, they are not men at all.[8]

The last sentence is quite jarring. Taken literally, this suggests that we should understand that beings who consume soma are not members of the human species. This may seem a little over the top given that genetically there would be no discernible differences between our genomes and theirs. So, it may be thought that Kass is being slightly hyperbolic here in saying "they are not men at all."

But Francis Fukuyama in *Our Posthuman Future* takes seriously the idea that ushering in *Brave New World* would constitute a speciation event. He argues that if we were to deploy advanced pharmacology for the purposes of mass enhancement, we would alter human nature and create a posthuman nature:

> Since the novel's publication, there have probably been several million high school essays written in answer to the question, "What's wrong with this picture [i.e., *Brave New World*]?" The answer given (on papers that get A's, at any rate) usually runs something like this: the people in *Brave New World* may be healthy and happy, but they have ceased to be *human beings*. They no longer struggle, aspire, love, feel pain, make difficult moral choices, have families, or do any of the things that we traditionally associate with being human.[9]

This answer seems to raise its own questions. As Fukuyama notes, it may be good enough for a high school paper, but "it does not (as Kass goes on to note) probe nearly deeply enough. For one can then ask, What is so important about being a human being in the traditional way that Huxley defines it?"[10]

As Mary Winkler observes, " . . . the novel is Aldous Huxley's contemplation of a great and ancient question: What is the good life?"[11] In this light, the novel can be seen as following the refrain, "Ultimately I just want to be happy," through to its logical consequence. Huxley's answer is: be careful what you wish for. A world like *Brave New World* where happiness is the dominant goal is a world where we have lost much of what is valuable in life.

A number of the earlier commentators on the novel understood Huxley as interrogating the question of the good life in just this way, including Bertrand Russell. In his review, "We Don't Want to Be Happy," Russell found himself puzzling over why we instinctively recoil in horror from *Brave New World* despite the high level of happiness and material prosperity portrayed in the novel:

> In spite of these merits, the world which Mr. Huxley portrays is such as to arouse disgust in every normal reader, and obviously in Mr. Huxley himself. I have been asking myself why, and trying hard to think that his well-regulated world would really be an improvement upon the one in which we live. At moments I can make myself think this, but I can never make myself feel it. The feeling of revulsion against a well-ordered world has various sources: one of these is that we do not value happiness as much as we sometimes think we do.[12]

Russell's suggestion is quite poignant: "we do not value happiness as much as we sometimes think we do." As Russell was well aware, it is not simply that they are happy in *Brave New World*; it is that they are much happier. If happiness were our sole value, then remaking our world to be like *Brave New World* where there is so much happiness ought to be a no-brainer.

Russell's thought, that there is more to the good life than happiness, is expressed eloquently by John the Savage when his disagreement with Mustapha Mond reaches its climax:

> "But I don't want comfort. I want God, I want poetry, I want real danger, I want freedom, I want goodness, I want sin."
>
> "In fact," said Mustapha Mond, "you're claiming the right to be unhappy."
>
> "All right then," said the Savage defiantly, "I'm claiming the right to be unhappy."
>
> "Not to mention the right to grow old and ugly and impotent; the right to have syphilis and cancer; the right to have too little to eat; the right to be lousy; the right to live in constant apprehension of what may happen tomorrow; the right to catch typhoid; the right to be tortured by unspeakable pains of every kind." There was a long silence.
>
> "I claim them all," said the Savage at last.
>
> Mustapha Mond shrugged his shoulders. "You're welcome," he said.[13]

The argument leading up to this famous passage initially has John asking whether the happiness of *Brave New World* could have been achieved at a smaller cost to other values, such as truth, beauty, and a relationship with the divine. The Controller argues that ultimately these are incompatible with happiness. For example, if the pursuit of truth through scientific investigation were unconstrained, this would lead to a destabilization of society, and to unhappiness.

Interestingly, Mustapha *never* suggests that truth is not valuable. Indeed, as a young man the Controller had once pursued truth and science too vigorously for the likings of those who held political power in his youth. When asked by Helmholtz why the Controller did not land on one of the islands for dissidents, we are told that the Controller had to choose. So, both the Controller's own life and the history of *Brave New World* are described in terms of a tragic dilemma. The Controller faced the choice between a life devoted to science and a life devoted to happiness: he couldn't have both. The political situation of *Brave New World* itself is predicated on a similar choice. If the pursuit of science is not sufficiently curtailed, says Mustapha, scientific progress would cause much unhappiness: society cannot have both scientific progress and happiness. So too for art, philosophy, and religion: serious pursuit of any of them would undermine the goal of happiness. They too are banished in all but the most truncated forms in order to maintain *Brave New World*'s high levels of happiness.

The upshot of this line of thought is that the price of happiness in the *Brave New World* comes at too high a price: it requires the sacrifice of far too much for the sake of happiness. The title of Russell's review is a little bit of hyperbole: it is not that we don't want to be happy; it is just that *Brave New World* looks like too high a price to pay.

The main theme of bioconservatives who cite *Brave New World* as an objection to happy-people-pills is that turning our world into *Brave New World* would involve a catastrophic loss of the higher aspects of our humanity: love, deep friendships, art, religion, scientific progress and the like. So, *Brave New World* does not offer more of the good life, it offers less. Let us see what can be made of these claims.

2.4   Alcohol Stunting, Indoctrination, and Other Pernicious Means of Soul Crafting

Brave New World employs a salmagundi of technologies and techniques for soul crafting, which complicates the question of how we should understand the novel as an objection to happy-people-pills. The problem, in a nutshell, is that the novel interweaves many objectionable uses of technology that have nothing to do with happy-people-pills. A proper assessment requires that we disentangle happy-people-pills from the extraneous uses of technology.

Consider first the biological class system of *Brave New World*. Readers quite rightly find morally objectionable the idea of purposely creating a class system using alcohol in vitro to stunt the intellectual capacities of many of its citizens. Of all the morally objectionable policies in *Brave New World*, surely this has to be the most objectionable. But notice that alcohol stunting has absolutely nothing to do with happy-people-pills. There is nothing inconsistent in advocating for happy-people-pills and being adamantly against alcohol stunting. Nor is there the slightest reason to suppose that if we were to take mood boosters, we would inevitably start stunting our offspring with alcohol.

Indeed, there is also a certain irony in citing *Brave New World* as an example of a scientifically advanced dystopia, since inflicting fetal alcohol syndrome on children is something that can be done today. We could encourage this "advanced technology" simply by encouraging pregnant mothers to drink copious amounts of alcohol. Of course, it is done in a much more purposeful and systematic way in *Brave New World*, but in itself the procedure is hardly cutting-edge technology.

Since no one thinks we should use alcohol to limit human intelligence in vivo or in vitro, if *Brave New World* is to be used as an objection to happy-people-pills, this aspect must be factored out. But we need to wonder whether the story could survive if this aspect were excised. In the novel we are told about the "Cyprus experiment" where the Controllers experimented by populating the island of Cyprus exclusively with members of the intellectual Alpha class. According to Mustapha, the experiment quickly devolved into anarchy and mass murder. The reason offered is that no one wanted to perform the more menial tasks, and could not abide by agreements to divvy these tasks equitably amongst the Alphas. One can only smile at the colossal inconsistency here: the Alphas – the most intelligent class – were incapable of seeing that it was in their own best interests to abide by the agreement to distribute menial tasks in an equitable fashion, and so resorted to violence. They couldn't reason that this might work as a stopgap measure until more labor-saving devices could be implemented.

In fact, the whole issue of labor-saving devices in the novel is somewhat perplexing. We are told that the Controllers banned many labor-saving devices in *Brave New World* precisely because they would save on menial labor, and the lower classes need to keep working or they would become unhappy. For instance, as noted above, one of the jobs assigned to members of the Epsilon class is to operate elevators. But which is it? Are the menial jobs to keep the lower classes occupied or are the lower classes created in order to do the menial jobs? It seems that if Huxley had taken seriously the idea of labor-saving devices, he could have eliminated at least the very lowest classes from his society. And even if the menial jobs are simply to keep the lower classes employed, it is a mystery why the Alphas in the Cypress experiment did not employ such advanced technology to save themselves a violent death. Moreover, Huxley has us imagine that social engineering is strong enough to remake humans to do away with familial relations – including monogamy and child rearing – despite the fact that there is probably a strong genetic basis to this behavior. Yet at the same time we are to believe that the very same powerful techniques of social engineering are not strong enough to make people work part-time at menial tasks. If the indoctrination techniques are as powerful as Huxley imagines, it is hard to believe that the Cypress experiment could not have created the classless society famously envisioned by Marx in the *German Ideology*:

> In communist society, where nobody has one exclusive sphere of activity but each can become accomplished in any branch he wishes, society regulates the general production and thus makes it possible for me to do one thing today and another tomorrow, to hunt in the morning, fish in the afternoon, rear cattle in the evening, criticise after dinner, just as I have a mind, without ever becoming hunter, fisherman, herdsman or critic.[14]

It is understandable why Huxley envisioned biologically differentiated classes: he was trying to paint a morally repugnant world. But it is only pretense to think that there is any other motivating factor. The internal logic of the novel itself betrays Huxley on this point.

Since alcohol stunting is not linked to the happy-people-pills proposal other than in the imagination of a famous author, this aspect must be deleted from consideration. If we were to edit out alcohol stunting from the novel, then we would have to imagine John arriving in a world where there are no biologically differentiated classes. Admittedly this is a large edit, since so much of the novel is predicated on the class structure, which is tantamount to admitting that large portions of the novel are completely irrelevant to the happy-people-pills proposal.

Indoctrination via hypnopaedia is the other major technology of soul crafting employed by the Controllers; it is used to carefully manage all aspects of the *Brave New World*. Class antagonism is controlled through indoctrination, as is the rejection of monogamy, parenting, and any strong emotional attachments to others, the rejection of experiences of negative emotions, and the enjoyment of solitude, of not seeking to gratify every "infantile" desire, and so on. Of course we find the process of indoctrination and its result – lives that are uniformly stunted and shallow – morally repugnant. But hypnopaedia has nothing to do with happy-people-pills; and there is nothing inconsistent in advocating for happy-people-pills and being adamantly against indoctrination. Nor is there the slightest reason to suppose that if we were to take mood boosters, we would inevitably start indoctrinating our children.

It is perhaps worth pausing here to say something about indoctrination, since it may be thought that there is nothing unique about the indoctrination of *Brave New World*.[15] The objection might be put like so:

> *Every stable society ensures that the new generation adopts its beliefs, customs and practices. Certainly this is the case in* Brave New World. *But*

so too is it in our own world. So, there is no particular reason to suppose that there is a significant contrast here between the indoctrinated in Brave New World, *and those in our own world. Either both are indoctrinated, or neither society is indoctrinated.*

We should reject such skepticism. It is true that every known society socializes its young. There is no denying this. What I deny is that all forms of socialization are equivalent. Consider the contrast between education and indoctrination. Skeptics sometimes suggest that there is no significant difference here: 'education' is merely a euphemism for indoctrination of the youth, for in either case the intent is to socialize our children. However, there is a logical difference between these two concepts. One difference is what counts as a success criterion for education versus indoctrination. With education the goal is to inculcate understanding, with indoctrination the goal is belief. Consider an example. A student in an advanced evolutionary biology class has the highest mark in the class. His understanding of such diverse evolutionary biology notions as adaptation, selection, the unit of selection controversy, speciation, cladism, and convergent evolution is exemplary. Suppose when the student completes the course the professor says to him that he is the best undergraduate student he has taught and the professor hopes the student might consider doing graduate work with him. The student replies that he is off to do graduate work in theology. He says that although he enjoyed the course thoroughly he does not believe in evolutionary theory any more than he believes in Santa Claus. Both are fun stories but clearly they are not true, as they conflict with the Bible. Naturally the professor would be disappointed. But did the professor fail to educate the student properly? It is hard to see why we might claim this. The student showed greater understanding of the subject than other students.

On the other hand, it does seem clear that the student has not been successfully indoctrinated into evolutionary theory. The student, after all, rejects the claim that evolutionary theory is true. In other words, there is no inconsistency in saying that someone was successfully educated with respect to some subject, but does not believe it, whereas there is an inconsistency in saying that someone was successfully indoctrinated in some subject but does not believe it. For the Controllers of *Brave New World*, successful socializing means making sure the next generation believes that motherhood is pornographic, that solitude is bad, and so on. Our method of socializing is different: a high school student need only demonstrate understanding of subjects like history, English, and algebra; there is no belief requirement. I'm not saying that we never indoctrinate, nor that they never educate in *Brave New World*; rather, I'm saying that if we could draw a continuum from societies that use only indoctrination and societies that only educate, *Brave New World* is far to the indoctrination side while we are more to the education side.

Since hypnopaedia and indoctrination are irrelevant to the happy-people-pills proposal, this aspect must be deleted from consideration. If we were to edit out this aspect from the novel, then we would have to imagine John arriving in a world where indoctrination does not take place. Admittedly, this too is a large edit, since so much of the novel is predicated on the idea that hypnopaedia can form the beliefs and desires of the citizenry exactly to the specifications of the Controllers, which is tantamount to admitting that large portions of the novel are completely irrelevant to the happy-people-pills proposal.

Other technologies and techniques for soul crafting appear in the novel that are also of some importance. Many readers find repugnant the idea of ectogenesis as the obligatory means of procreation, but this seems more important for dramatic effect. It wouldn't change the novel significantly if women experienced maternity and then the newborns were voluntarily (because of successful indoctrination) placed in state nurseries. The Controllers also use some very traditional means of soul crafting: the exiling of dissidents and the banning of books. Again, none of this is connected with happy-people-pills and so must be excised if we are to imagine the novel provides a fair assessment of happy-people-pills.

To summarize, if we are to think seriously about *Brave New World* as an objection to happy-people-pills, then we must factor out extraneous elements such as alcohol stunting, indoctrination via hypnopaedia, ectogenesis, suppression of ideas and dissent. But if we try to factor out these elements from the story, it is not clear what we are asked to imagine, since these elements are critical to the fabric of the society envisioned in *Brave New World*.

2.5 Soma

Soma is of course relevant to the happy-people-pills proposal, but, as I shall explain, only to a limited extent. We will need to think about what is meant by 'soma' and how soma compares with the anticipated happy-people-pills.

The term 'soma' has made its way into the vernacular as a catchall for 'drugs' or pharmacological agents in general. So in this sense it may be used to refer to prescription drugs like Valium and antidepressants as well as street drugs; for example, people occasionally refer to marijuana and alcohol as 'soma.' It will help for us to reserve 'soma' exclusively for the pharmacological agent used in *Brave New World*.

This is important not only to avoid ambiguity, but because the drug used in *Brave New World* is really unlike any drug we know at present. The variable effects of *soma* were intimated above. Recall, at very low dosages it seems to work simply as a mood booster. At a medium dosage it seems to work much like a combination of Valium and alcohol. It emotionally blunts in the way that Valium does – "it takes the edge off" – and increases confidence in social situations as alcohol does for some. But like alcohol, *soma* seems to distort perception and impair cognitive functioning with increased dosage. Certainly the comparison between *soma* and alcohol is one that Huxley frequently draws, as in the famous adage that *soma* has "All the advantages of Christianity and alcohol; none of their defects."[16] In large dosages the effects of *soma* appear to be similar to hallucinogenics like LSD or magic mushrooms. So we are told " . . . there is always *soma*, delicious *soma*, half a gramme for a half-holiday, a gramme for a week-end, two grammes for a trip to the gorgeous East, three for a dark eternity on the moon . . . " Thus, the fact that soma can act like a mood booster, a stimulant, a sedative, and a hallucinogen (depending on what the plot requires) means that *soma* is unlike any drug we know at present.

This view seems to be endorsed by Huxley, who in 1958, a quarter of a century after the publication of *Brave New World*, wrote:

> We see then, that, though soma does not yet exist (and will probably never exist), fairly good substitutes for the various aspects of soma have already been discovered. There are now physiologically cheap tranquillizers, physiologically cheap vision-producers and physiologically cheap stimulants.[17]

Huxley's admission that there is no direct comparison between *soma* and any single drug we have now, or probably could concoct, is not too surprising; it is, after all, an entirely mythical drug. But the fact that *soma* has all these aspects rolled into one makes it difficult to assess. Consider the difference between taking a tranquilizer like Valium, a vision-producer like psilocybin mushrooms, and a mood booster like Reboxetine. The differences in terms of cognitive impairment are enormous. Should there be any doubt, just ask yourself this: would you rather the airplane's captain announce mid-Atlantic over the intercom that he was drinking, on Valium, on magic mushrooms or on the antidepressant Reboxetine?

The proposed happy-people-pills are intended as mood boosters, not as tranquilizers or as hallucinogenics. A careful reading of *Brave New World* reveals that *soma* is often mentioned in the story when the characters take larger doses, when they take enough to have some act like a tranquilizer or a hallucinogenic. So, again this aspect of the novel must be excised if we are to take seriously *Brave New World* as an objection to happy-people-pills.

It is interesting that for all its excesses, *Brave New World* offers only part-time happy-pills. The only character to take continuous doses of *soma* for any length of time is Linda when she returns to the civilized world. Recall that taking large continuous doses is said to be harmful to one's health, but the taking of copious quantities of *soma* is rationalized in Linda's case by the attending physician. For the rest of the population, *soma* is a recreational drug – something that one typically does after work hours. This means that for a good portion of most people's lives they are *soma*-less. Citizens of *Brave New World* are still required to work an eight-hour day, so workers have to remain without *soma* for their entire shift. This is underscored by the fact that workers receive their ration of *soma* after completing their shifts, in fact this plays a pivotal role in the story. It is John's attempt to destroy a group of Deltas' after-work ration that causes a riot, which brings him before the Controller.

So, the present proposal here is more radical, at least along this dimension: people would be constantly under the influence of happy-people-pills. One need not wait like the unfortunate *Brave New World*ers to get off work before partaking. *Soma* provides merely a 'holiday' – it is not a fulltime pill like the happy-people-pill proposal.

It is easy to see why Huxley wrote *soma* into the story, if for no other reason than that it is central to the crisis that brings John to the attention of the Controller. Still, there is a real strain in the logic of the story. We are told that the Controllers serve the sovereign good of happiness. *Soma* is said to serve this end. But the following, almost throw-away comment about one of the minor characters in the novel looks to undermine much of this internal logic:

> Benito was notoriously good-natured. People said of him that he could have got through life without touching *soma*. The malice and bad tempers from which other people had to take holidays never afflicted him. Reality for Benito was always sunny.[18]

This is quite striking: Benito is *naturally* happier than most. His sunny disposition carries through at work, so, unlike so many others in *Brave*

New World, his sunniness is not part-time. Since Benito had the same environmental influences as everyone else, it seems plausible to infer that Benito's sunny disposition has a lot to do with genetics. But, given the sovereign value of happiness, it is a wonder that the Controllers didn't use their advanced technology to make more people like Benito and do away with *soma*. I'm not sure why this option wasn't taken, but it is worth speculating for a moment.

One possibility is that it simply did not occur to Huxley that genetic technologies could be used to such ends; for example, pre-implantation genetic diagnosis was unknown in his time, as was genetic engineering. Indeed, DNA was unknown in 1933. While the novel never mentions any more sophisticated technology than cloning, it seems that Huxley must have been assuming that some genetic technology was employed by the architects of the world. The Alpha class, for instance, is described as nearly uniform in height. It is true that alcohol stunts the physical growth of the lower classes, but the fact that Bernard was three inches shorter than the average Alpha should not have seemed particularly surprising if some genetic technology was not used to ensure uniform height. Furthermore, like his brother Julian Huxley and many of his contemporaries, Huxley was a proponent of eugenics. He feared that civilization might slide into barbarism because the lower classes, with their inferior intelligence, bred much faster than the upper classes who (of course!) had superior intelligence. Since Huxley believed it was possible to use scientific knowledge to promote intelligence, it is difficult to see why he would resist the same conclusion when it came to temperament. And so it seems puzzling that Huxley did not have the Controllers use genetic technologies to create people with a sunny disposition like Benito's. This seems to violate their sworn mission to make the world as happy as possible. We can only surmise that the Controllers ought to have been fired for not carrying out their duty to promote the sovereign good of happiness. Perhaps it is too much to ask for this level of internal consistency in the story, or perhaps Huxley thought that using *soma* rather than giving people an innate disposition for happiness was a better means to ensure political stability: the Controllers could use *soma* as punishment and reward. As I said, this is all speculative, we may never know.

So, we can see why much of the novel's discussion of *soma* is irrelevant. At least in comparison to *soma*, happy-people-pills are quite modest: they would provide the rest of us with the cheeriness that people like

Benito experience naturally. It has nothing to do with intoxication or hallucination.

2.6 A Tragic Dilemma or a False Dilemma?

There are probably good literary reasons to write a tragic choice into the novel: making it so that the architects of *Brave New World* had to choose between happiness and the higher aspects of humanity: love, friendship, science, art, religion, etc. But is a choice inevitable? If the choice is inevitable, then Huxley has illuminated a permanent feature of the human situation. If the choice is not inevitable, then the novel offers us a false dilemma: we need to consider the possibility of a world with greater happiness without the loss of the higher aspects of humanity. So which is it: a tragic choice or a false dilemma?

Ironically, perhaps the most trenchant statement that *Brave New World* offers a false dilemma was made by Huxley himself. In a preface written in 1946, Huxley wrote: "If I were to rewrite the book, I would offer the Savage a third alternative. Between the utopian and the primitive horns of the dilemma would be the possibility of sanity . . ."[19] Huxley describes this sanity as a society devoted to the pursuit of

> man's Final End, the unitive knowledge of the immanent Tao or Logos, the transcendent Godhead or Brahman. And the prevailing philosophy of life would be a kind of High Utilitarianism, in which the Greatest Happiness principle would be secondary to the Final End principle – the first question to be asked and answered in every contingency in life being: 'How will this thought or action contribute to, or interfere with, the achievement, by me and the greatest possible number of individuals, of man's Final End?' [20]

Huxley goes on to say that in this revised version John the Savage would not be brought to *Brave New World*

> until he had had the opportunity of learning something at first hand about the nature of a society composed of freely co-operating individuals devoted to the pursuit of sanity. Thus altered, *Brave New World* would possess an artistic and (if it is permissible to use so large a word in connection with a work of fiction) a philosophical completeness, which in its present form it evidently lacks.[21]

Interestingly, Huxley's last novel, *Island*, actually offers something like this "sanity" alternative.

Rather than look at the details of Huxley's *Island*, it will be more advantageous to imagine a sequel: *Mark's Braver New World*. It turns out that John the Savage did not die after the lighthouse incident – he was only in a coma. (I didn't say the sequel was a good or original literary work.) Mustapha relents and allows John to visit the island of dissidents where Bernard and Helmholtz are exiled. Here John finds a classless society: there are no Alphas, Betas, Gammas, etc. Art, science, and religion have not been banished or severely curtailed, but are pursued with even greater vigor than in our world. Helmholtz is no longer forced to write mindless ditties to educate his students at the College for Emotional Engineering, but is a poet of some skill. John meets scientists who are pursuing the scientific work started by Mustapha before this line of enquiry was banned in *Brave New World*. Citizens of *Mark's Braver New World* do not take *soma* as a holiday from reality. However, many choose to incorporate happy-people-pills into their everyday lives: they get in pill form what Benito has naturally. Since no one is forced to take the mood boosters, some do not. Their reasons are typically philosophical or religious. But most do take happy-people-pills, even Bernard. Bernard enjoys the better moods they put him in while allowing him to maintain his complete cognitive faculties. The pills have helped Bernard become more sociable. In fact, he has found himself a wife and a fulfilling career as a child psychologist.

So, John finds that *Mark's Braver New World*, like the *Brave New World*, has considerable advantages over our world in terms of happiness. But *Mark's Braver New World* also has more of the higher aspects of humanity than either our world or the *Brave New World*. If we are hoping for as much happiness and achievement as possible in terms of the higher aspects of humanity, then *Mark's Braver New World* is the clear choice over our world and the *Brave New World*.

Let me hasten to add that I do not take this as proof that greater happiness and higher achievement can both be had. After all, it is simply a story (with, no doubt, little literary merit). To think that *Mark's Braver New World* shows that the two can be combined is to make the same mistake as those who think the *Brave New World* shows that the two cannot be combined. My point here is simply that a work of fiction can be written to show that there is no tragic dilemma just as easily as writing fiction like *Brave New World* can be written to show that there is a tragic dilemma.

The upshot is this: it is possible to write a work of fiction that makes the choice between greater happiness than we now experience and the higher aspects of humanity a tragic choice, and it is possible to write a work of fiction that says that this is a false dilemma: it is possible to have much greater happiness and more of the higher aspects of humanity. Works of fiction cannot adjudicate which alternative is correct. This is an empirical matter, or at least this is what I shall argue. We need to look to our best science to tell us about the relationship between happiness and the higher aspects of humanity to see whether they are necessarily antagonistic, as the Controllers of the *Brave New World* claim, or whether the two are in fact compatible.

In Chapter 6 we will review some of the scientific evidence suggesting that happiness and the higher aspects of humanity are in fact linked, that they are not antagonistic. In the meantime, we will explore some of the philosophical questions raised by the *Brave New World*: What is happiness? How does happiness contribute to the good life?

Notes

1. Fukuyama, *Our Posthuman Future*, 7.
2. Huxley, *Brave New World and Brave New World Revisited*, 129.
3. Ibid., 60.
4. Ibid.
5. Ibid., 148.
6. Ibid., 53.
7. Winkler, "Devices and Desires of Our Own Hearts," 246.
8. Kass, *Toward a More Natural Science*, 34–5.
9. Fukuyama, *Our Posthuman Future*, 5–6.
10. Ibid., 6.
11. Winkler, "Devices and Desires of Our Own Hearts," 246.
12. Russell, "We Don't Want to Be Happy," 211.
13. Huxley, *Brave New World and Brave New World Revisited*, 225–6.
14. Marx and Engels, *The German Ideology*, 53.
15. Bertrand Russell considers something analogous to this point ("We Don't Want to Be Happy," 211–12).
16. Huxley, *Brave New World and Brave New World Revisited*, 60.
17. Ibid., 343.
18. Ibid., 65–6.
19. Ibid., 7.
20. Ibid., 7.
21. Ibid., 7–8.

References

Fukuyama, F. *Our Posthuman Future: Consequences of the Biotechnology Revolution.* London: Profile, 2003.

Huxley, A. *Brave New World and Brave New World Revisited.* Toronto: Vintage Books, 2007.

Kass, L. R. *Toward a More Natural Science.* New York: Free Press, 1988.

Marx, K. and F. Engels. *The German Ideology Part One: With Selections from Parts Two and Three and Supplementary Texts,* edited, with an introduction, by C. J. Arthur. New York: International Publishers, 1970.

Russell, B. "We Don't Want to Be Happy." In *Aldous Huxley: The Critical Heritage,* edited by D. Watt, 210–12. New York: Psychology Press, 1997.

Winkler, M. "Devices and Desires of Our Own Hearts." In *Enhancing Human Traits: Ethical and Social Implications,* edited by E. Parens, 238–50. Washington, D.C.: Georgetown University Press, 1998.

3

What Do We Mean by `Happiness´?

As noted in the Introduction, Chapters 3, 4, and 5 are the most philosophically dense. Some readers may wish to skip ahead to Chapter 6 where they will find a brief summary of the conclusions reached in these chapters, and perhaps return later to examine the arguments for these conclusions.

The aim of this chapter is to provide at least a partial analysis of the word 'happiness' as it is used in everyday language. The analysis is "partial" because there are several questions which we need not answer for present purposes. On the other hand, there are several reasons we must pursue at least a partial analysis. First, it is important to ensure that 'happiness' is not being redefined. There is a perfectly good sense in which you might describe your slightly intoxicated co-worker as "happy," but clearly this is not the intended usage when parents say they "just want their children to be happy." In attempting to be clear about what is meant by 'happiness,' we can avoid more subtle forms of the same error. Second, as previously mentioned, we will be drawing on social and natural scientific investigations into happiness. As we shall see, these theorists employ several different understandings of happiness. It is important that we get clear about the relevant understandings of 'happiness' upon which this research is built. Third, we will investigate the relationship between happiness and the good life in Chapter 4, and so again it is important that we understand exactly what happiness amounts to.

Happy-People-Pills For All, First Edition. Mark Walker.
© 2013 John Wiley & Sons, Inc. Published 2013 by John Wiley & Sons, Inc.

In the first few sections of this chapter I will try to make clear exactly what we are looking for in a theory of happiness and then go on to argue for a particular theory. The theory I shall endorse is a composite of affective and cognitive elements.

3.1 Two Senses of 'Happiness': Wellbeing and a Psychological State

It will help to locate our subject matter by observing the frequently made distinction between 'happiness' as a synonym for wellbeing and 'happiness' as a psychological term.[1] To say that persons had a 'happy life' in the wellbeing sense is to say that their life went well for them. In this sense, 'happy' is clearly an evaluative term. It is, in effect, a place-holder for answers to the question: "What is the good life?" The question seeks an account of what, in self-interested terms, makes a life good for the person whose life it is.[2] Other synonyms include 'welfare' and 'prudential value.'[3] In contrast, the psychological sense of 'happiness' refers to a mental state. To describe persons as happy in this sense is to say something about their state of mind in just the way that 'melancholy' and 'depressive' are descriptive of mental states.[4] Thus, happiness in its psychological sense is a descriptive term.[5]

Although these two senses of happiness are distinct, there are three possibilities for connecting them. One option is to say of identity that to be happy in the wellbeing sense just is to be happy in the psychological sense.[6] Fred Feldman has recently argued in support of the view that one is happy in the wellbeing sense to the extent that one is happy in the psychological sense.[7] A second view is that happiness in the psychological sense is a proper part of happiness in the wellbeing sense. Wayne Sumner has supported this position, saying that wellbeing requires, in addition to psychological happiness, that subjects must also be informed and autonomous. So, happiness in the psychological sense is a necessary but not sufficient condition for happiness in the wellbeing sense according to Sumner.[8] Finally, there is the view that there is no substantive relationship between the two concepts of happiness. Perfectionists of the sort outlined by Thomas Hurka believe that happiness is not a component of the good life.[9] For perfectionists, wellbeing includes such items as knowledge or intellectual excellence, physical excellence, virtue, and so on. Perfectionists might value happiness instrumentally, if happiness helps subjects realize perfectionist goods like intellectual excellence, but happiness is not intrinsically valuable.

In Chapter 4, I will argue for the second position: psychological happiness is a part of the good life, but there is more to the good life than happiness. In this chapter our focus is on the psychological sense of happiness, so, to avoid confusion, hereafter 'happiness' refers to the psychological sense unless otherwise noted.

We are about to look at four monistic theories of happiness. They are monistic in the sense that each says the term 'happiness' can be analyzed in terms of a single constituent. I will briefly review the four theories before showing why each is insufficient on its own to capture what we mean by 'happiness.'

3.2 Affective Theories of Happiness

In this section we will consider two affective accounts of happiness: sensory hedonism and emotional state theory. For sensory hedonism, the basic unit of analysis of happiness is sensory pleasure and sensory pain. Paradigmatic instances of sensory pleasure include the experience of an orgasm and the sensation of a refreshing beverage on a hot summer's day; paradigmatic instances of pain include the experience of a headache or the stubbing of a toe. The sensory hedonistic account says that happiness is some positive surplus of sensory pleasure over sensory pain; and unhappiness is some surplus of sensory pain over sensory pleasure.[10] The happiness of individuals can be ascertained by adding up the "atoms" of happiness over any arbitrary length of time.[11] So, Aristippus is happy at sunrise on his twentieth birthday if he has some positive balance of sensory pleasure over sensory pain at sunrise on this day. He is happy in his twentieth year if he has some positive balance of sensory pleasure over sensory pain in that year. Aristippus has a happy life if, over the course of his life, he has some positive balance of sensory pleasure over sensory pain throughout his life.

The emotional state view of happiness is one of the major views of happiness in the social science literature[12] and has been defended by philosopher Daniel Haybron.[13] In a landmark study on the relationship between happiness and achievement, which we will examine in some detail in Chapter 6, psychologists Sonja Lyubomirsky, Laura King, and Ed Diener describe their focus on "happy individuals – that is, those who experience frequent positive emotions, such as joy, interest, and pride, and infrequent (though not absent) negative emotions, such as sadness, anxiety, and anger."[14] So, on the emotional state view, 'happiness' is understood as the antipode to the negative moods and emotions, such as sadness, anxiety, and anger, frequently studied in psychology.[15]

The basic unit of analysis for emotional state theorists is positive moods and emotions. To be happy on this view is to have some favorable balance of positive moods and emotions over negative moods and emotions; to be unhappy is to have some unfavorable balance of negative moods and emotions over positive moods and emotions. As with sensory hedonism, happiness can be ascribed for any arbitrary interval of time by simply substituting "positive moods and emotions" and "negative moods and emotions" where we previously had "sensory pleasure" and "sensory pain": Aristippus is happy at sunrise on his twentieth birthday if he has some positive balance of positive moods and emotions over negative moods and emotions at sunrise. He is happy in his twentieth year if he has some positive balance of positive moods and emotions over negative moods and emotions in that year. Aristippus' life is a happy one if over the course of his life he has some positive balance of positive moods and emotions over negative moods and emotions throughout his life.[16]

As Haybron notes, it may be that some of the classical hedonists, such as J. S. Mill, have not fully distinguished sensory pleasure from emotional state theory.[17] However, it seems there are good reasons to think the two distinct. It is possible to experience sensory pleasure but not be in a positive mood. Imagine you have sex with your spouse at the regularly appointed time despite not being in a good mood: you suspect he has been cheating on you. You experience sensory pleasure during orgasm, but this in itself does not put you in a good mood. Of course, sensory pleasure and pain may often influence our moods: a delicious dinner may buoy our spirits and chronic or intense pain can negatively influence moods and emotions. So, sensory pleasure and positive moods and emotions are conceptually distinct even if causally connected.

3.3   Cognitive Accounts of Happiness

In this section we will look at two cognitive accounts. The "whole life satisfaction view," the idea that happiness is a positive judgment about one's life; and Fred Feldman's attitudinal hedonism account of happiness.

The "whole life satisfaction" view of happiness, as its name suggests, is one in which individuals judge the overall quality of their lives as favorable.[18] Ed Diener and his colleagues formulated a comprehensive tool to investigate this sense of happiness:

The Satisfaction with Life Scale

DIRECTIONS: Below are five statements with which you may agree or disagree. Using the 1–7 scale below, indicate your agreement with each item by placing the appropriate number in the line preceding that item. Please be open and honest in your responding.

1 = Strongly Disagree
2 = Disagree
3 = Slightly Disagree
4 = Neither Agree or Disagree
5 = Slightly Agree
6 = Agree
7 = Strongly Agree

_____1. In most ways my life is close to my ideal.
_____2. The conditions of my life are excellent.
_____3. I am satisfied with life.
_____4. So far I have gotten the important things I want in life.
_____5. If I could live my life over, I would change almost nothing.[19]

Happiness, on this view, is having a reasoned positive global judgment about the course of your life. It is important to understand that whole life satisfaction is not used to indicate whether someone is happy or unhappy, but, on this view, happiness *is* whole life satisfaction.[20]

A number of philosophers have recommended the life satisfaction view.[21] Wayne Sumner claims happiness is

> a positive evaluation of the conditions of your life, a judgment that, at least on balance, it measures up favourably against your standards or expectations. This evaluation . . . represents an affirmation or endorsement of (some or all of) the conditions or circumstances of your life, a judgement that, on balance and taking everything into account, your life is going well for you.[22]

Let us note a few features about whole life satisfaction accounts. The basic unit of analysis is a propositional attitude. Propositional attitudes have an object – a proposition that describes some state of affairs – and an attitude – a mental state connecting a person to the proposition. Consider a proposition such as: "It will rain tomorrow." I might have various propositional *attitudes* to this proposition, for example "I *believe* that it will rain tomorrow," or "I *desire* that it will rain tomorrow." In the case of life satisfaction accounts, the proposition is some global statement about the relationship between one's "standards or expectations" and one's life. The first item on Diener's survey nicely illustrates this: "In most ways my life is close to my ideal." The propositional attitude is one of (degrees of) agreement or disagreement. Thus, the happiest persons are those who would say, "I strongly agree that in most ways my life is close to my ideal"; the unhappiest persons are those who would say, "I strongly disagree that in most ways my life is close to my ideal."[23] For whole life satisfaction accounts of happiness, the relevant domain of propositions deals with a person's life, or some important domain thereof, for example one's work or family life.

Our fourth and final account of happiness has recently been formulated by Fred Feldman. Rather than thinking of pleasure as experiential with the sensory hedonist, Feldman understands the basic unit of analysis of happiness in terms of the propositional attitude of being pleased. One is happy, on Feldman's view, to the extent that one takes attitudinal pleasure in things, and less happy to the extent that one takes attitudinal displeasure in things.

More formally, Feldman defines momentary happiness as "S's momentary happiness at t = the sum, for all propositions, p, such that S is occurrently intrinsically (dis)pleased about p at t, of the degree to which S is occurrently intrinsically (dis)pleased about p at t."[24] A few of his terms need unpacking. To be intrinsically pleased with something is to be pleased with it for its own sake, not for the sake of something else. You might be pleased to be driving, but not intrinsically so. You are heading over to a friend's for dinner. You are pleased to be driving only for the sake of getting to your dinner destination; driving in traffic is not something that you would find pleasing independently of its instrumental value as a means to get where you want to go. Dinner at your friend's, however, is intrinsically pleasing: it is pleasing for its own sake.

To be occurrently pleased is to be thinking about something and to have the attitude of being pleased with respect to what is being thought. The contrast with occurrent pleasure is with dispositional pleasure: you may not be thinking about it at the moment but, if asked, you might say that you are pleased the Allies won World War II. For Feldman, happiness is tied to what we are thinking about; it is not defined in terms of what we *would* think about.

Finally, being pleased about something comes in degrees; for example, most people would be more pleased about receiving a promotion at work than about the weather being particularly pleasant on some particular day. So, being pleased about the former adds more to your happiness than being pleased about the latter. Indeed, the degree of being pleased (or displeased) is as important as the number of thoughts that an individual is pleased or displeased about. Suppose we want to ascertain whether you are happy or unhappy during your drive to work. We ascertain that you had ten thoughts relevant to attitudinal hedonism. Nine of these thoughts involved attitudinal pleasure, and one attitudinal displeasure. It would be hasty to suppose that you must be rated as happy during that period by attitudinal hedonism. Suppose your first thought is one of attitudinal displeasure: you recall that your husband left you two days ago for his mistress. Determined not to let this affect you too much, you try to take your friend's advice and count your "small blessings." You take pleasure in the facts that the traffic is unusually light, that the new coffee your friend recommended tastes particularly good, a song on the radio reminds you of happier times, and so on. We can imagine on some attitudinal happiness scale that each of these small blessings count for three units of attitudinal pleasure, for a total of twenty-seven units of attitudinal pleasure. The thought about your husband leaving you, however, yields one thousand units of attitudinal displeasure, so your "net happiness" is nine hundred and seventy-three units of displeasure. Despite a greater quantity of happy thoughts, attitudinal hedonism would say that you are unhappy overall during your drive to work. This verdict seems intuitively plausible: we should allow for qualitative matters; the extreme unhappiness caused by your husband leaving is not adequately compensated for by the counting of the small blessings. (Counting small blessings may soften the pain, but they do not fully compensate for the pain of betrayal.)

It is worth thinking about the difference between sensory and attitudinal hedonism, and Feldman's Stoicus example is a good means to illustrate the difference. Stoicus enjoys his life immensely, but he eschews sensory pain and pleasure. He seeks a life of tranquility; he enjoys *not* experiencing sensory pain and pleasure. "Suppose Stoicus eventually dies a happy man. He lived 90 years of a somewhat boring but on the whole quite enjoyable peace and quiet. Stoicus thinks (right before he dies) that his has been an outstandingly good life."[25] On the sensory hedonism view of happiness, Stoicus did not have a happy life, because he did not have some positive surplus of sensory pleasure over sensory pain. (Of course it is practically impossible to avoid all sensory pleasure and pain, so let us assume that Stoicus had unusually small amounts of both and that the balance of sensory pleasure versus sensory pain was neutral over the course of his life.) On Feldman's attitudinal hedonism view, Stoicus has had a happy life, since he was immensely pleased by his peace and quiet: Stoicus has an impressive positive surplus of attitudinal pleasure over attitudinal displeasure over the course of his long life.

I have termed Feldman's account a "cognitive account," but it may seem that there is an affective component. Even if Stoicus does not have much in the way of sensory pleasure, it seems that if he is pleased by the course of his life he must be affectively moved. It may seem hard to imagine Stoicus not having what Feldman describes as "cheery feelings" when he reflects on how well his life has gone. It may seem, then, that the affective component of emotional state theory has surreptitiously been reintroduced.

However, Feldman offers an example to show how the affective component of emotional state theory is not an essential constituent of happiness. His example involves a researcher who hopes to investigate the "cheery feelings" associated with happiness and who has a conjecture about where in the brain the cheery feelings are located:

> Let us imagine that this researcher finds a way to disable the relevant area of his own brain. Imagine that he then spends some quality time with his children. He has a lot of fun with them, but feels decidedly strange: though he is enjoying the time spent with his children, something is missing. He cannot feel any cheery feelings. The sensory background normally associated with happy times is simply gone. The researcher is delighted. This is good news. His hypothesis [concerning the location of cheery feelings] is confirmed. He will now be able to publish a paper in which he announces the neural basis of cheery feelings.[26]

Feldman says that it is plausible to think that the researcher is happy when playing with his children and with the thought that he will publish his findings. This shows that cheery feelings are not necessary for happiness. Feldman clarifies this thought: "Of course, I am not denying that there are such feelings; nor am I denying that happy people often feel them. I am just saying that they are not essential constitutive elements of happiness."[27]

This completes our rapid survey of four theories of happiness. We will now turn to the question of their adequacy.

3.4   Counterexamples to Monism About Happiness

The fact that we have both affective theories and cognitive theories of happiness makes it sound like another skirmish in the timeless battle between the emotional and the cognitive elements of our psyches: which aspect is happiness associated with – emotion or cognition? An obvious move is to reject the dilemma and embrace a view that comprises a cognitive and an emotional element. As noted above, this is precisely what I want to urge: a composite view that combines both emotional state theory and attitudinal hedonism. To this end, I will attempt to show why each of these theories fails when understood as a complete theory of happiness.

Consider first the cases of Harry and Harriet:

HARRY: *Harry is a slave in the South in pre-Civil War America who is often in a positive mood. He whistles while chopping wood, tilling, planting, and harvesting for his master. Imagine someone observes Harry and remarks that he seems very happy. Harry replies: "How can you say that? Can't you see I am a slave? My master treats me as a mere tool for his every whim. You are sorely mistaken: I am not pleased about things. Think about my day: I must attend a meeting where we are given work orders for the day. So, each day I am reminded that I am a slave. Each day my master beats at least one of his slaves, usually for no reason but to instill fear and compliance. So, I estimate I have at least 2,000 units of attitudinal displeasure before we even get our orders.* Typically, my master's orders are so asinine that I am further displeased; for example, today he has ordered us to plant seeds when it is clearly too wet to do so. He knows nothing about farming, but he is in charge. This adds another 200 units of displeasure, for much of my labor goes to complete waste. Yes, in the field away from my master I may take pleasure in small things. I may take pleasure in hearing the birds sing, and I may take pleasure in the warm sun. Perhaps these things will give me 10 units of attitudinal pleasure each. On a good day perhaps these small pleasures may add up to a few hundred units of positive attitudinal pleasure. Obviously, this pleasure is overshadowed by the displeasure of being treated as a mere thing. You can hardly say that I am pleased about things overall." When the observer protests that Harry often seems in a positive mood when he is doing his master's bidding, Harry responds: "What use would it be to be constantly in a negative mood? Of course, when I was first captured I was often in a negative mood. But*

---

*   Readers may wonder how Harry learned about Feldman's attitudinal hedonism more than a century before Feldman formulated it. So do I.

> *I realized that this would not change my situation. My small revenge against the*
> *displeasure of being treated as a tool by my master and an unjust society is that I*
> *stay upbeat: I maintain positive moods through it all even though my displeasure*
> *at being a slave has remained steadfast."*

HARRIET: *Harriet is an artist who experiences many negative moods. Sometimes her moods*
            are so negative she spends most of the day just lying in bed. A psychologist friend
            has suggested that she has chronic negative affect: a preponderance of negative
            moods and emotions. The psychologist suspects Harriet meets the criteria for
            clinical depression. When asked how happy she is, she says she is very happy. Her
            friends are surprised to hear this, but she says that she is very pleased with her
            art, and she sees her propensity for negative moods as a positive: it helps with
            her painting. According to Harriet, without the negative moods her art would
            suffer, so she is pleased with her negative moods as a means to further her art.
            Yes, this means that her attitudinal pleasure about many things is reduced so
            often it has a negative valence. For example, she does not take as much pleasure
            in the company of her friends as a typical non-depressed person might. But the
            fact that she experiences great attitudinal pleasure in her art, say 2,000 units
            a day, more than makes up for the loss in what she sees as a less important
            aspect of her life. Her psychologist wonders whether, when she gets attitudinal
            pleasure, it puts her in a good mood. She said sometimes this used to happen.
            Sometimes she would look at a painting she was working on and be pleased by
            her progress, which in turn would lead to a boost in her mood. But over time she
            has disciplined herself not to let being pleased with her work affect her in this
            way, for it is counterproductive.

On the attitudinal hedonism model of happiness, Harry is unhappy despite his positive moods and Harriet is happy despite her borderline emotional depression. Using the emotional state model of happiness, we get precisely the opposite result: Harry is happy despite his enslavement and Harriet is unhappy despite her great art. Which notion better captures our understanding of happiness? The fact that in both examples we might be reluctant to say Harry or Harriet is happy or unhappy without further qualification – the obvious thing to say is that they are happy in certain respects and not in others – provides some intuitive support for the composite view.

A much greater challenge for monism comes from the continuing sagas of Harry and Harriet.

HARRY PART II: *Harry gains his freedom at the end of the Civil War. Naturally, he is*
                  pleased about this. Most days the first thing he thinks about is how great
                  it is to be free. And often this is his last thought before he falls asleep. His

attitudinal pleasure has risen dramatically, but there is, as in all human life, some attitudinal pain. After all, he has new things to worry about. When he was a slave he knew where his next meal would come from, and what his future looked like. With this newfound freedom Harry has more to worry about. Yes, he takes great attitudinal pleasure in not being a mere tool for his master's whims, yet his overall emotional state has not risen. Let us suppose that the pleasure he takes in his freedom causes X units of increased positive moods, but this increase is exactly cancelled by X units lost in positive moods caused by an uncertain future. It should be emphasized that Harry is just as emotionally upbeat as before – he still whistles while he works, and is quick to smile. It is just that he is not more *emotionally upbeat. So, Harry's attitudinal pleasure has risen dramatically, but his emotional state remains unchanged on balance.*

HARRIETT PART II: *Under pressure from her friends, Harriet relents and sees a psychother- apist, who helps her explore the basis of her negative emotions. It is discovered that bad toilet training as an infant is the cause of her neg- ative emotional states, and Harriet begins a therapeutic journey that dramatically changes her. As a result of this therapy and prescribed mood-boosting drugs, her moods are now upbeat much more frequently than before. According to her friends, her art has not suffered in the least for her cathartic experience on the psychiatrist's couch and taking antidepressants. Some maintain that her art is even better than before. Harriet rates the pleasure she takes in things the same as before. It is true that her positive moods have made much of her everyday life much more pleasant, and so she takes greater pleasure in this aspect. However, despite what her friends say, she has lingering doubts about her art. She is not entirely convinced that her art has not suffered, although sometimes she thinks it has taken a turn for the better. Certainly, the fact that some of her friends say it is better seems to indicate that it has changed, so she cannot entirely dismiss the thought that it may not have changed for the better. Her therapist says that she shouldn't have these doubts, and that she needs to free herself of the idea that she must suffer for her art. This is a lingering effect of the bad toilet training. Still, she is not as pleased with her art as she once was. Her greater attitudinal pleasure in the rest of her life is exactly offset by the reduced pleasure in her art. Let us suppose that she takes X units of attitudinal pleasure in not being constantly in negative moods in her daily life, but this increase is exactly cancelled by X units lost in attitudinal pleasure about her art. It should be emphasized that Harriet is just as pleased about things it is just that she is not* more *pleased about things overall. So, Harriet's emo- tional state has risen dramatically, but her attitudinal pleasure remains unchanged.*

Let us think about what attitudinal hedonism and emotional state theory must say about these cases. If attitudinal hedonism is correct, then Harry is happier after being released from slavery. He is very pleased about not being treated as a tool. He is very pleased to be in charge of his life. These attitudinal gains completely overshadow the attitudinal displeasure in being uncertain about his future. And, if attitudinal hedonism is correct, then Harriet is not happier after receiving psychiatric help. She takes attitudinal pleasure in not being subject to so many negative emotions, but she takes less attitudinal pleasure in her art. Since there is no gain in her overall balance of attitudinal pleasure, she is not happier. It is worth emphasizing that this result turns on the fact that attitudinal hedonism says we must rate attitudinal pleasure in both its quantity and quality. After her therapy, we imagine that the quantity of things that Harriet takes pleasure in has risen dramatically. She feels pleased when visiting with friends, and takes new-found pleasure in cooking and shopping. However, the attitudinal pleasure of these things is minor compared to the one thing that she thinks about and that matters to her most: her art. And because of this qualitative difference, her net attitudinal pleasure is the same.

If the emotional state theory of happiness is correct, then Harry is not any happier after being released from slavery. Since his emotional state remains unchanged overall, he cannot be said to be happier. And if the emotional state theory is correct, then Harriet is much happier after psychiatric intervention. Her preponderant negative moods and emotions have been lifted and replaced by positive moods and emotions like joy and excitement.

The trouble of course is that the ordinary use of 'happiness' is such that it seems entirely appropriate to describe both Harry and Harriet as happier in the second parts of their stories. If this is the case, then both attitudinal hedonism and emotional state theory must be rejected as theories that completely capture what we mean by 'happiness.' Attitudinal hedonism gives us the right verdict in Harry's case – it says that Harry is happier – but gives us the wrong verdict in Harriet's case – it does not permit us to say that Harriet is happier. Conversely, emotional state theory gives us the wrong verdict in Harry's case – it says he is no happier upon being released from his bonds – but gives us the right verdict in Harriet's case – it permits us to say that Harriet is happier after her therapy.

The composite view advocated here – the view that combines attitudinal hedonism and emotional state theory – gives the right verdict in both of these cases. It allows us to say Harry is happier after his release because he is pleased about more things, and it permits us to say Harriet is happier after her therapy because of the improvement in her emotional condition.

3.5   Methodological Remarks

The initial defense of this composite account is simply that it can successfully deal with the aforementioned counterexamples. In this section, I hope to bolster this result by making some remarks about different concepts of happiness, the aims of the present analysis, and appropriate methodology for arguing for or against different theories of happiness. The upshot will be that a very common argumentative pattern used is, in fact, faulty. I offer an alternative.

Initially, it is worth noting that the aim of these counterexamples is to argue *to* compositism, not *from* compositism. The examples ask fair-minded readers how the word 'happiness', as we ordinarily understand it, should be applied to these cases. It is an argument *to* compositism because it has this structure: it asks how we would apply our everyday understanding of happiness to Harry and Harriet in the second part of the examples. Untutored judgments suggest both are happier, and so this is some reason to believe compositism. An argument *from* compositism would say that since compositism is correct, we ought to judge Harry and Harriet as happier in the second part of each example. Similarly, one can argue *from* emotional state theory to the conclusion that Harry is not happier upon being granted his freedom, and one can argue *from* attitudinal hedonism to the conclusion that Harriet is not happier after her psychiatric intervention. Any argument *from* a particular conception of happiness begs the question in this context, since we are seeking to establish a theory of happiness. To adjudicate, we must appeal to pre-theoretic judgments about how we would normally use the word 'happy.' I have argued that these judgments favor the composite conception.

We can understand the methodological issues further by considering a commonly employed argumentative strategy, which we will think of as the "necessary/sufficient" strategy. I hope to demonstrate that this strategy will not work, even in principle, to show that some forms of pluralism are wrong. This is the familiar strategy that says theory T does not work as an analysis of some concept C, because T is neither necessary nor sufficient for C. Thus, recall Feldman's example of Stoicus. Using the necessary/sufficient strategy it could be argued that sensory pleasure is not necessary for happiness, since Stoicus is happy, but experiences very little sensory pleasure.

Feldman's orgasm enhancer example below shows why sensory pleasure is not sufficient for happiness. In the following example, 'hedons' and 'dolors' are units of pleasure and pain respectively:

> Suppose that, after being endlessly bombarded by email advertisements, Wendell has purchased a highly touted orgasm enhancer. Suppose he has paid for, and is expecting a monster 400 hedon orgasm. Suppose when the orgasm comes, it is a pathetic little 12 hedon orgasm. Wendell is disappointed. He thinks he has wasted his money. He is also somewhat embarrassed, since he had been warned that the email advertisements were just scams. However, at the moment of orgasm, his hedonic-doloric balance is definitely positive. He feels 12 hedons of sensory pleasure, and no dolors of sensory pain. Yet he is not happy.[28]

The example seems plausible enough: it seems we can quite easily imagine someone experiencing some pleasure but not being happy. What does this tell us about the relationship between happiness and pleasure? According to Feldman, the example helps support the conclusion that the hedonic theory of happiness is false.[29] The strategy works if sensory hedonism is offered as a monistic theory; and since Feldman understands sensory hedonism as a monistic theory, as offering necessary and sufficient conditions for 'happiness', his argument is successful.

However, Feldman's use of the necessary/sufficient strategy does not work against a composite conception of happiness. Since compositism says that happiness must be analyzed in terms of the units of analysis of two or more theories – T1 *and* T2, etc. – a composite conception, by definition, is committed to the insufficiency of T1 in isolation, and the insufficiency of T2 in isolation, etc.

Still, it may be thought that if pluralism says that some concept C is to be analyzed in terms of two or more theories, T1, T2, etc., then each theory itself must be necessary. For example, suppose one philosophical apprentice suggests that the concept of 'bachelor' can be analyzed solely in terms of being a male, and another suggests 'bachelor' can be analyzed solely in terms of being unmarried. The philosophical master will hardly need to break a philosophical sweat to show that these monistic theories are wrong, that is, bachelor is a composite concept: neither is sufficient on its own, and both are necessary. Analogously, it seems that Feldman still has some argument against compositism because he attempts to show that a number of theories of happiness are not even a necessary component of happiness. Thus, Feldman's Stoicus example seems to show that sensory pleasure is not necessary for happiness: Stoicus is happy without sensory pleasure. And so it seems that we can conclude that sensory hedonism is not part of a composite theory of happiness.

There are several reasons for thinking that this line of argument is suspect. To see why, we will need to draw a few distinctions.

First, we should be clear about the inventory and logical questions concerning the units of analysis offered by different theories of happiness. The inventory question asks: What are the basic constituents of X? The basic constituents of the concept 'bachelor' are 'male' and 'unmarried.' The logic question asks about the logical relationship between the basic constituents in terms of explicating the target concept. In the case of the concept of bachelor, male and unmarried are each necessary, and jointly sufficient. But consider the concept of 'zachelor.' Someone is a zachelor if unmarried or a male. Notice then the concept of zachelor shares the same basic constituents as that of bachelor. So, the inventory question yields the same answer when asked of both bachelor and zachelor: the basic (non-logical) units of analysis are 'male' and 'unmarried' for both concepts.

The logical difference between 'bachelor' and 'zachelor' is that the former offers a conjunctive theory whereas the latter is disjunctive.[†] If Chris is a bachelor, it must be the case that Chris is both male and unmarried. If Chris is a zachelor, it must be the case that Chris is either a male or unmarried, but Chris could be a married male or an unmarried female and be a zachelor. So, it is enough to show that Chris is not a bachelor if it can be demonstrated that Chris is not a male. It is not enough to show that Chris is not a zachelor if it can be demonstrated that Chris is not a male or that Chris is married. So, Feldman's Stoicus example works as a counterexample to a conjunctive analysis of happiness that invokes sensory pleasure as an additional element, but it is not a counterexample to a disjunctive analysis that invokes sensory pleasure.

Another thing we should notice is that there is a sense in which happiness is gradable. This is apparent when we use it in its comparative sense. In this respect, happiness is like being tall: just as we can say that X is taller than Y, it is appropriate to speak about X being happier than Y. We can

---

[†]   A less artificial disjunctive concept is that of 'legally in the country': one can be legally in the country if one is a citizen, or has permanent resident status, or has a valid visa. No disjunct is necessary for being in the country legally.

speak about Jack being happier than Jill, or Jack being happier before he fell down and broke his crown.

Like many gradable concepts, happiness can be understood in a threshold and a superlative sense. Using the threshold sense we can classify people as happy or not happy. The threshold sense and the gradable sense of happiness are related but distinct. Jack can be happier than Jill, but Jack may not be happy. He may simply be less unhappy. Alternatively, if we describe Jack and Jill as both meeting the threshold for happiness, then the gradable concept is still relevant: Jack may be happier than Jill (or vice versa) even though they are both happy. The two concepts are not without some logical relationship. If we know that Jill is happier than Jack, and Jack meets the threshold to be described as 'happy', then we can infer that Jill is happy too.

We can think of the superlative sense of happiness in terms of ideal happiness or as membership amongst the happiest. Many people are happy in the threshold sense, but few are superlatively happy. If we were to imagine rating happiness on a scale of 1–10, then the superlatively happy would be at the ten end of the scale. The threshold sense might demand that to be happy one is above six on the happy scale. Again, there are logical relations between the two concepts: if someone is superlatively happy, then he or she is also happy in the threshold sense.

These distinctions permit a more precise statement of our aim: the aim here is to answer the inventory question and the logical question as applied to the superlative conception: what are the basic units of superlative happiness and how are these units logically related? The proposal offered is that the superlative pluralistic conception is conjunctive: ideal happiness has both an affective and a cognitive component. I will not argue the question of the threshold sense of happiness, as it is not important for present purposes. At least one answer to the threshold question, and to my mind quite a plausible answer, is that threshold happiness may be disjunctive. Consider the initial versions of the Harry and Harriet examples. Harry might be happy despite lacking positive overall attitudinal pleasure, and Harriet may be happy despite lacking an overall positive emotional state. On this view, a certain positive balance of attitudinal pleasure *or* emotional state is sufficient for threshold happiness, but neither is necessary.

A critical point here is that a conjunctive understanding of superlative happiness does not logically necessitate a conjunctive threshold conception of happiness. We can see the relevance of this by considering again Feldman's example of the researcher who is investigating the neural basis of happiness. Recall he says that the putative affective components of happiness, the "cheery feelings," "are not essential constitutive elements of happiness,"[30] since it still seems appropriate to call the researcher happy while the neural basis for cheery feelings have been knocked out. Notice that the example seems to be addressing the threshold sense of happiness: Feldman is asking whether we would still call the researcher happy under these circumstances. This is further confirmed when we realize that Feldman never asks whether the researcher would be *happier* if he had the cheery feelings. In the latter case, his attitudinal pleasure is conditional upon lack of cheery feelings. In effect, Feldman has built into the example the stipulation that at most the researcher can have cheery feelings or attitudinal pleasure. This does not threaten a composite superlative conception; it merely shows that in some cases it may be impossible for individuals to achieve superlative happiness. As further evidence we can imagine adapting the example. Suppose if the experiment confirms the location of cheery feelings, the researcher will have 100 units of attitudinal hedonism. As before, the researcher is pleased to confirm his theory. Suppose that if the experiment does not confirm the location of cheery feelings, the researcher will have 100 units of attitudinal pleasure. In this case, we imagine that the researcher wins a significant cash prize for failure to confirm the location of cheery feelings. He intends to use the money to buy shoes for his children. The example thus modified allows us to ask a question about superlative happiness that Feldman's original example does not: is he happier with cheery feelings? According to Feldman's attitudinal hedonism, the researcher must be equally happy whether the experiment confirms the location of cheery feelings or not, since the attitudinal pleasure is exactly equal. Of course the composite view says that the addition of the cheery feelings, the positive mood, adds at least a little to his happiness.

This suggests a methodology for investigating the inventory question of a conjunctive analysis of superlative happiness. Rather than asking whether some putative part of happiness X is required for happiness, we ask whether the addition of X adds any additional happiness, that is, whether the addition of X makes subjects *happier*. There are two potential pitfalls with this strategy, one of which is easy to control for, the other less so.

We have to be careful when thinking about the addition of X that it is not adding to happiness merely in an instrumental fashion. Suppose it is agreed with Feldman that attitudinal hedonism is an essential component of superlative happiness, and now we want to investigate whether money is an additional part of superlative happiness. It won't do simply to imagine giving money to subjects and asking whether they are happier, because their attitudinal enjoyment is likely to rise. If we judged subjects as happier after receiving money, we would have no idea whether money is a constituent element of happiness or whether it is merely instrumental: it causes people's attitudinal pleasure to rise. We need to control for this by stipulating that their attitudinal pleasure remains the same after receiving money. This way we can be sure that the additional factor is not simply causally affecting the non-disputed elements of happiness. This is what we might think of as the "method of difference":[31] we compare two lives (or two versions of the same life) which are equal in some non-disputed part of happiness and see whether the addition of some putative part of happiness adds happiness to one life (or to one version of a life).

The method of difference is by no means a perfect test. The aforementioned problem that is harder to control for is whether the addition of X is itself a constituent of happiness, or whether it is causally contributory to some unrecognized element of happiness. Suppose we run the experiment just mentioned where we give subjects money but control for their attitudinal enjoyment; and it is agreed by observers that subjects are happier. We would be hasty in concluding that money is a constituent element of happiness, for money may causally contribute to something else that is a constituent of happiness that we have not recognized in our experiment. For example, suppose giving subjects money boosts their emotional state. It may then be that it is a positive emotional state rather than money that is a constituent of happiness.

It is worth emphasizing here that the problem is not testing whether it is a boost in emotional state or money that leads us to say that the subjects are happier. The method of difference would allow us to tease these apart. The problem is making sure that we have identified all the relevant candidates or theories. Consider that one of the candidates we are investigating, Feldman's attitudinal hedonism account of happiness, has only been explicitly formulated in the last decade or so.

I have no general answer as to how to avoid this difficulty, as it requires an answer to the question of how we know we have considered all the theoretically relevant options.[32] In practice, it should be sufficient to have identified the most plausible candidates for constituents of happiness, and test them out in the manner suggested by the method of difference. This is no guarantee that there is not some better unconsidered theory, only that this is the best we can do, given our epistemic limitations.

It should be apparent that the method of difference was used in the cases of Harry and Harriet: we imagined adding positive emotions while controlling for attitudinal pleasure, and adding attitudinal pleasure while controlling for emotional state. As argued in this section, the method of difference is well suited to answering the inventory question about superlative happiness.

3.6   Sensory Hedonism

We have seen that, using the necessary/sufficient strategy, Feldman's Stoicus example cannot demonstrate that sensory pleasure is not part of superlative happiness. However, his example can be adapted using the more promising method of difference to show that sensory pleasure is part of happiness.

Imagine two versions of Stoicus' life. In the A version, he lives a life much as Feldman asks us to imagine: a life where he enjoys immense attitudinal pleasure but very little sensory pleasure. We will add that he also experiences positive emotions: Stoicus is usually upbeat. For the purposes of illustration we can imagine that he receives a daily average of exactly 100 units of attitudinal pleasure, 100 units of positive emotions, and 0 units of sensory pleasure. In the B version, Stoicus receives a daily average of 100 units of attitudinal pleasure, 100 units of positive emotions, and 200 units of sensory pleasure. The explanation for the difference is this: in the B version, Stoicus is captured by Aristippus and his band of merry sensory hedonists. They force Stoicus to indulge in a life full of bacchanalian pleasures: sex, rich food, and wine. At first, Stoicus' attitudinal pleasure and emotional state take a sharp drop – he takes little pleasure in being kidnapped and is emotionally depressed. But over time, Stoicus takes less displeasure in being kidnapped. In fact, after a while, Stoicus begins to enjoy it somewhat: he enjoys the carefree life of a captive. Eventually he begins to take great attitudinal enjoyment in the various sensory pleasures presented to him. So much so, that the initial loss in attitudinal pleasure and positive emotional state is made up for by increased attitudinal pleasure and positive emotions later on to the extent that the averages of the two versions of his life are exactly the same: he enjoys 100 units of attitudinal pleasure and 100 units of positive emotional state on average.

In thinking about these two versions of Stoicus' life, we must be careful that the causal influences of sensory pleasure on attitudinal pleasure and emotional state are not clouding our judgment. Some attitudinal pleasure may be the same between the two versions of his life: for example, perhaps

Stoicus takes attitudinal pleasure in being alive in both the A and the B version. So let us suppose that there are 25 units of attitudinal pleasure and positive emotional state common to the A and B versions. Let us suppose further that in the A version Stoicus gets 75 units of attitudinal pleasure and 75 units of positive emotions from teaching, writing, and discussing philosophy. As per his wish, his philosophical life in the A version is not often marred by intense pain or pleasure. In the B version of his life, he receives 75 units of attitudinal pleasure and 75 units of positive emotions from his life of intense sensory pleasure: his bacchanalian revelry involving wine and orgies.

In thinking about whether Stoicus is happier in either of these two cases, we must be careful here to be sure that we are asking about the psychological sense of 'happiness.' We can ask two questions of Stoicus:

1. Is Stoicus happier in the B version than in the A version of his life?
2. Is Stoicus better off in the B version than in the A version of his life?

Notice, question 2 is irrelevant for our purposes. I mention it because we need to be sure that in considering the difference between the A and B versions we are focusing on whether he is happier in the psychological sense. For example, some might be tempted to say that Stoicus is better off in the A version because he has more knowledge. We don't need to adjudicate this question; we must merely note it is a different question than the question of the psychological sense of happiness.

I believe that Stoicus is happier in the B version; a superabundance of sensory pleasure adds happiness to Stoicus' life, even if only marginally so. Recall that even if we rank Stoicus' life as just the tiniest bit happier in the B version, this is enough to say that emotional state theory and attitudinal hedonism do not comprise the totality of superlative happiness. Admittedly, the increased happiness of Stoicus in the B version is not as easy to see as in the cases of Harry and Harriet. I suspect in part this may be because we are imagining Stoicus to be quite happy in both versions, so the additional happiness that results in the B version from sensory pleasure is overshadowed by his positive emotional state and attitudinal hedonism.

One means to bring the role of sensory pleasure in happiness into greater relief is to exaggerate the difference. Imagine the C version of Stoicus' life. It is like the A version except that he experiences a nagging toothache for much of his life. Suppose he has 10 dolors of sensory pain per day on average. Of course, this brings some attitudinal displeasure: let us suppose that the awareness of his pain leads to 10 units of attitudinal displeasure. Let us suppose, however, that Stoicus is pleased by his self-control: he does not let the pain "get to him" in the way that lesser folks, like Aristippus, would. The self-congratulatory attitude yields him exactly 10 additional units of attitudinal pleasure for a daily total of 100 units. Assuming too that his average mood is identical we can see that the only difference between the A and C version is 10 units of pain. Comparing the C version with the B version, we see the temptation is to say that sensory pleasure contributes to happiness, otherwise we have to admit that Stoicus is equally happy in the A, B, and C versions of his life. The contrast between the B and C versions says this is implausible. So, again, we must conclude that sensory hedonism must be part of a composite theory of happiness.[33]

3.7 Not Life Satisfactionism

We can use the same methodology to see that whole life satisfaction is not a constituent of superlative happiness. This conclusion may sound somewhat radical in that whole life satisfaction is perhaps the most common understanding of happiness in both social science and philosophical literature. As I hope to show, interpretation ought to be somewhat tempered by the fact that there is some significant overlap between attitudinal hedonism and whole life satisfaction accounts of happiness.

It is time to give poor Stoicus a rest: this time we will compare the lives of Stoicus' identical twin sons, Adventurous and Unadventurous. Unadventurous lived a life much like the A version of his father's life we discussed above: he lived a very quiet and uneventful life devoted to philosophical study. Adventurous had hoped for a life of peace and quiet, as was his family's tradition, but had neither. As a young man, Adventurous was kidnapped by Aristippus and his band of merry sensory hedonists. Adventurous managed to escape his captors, which led to a series of action-packed adventures that make the tales of Ulysses, Don Quixote, and Candide pale in comparison. Along the way, he started a family that he thought he never would have, and he accumulated far more friends than he ever thought possible. He made such stunning discoveries in philosophy, science, and mathematics that he was universally hailed as a genius. Adventurous also became rich beyond compare. He was known as a hero far and wide for saving countless drowning puppies and babies. He was made emperor of an empire larger than Alexander the Great's, and was beloved by all his subjects for the judicious manner in which he ruled.

Adventurous took attitudinal pleasure in his adventures, family, fortune, fame, learning, and empire. But they are equal in non-life satisfaction components of happiness. That is, Adventurous and Unadventurous both had 100 units attitudinal pleasure, 100 units of positive emotional state, and 1 unit of sensory pleasure per day.[‡]

Where the brothers differ is in their whole life satisfaction. We can imagine that near the end of his life Unadventurous was interviewed by Ed Diener and Unadventurous strongly agreed with the survey statements: "In most ways my life is close to my ideal" and "If I could live my life over, I would change almost nothing." So, solely on the basis of the whole life satisfaction view, then, Unadventurous was superlatively happy.[34] He sought to live a quiet life of philosophical study and contemplation, and he succeeded in doing so.

Adventurous disagreed with the survey statement: "In most ways my life is close to my ideal" and "If I could live my life over, I would change almost nothing." Adventurous said that he was pleased with his life, but his life was based on an extraordinary amount of good luck. He still recommended the quiet life of contemplation, recommended by his father, to his philosophical followers; and he would follow the quiet life advice if he could do his life over again. Circumstances forced him to stray far from his ideal; and circumstances permitted him to have a great life; but circumstances did not permit him to have the ideal life of quiet contemplation. Clearly his life is not anywhere near this ideal. So, solely on the basis of the whole life satisfaction view, Adventurous is not happy.

It may be thought that Adventurous is being disingenuous in claiming that his life is nowhere near his ideal. With all the power he had amassed, it seems he could have easily changed his life at some point to that of quiet contemplation. The fact that he didn't seems to suggest that this is not really his ideal. However, we can easily imagine him responding that he felt compelled out of a sense of duty to adopt his less than ideal life: he had incurred obligations to a family and to an empire that prohibited him from adopting his ideal life. Unless we insist that whatever life people freely choose is the one that is their ideal, the objection will have little weight. And Adventurous's explanation makes it abundantly apparent why we should not so insist: people might act in ways that are in contradiction to their

---

[‡] For ease of discussion, and since the amount of sensory pleasure is so minute, unless otherwise noted, I will drop consideration of sensory pleasure from consideration as components in Adventurous and Unadventurous's lives.

ideals because of a sense of duty to others. We can't read off a person's ideal life simply from what they freely choose to do.

So, at least in the case of Adventurous, a monistic conception of whole life satisfaction gives the wrong result. Those not already persuaded by the whole life satisfaction account who met Adventurous would be inclined to say that he is not completely unhappy: his buoyant moods and the fact that he was pleased about so much suggests that he was not maximally unhappy. After all, it seems that we can easily imagine greater unhappiness: someone who fails to live up to their life's ideal in the way that Adventurous did, but who is also attitudinally displeased to a great extent and who experiences many negative moods and emotions. So, a monistic conception of whole life satisfaction cannot be the complete story about the psychological state of happiness.

This still leaves unanswered the question of whether a whole life satisfaction account of happiness is part of a composite account of superlative happiness. To resolve this question, we can apply the method of difference to the lives of Unadventurous and Adventurous. If our previous argument is correct, that attitudinal pleasure and positive emotional states are constituents of happiness, then we need only ask whether the fact that Unadventurous had high life satisfaction adds to his happiness as compared with that of Adventurous, for Adventurous and Unadventurous are otherwise equal in the non-disputed aspects of happiness.

In fact, it may be thought that Unadventurous was happier than Adventurous, at least in respect of having reached his life's ideal. Notice we do not need to take any position on the relative degree that whole life satisfaction contributes to happiness to say that Unadventurous was happier than Adventurous. It is sufficient to say that even if whole life satisfaction contributes the smallest amount of happiness, Unadventurous was happier than Adventurous.

To assess this argument, we will need to examine the relationship between whole life satisfaction and attitudinal hedonism in a bit more detail. I shall argue that there is considerable overlap between the two theories, and that where they overlap, whole life satisfaction adds nothing. Where they don't overlap, whole life satisfaction is not a plausible aspect of superlative happiness.

As noted above, whole life satisfaction and attitudinal hedonism are both propositional attitude accounts of happiness. This means that they can differ in (1) the domain of admissible propositions, and (2) the propositional attitudes that they countenance. We will take these in turn.

If whole life satisfaction is part of a superlative conception of happiness, it cannot be because whole life satisfaction countenances propositions overlooked by attitudinal hedonism; for in Feldman's attitudinal hedonism, there are no restrictions on the domain of propositions that one might be pleased about. On Feldman's view, attitudinal pleasure can come from small inane matters – you are a tiny bit pleased that there is a sale on coffee at your local coffee shop that will reduce the price by 1 cent – to larger matters such as one's life considered as a whole. The whole life satisfaction view, in contrast, restricts the domain of relevant propositions precisely to statements about one's life considered as a whole.§ So, any argument for including whole life satisfaction in a pluralistic account cannot be based on the idea that it includes propositions that are beyond the reach of attitudinal hedonism, because attitudinal hedonism puts no bounds on admissible propositions.

So, if there is a difference between the whole life satisfaction view and attitudinal hedonism, then it must be about the attitude to whole life propositions, not the propositions themselves. But this reveals the problem for the whole life satisfaction view: it does not show how the seemingly "sterile" question of whether your life meets with your ideal connects with the psychological state of happiness. In effect, asking to what extent you agree or disagree that your life has met with your ideal is to ask to what extent you *believe* that your life has met with your ideal. This does not tell us anything directly about whether you view this positively or negatively. The point about sterility, then, is that without any indication of your view – if you view the fact that your life has or has not met your ideal positively or negatively – it is hard to see the relevance to happiness. In comparison, attitudinal hedonism does tell us directly how one views the state of affairs depicted by the proposition, for it asks whether one is pleased (or displeased) that one's life has (or has not) met one's ideal.

One way to illustrate this point about sterility is to imagine that Unadventurous strongly agrees that his life is close to his ideal, but he is not pleased about the fact that his life has met his ideal. Suppose he is jealous of the extraordinary luck and success of his brother. Philosophically he is still committed to thinking that the life of peace and quiet is the surest means to a good life, but he can't help feeling a certain amount of envy at his brother's good fortune in having such an exciting life. Now it might be thought that

---

§ As noted above, sometimes important domains of one's life are interrogated individually, for example, whether one's work or family life meets up with one's ideal. I will ignore this wrinkle as it adds nothing of substance to the discussion.

his ideal really is to live like his brother, since he is not pleased with his lot. Unadventurous rejects this notion because it would make a mockery of having a life's ideal. Almost everyone would choose as part of their ideal to have extraordinary good luck like his brother Adventurous, but then almost everyone would end up being extremely unhappy, for almost no one has the good luck of his brother. Unadventurous, then, interprets Diener's question as asking whether one's life meets a "realistic ideal," not some almost impossible to obtain ideal. So, thinking in these terms, Unadventurous can consistently think that his life is meeting a realistic ideal, but not be pleased that his life has only met this ideal. Contrariwise, it is easy to imagine Adventurous saying that his life did not meet his ideal, but he is pleased with his life.

Naturally we must be careful that we haven't violated the method of difference in considering the idea that Unadventurous is displeased with his life as a whole, even though it meets his ideal, and Adventurous is pleased with his life as a whole, even though it does not meet his ideal. Since the method of difference requires in this instance we keep the non-disputed aspects of happiness, attitudinal pleasure, and emotional state equal between the brothers, we must imagine that Unadventurous gets more attitudinal pleasure from consideration of propositions about things other than his whole life in order to ensure that each brother receives 100 units of attitudinal pleasure per day on average.

We are now in a position to ask: is Unadventurous happier than Adventurous? I see no reason to suppose that Unadventurous is happier. True, his life meets with his ideal in a way that his brother's does not, but this does not "move" Unadventurous, since he does not view this in a positive manner. So, I think the appropriate conclusion here is that Unadventurous is not happier than Adventurous.

As a number of authors have noted, whole life satisfaction theories constitute a family of views rather than a single agreed-upon theory.[35] This is important because some forms of whole life satisfaction are impervious to the sterility criticism. Consider, for example, the "Delighted – Terrible" scale developed by Andrews and Withey.[36] Their instrument offers seven options from which participants may choose: " 'Delighted', 'Pleased', 'Mostly satisfied', 'Mixed – about equally satisfied and dissatisfied', 'Mostly dissatisfied', 'Unhappy', 'Terrible'."[37] Applying this scale to a whole life proposition such as "This is how my life has turned out," a survey might take this form, "I am _____ that this is how my life has turned out," where subjects are asked to fill in the blank using the seven-point scale. A second example is the instrument developed by Diener et al., mentioned above. Recall, it has an item that indicates how subjects feel about their lives: the third item asks subjects to record their degree of agreement or disagreement with the claim "I am satisfied with my life."[38]

A few points about these different measures are in order. Both scales permit an expression of one's view about the course of one's life: to be "delighted" on the Andrews and Withey scale, or "very satisfied" on the Diener et al. scale, both suggest a positive view. Second, there is a clear overlap between the Delighted–Terrible inventory and Feldman and Diener et al.'s scales. The Delighted–Terrible scale permits expression of happiness in terms of being pleased about one's life as a whole, as does Feldman's attitudinal hedonism. Likewise, the Delighted–Terrible scale permits expression of satisfaction with one's life, as does the third item on Diener et al.'s scale. Third, it may be that one or more of these scales are redundant. Consider that the degree of satisfaction expressed on Diener et al.'s scale can be captured by the Delighted–Terrible scale, but not vice versa. To be delighted by X seems to express greater positive feeling towards X than to be satisfied with X, or even very satisfied with X. So, Diener et al.'s scale seems to lack the range that the Delighted–Terrible scale offers.

It may be that there is no significant difference on this score between the extremes of the Delighted–Terrible scale and Feldman's attitudinal hedonism. Admittedly, I suppose I would rather have my boss express the view that he is delighted by my work than that he is (merely) pleased with it. So, this suggests that Feldman's attitudinal pleasure model has less range. However, I am not sure if any significant difference remains if the choice is between "very delighted" and "very pleased." Furthermore, if we were to construct an ordinal scale like Feldman suggests, any residual difference may disappear.[39] In any event, the conclusion here can be put conditionally: if being "very delighted with X" expresses a more positive view than being "very pleased with X," then Feldman's attitudinal hedonism should be revised to accommodate this to capture a greater range of attitudinal happiness.

So, those forms of whole life satisfaction that permit the expression of a positive (or negative) view about one's life as a whole will not differ significantly from attitudinal hedonists' assessment of the same. This still leaves the question of scope: life satisfaction views restrict the scope of relevant propositions to global areas such as one's entire life (or sometimes finer distinctions are allowed: work life, family life, etc.).

We can use the method of difference to show that the restriction on the domain of admissible propositions is not justified. Consider two subjects,

Ed and Fred. Ed and Fred both express the thought that they are very happy about their lives taken as a whole. Who is happier? When the domain of propositions is restricted to whole life considerations, then we must say they are equal. But suppose it turns out that 95 percent of all days Fred is overall more pleased than displeased about many local propositions that he is thinking about. Ed is more displeased than pleased about local propositions 80 percent of all days. Now it may be thought that Ed wouldn't express as much pleasure about his whole life as Fred. But we can easily imagine that Ed expected, perhaps with good reason, things to go much worse, and so the fact that things are not quite as bad as he expected leads him to be pleased with the course of his life. The fact that whole life satisfaction can't capture these more local aspects of Ed and Fred's mental states suggests that including our feelings about local matters must be part of a superlative conception of happiness.

It should be noted too that nothing said indicates how much happier Fred is than Ed. One might develop a view in which pleasure or displeasure about one's life as a whole counts for the overwhelming majority of happiness. In which case, Fred and Ed will be very close in terms of their happiness levels. However, if the argument above is sound, it must be admitted that Fred is ever so slightly happier than Ed.

To summarize, there is considerable overlap between attitudinal hedonism and whole life satisfaction accounts of happiness: both countenance expressions of positive views – being pleased or delighted, for example – about the course of one's life. Where they differ is in whether one's life has met one's ideal, and whether thoughts about more local matters should count towards one's happiness. In both cases, attitudinal hedonism is more plausible. One could believe that one's life has met one's ideal, and not be pleased about this, and one could believe that one's life has not met one's ideal and be pleased about this. The fact that attitudinal hedonism permits being pleased or delighted about local matters in addition to global life judgments permits intuitively plausible judgments about how individuals might differ in their happiness even though they are equally pleased or displeased about their lives considered as a whole.

3.8   Folk Psychology

I have argued for a composite view of happiness that includes sensory pleasure, positive emotional states, and positive propositional attitudes. It should not strike us as the least bit surprising that our everyday understanding of happiness, that is, the "folk psychology" of happiness, is composite. Folk psychology divides our mental life into cognitive and emotional faculties, and folk psychology describes both of these in terms of a positive or negative valence. It seems likely that for most people, most of the time, these two co-vary: those in a positive mood or experiencing sensory pleasure often will have positive thoughts, and those in a negative mood or sensory pain will be more likely to take attitudinal displeasure in the objects of their thoughts. We had to think of extreme cases, like that of Harry and Harriet, to disentangle these two. The fact that they are so intimately interconnected explains why a single word 'happiness' in folk psychology would refer to these two phenomena.

As noted above, it seems a reasonable expectation that a book devoted to boosting happiness should offer an account of happiness, and so this is why we have spent a chapter on this task. I hope to show in Chapter 6 that the argument of this work can survive if I am wrong about the composite view of happiness. So, objections to the composite view may not be devastating. In the meantime, we need to consider the role of happiness in a good life.

Notes

1. Feldman, *What Is This Thing Called Happiness?*; Sumner, *Welfare, Happiness, and Ethics*; Haybron, "Happiness."
2. As Fred Feldman points out (*Pleasure and the Good Life*), the question about the good life can be asked about other values as well, e.g., the morally good life or the aesthetically good life. As noted below, the question we want to ask is about prudential value.
3. I borrow the term 'prudential value' from Griffin (*Well-Being*).
4. Haybron, "Happiness."
5. See Haybron (ibid.) for several references to skepticism about the descriptive/ evaluative distinction in this context.
6. Perhaps 'extensional equivalence' is a more apt technical term here than 'identity.'
7. Feldman, *What Is This Thing Called Happiness?*
8. Sumner, *Welfare, Happiness, and Ethics.*
9. Hurka, *Perfectionism.* Hurka does not specifically address the question of the relationship between prudential value and perfectionism, but others have made the connection noted in the text (Sumner, "Two Theories of the Good"; Griffin, *Well-Being*; Hooker, "Does Moral Virtue Constitute a Benefit to the Agent?").

10. The idea of 'some surplus' is intentionally left vague to allow that sensory hedonists might argue that not just any amount of surplus is sufficient for happiness. For example, the hedonist may want to leave a midrange where people are neither happy nor unhappy, and this range may include instances where there is just the smallest surplus of pleasure over pain. Nothing here or below depends on exploiting this issue, so I leave the question of the "threshold" for happiness undecided. For discussion of this issue see Haybron, *The Pursuit of Unhappiness*.

11. The metaphor of "atoms of happiness" comes from Feldman, *What Is This Thing Called Happiness?*

12. Lyubomirsky, King, and Diener, "The Benefits of Frequent Positive Affect."

13. The term 'emotional state view' comes from Haybron ("Happiness and Pleasure", *The Pursuit of Unhappiness*). Haybron does not offer the emotional state view as a monistic conception of happiness. He suggests that happiness is a "mongrel" concept that defies such analyses.

14. Lyubomirsky, King, and Diener, "The Benefits of Frequent Positive Affect."

15. Haybron, "On Being Happy or Unhappy." Haybron (*The Pursuit of Unhappiness*) offers a detailed and slightly different inventory of positive moods and emotions from Lyubomirsky, King, and Diener's "The Benefits of Frequent Positive Affect." This is one of the "details" that we will hope a sufficiently robust emotional state theory will resolve, but one which is not of present concern, since the present argument does not turn on how this question is adjudicated.

16. Lyubomirsky, King, and Diener allow the short-term and long-term understandings of happiness. Haybron emphasizes the long term in his argument that we ought to understand happiness as a disposition for positive moods and emotions. Feldman (*What Is This Thing Called Happiness?*) criticizes the appeal to dispositional claim. Nothing in the argument turns on whether we side with Lyubomirsky et al. in understanding the emotional state theory to require simply frequent positive moods and emotions or whether we must also understand it as having a dispositional aspect.

17. Haybron, *The Pursuit of Unhappiness*.

18. Veenhoven, "Is Happiness Relative?," "Happiness in Nations."

19. Diener et al., "The Satisfaction with Life Scale."

20. Feldman (*What Is This Thing Called Happiness?*) notes that there seem to be problems here for the whole life satisfaction theorist concerning whether the view about one's life is understood as actual or hypothetical. (But see Suikkanen, "An Improved Whole Life Satisfaction Theory of Happiness.")

21. Tatarkiewicz, *Analysis of Happiness*; Nozick, *Philosophical Explanations*; Telfer, *Happiness*; Sumner, *Welfare, Happiness, and Ethics*.

22. Sumner, *Welfare, Happiness, and Ethics*, 145.

23. A number of whole life satisfaction theorists add an affective element: ibid., 111. Tatarkiewicz, *Analysis of Happiness*, 12; Brandt, "Happiness." These views count among the composite in the sense discussed below.
24. Feldman, *What Is This Thing Called Happiness?*, 118–19.
25. Feldman, "The Good Life," 610. Stoicus has a return engagement in Feldman's later work, *Pleasure and the Good Life*, 50.
26. Feldman, *What Is This Thing Called Happiness?*, 145–6.
27. Ibid., 145.
28. Ibid., 32.
29. Ibid.
30. Ibid., 145.
31. The expression comes from Mill, *A System of Logic*.
32. An answer to this question would probably go a long way to answering underdetermination arguments in the philosophy of science.
33. Thanks to Nick Agar for this point.
34. I am ignoring the other questions on the survey instrument proposed by Diener et al., "The Satisfaction with Life Scale." See below for discussion of the similarities between whole life satisfaction and attitudinal hedonism.
35. This point is emphasized in Feldman's work *What Is This Thing Called Happiness?*, where he distinguishes hundreds of potential permutations.
36. Andrews and Withey, *Social Indicators of Well-being*.
37. Ibid.
38. One difference here is that Diener et al.'s instrument has the locution "satisfied" embedded in the proposition, rather than in the propositional attitude. To draw the parallel here we could imagine the survey question being changed slightly to: "I am _____ that the course of my life has been thus and so," where the blank would be filled in by 'very unsatisfied,' 'slightly unsatisfied,' 'slightly satisfied,' or 'very satisfied.'
39. Feldman, *What Is This Thing Called Happiness?*

References

Andrews, F. M. and S. B. Withey. *Social Indicators of Well-being: Americans' Perceptions of Life Quality*. New York: Plenum, 1976.

Brandt, R. B. "Happiness." *The Encyclopedia of Philosophy* (1972): 3, 413–14.

Diener, E., R. A. Emmons, R. J. Larsen, and S. Griffin. "The Satisfaction with Life Scale." *Journal of Personality Assessment* 49, no. 1 (1985): 71–5.

Feldman, F. "The Good Life: A Defense of Attitudinal Hedonism." *Philosophy and Phenomenological Research* 65, no. 3 (2002): 604–28.

Feldman, F. *Pleasure and the Good Life: Concerning the Nature, Varieties, and Plausibility of Hedonism*. Oxford: Clarendon Press, 2004.

Feldman, F. *What Is This Thing Called Happiness?* New York: Oxford University Press, 2010.

Griffin, J. *Well-Being: Its Meaning, Measurement, and Moral Importance.* Oxford: Clarendon Press, 1986.

Haybron, D. "Happiness." In *The Stanford Encyclopedia of Philosophy* (Fall 2011 edn.), edited by Edward N. Zalta. http://plato.stanford.edu/archives/fall2011/entries/happiness/.

Haybron, D. "Happiness and Pleasure." *Philosophy and Phenomenological Research* 62, no. 3 (2001): 501–28.

Haybron, D. "On Being Happy or Unhappy." *Philosophy and Phenomenological Research* 71, no. 2 (2005): 287–317.

Haybron, D. *The Pursuit of Unhappiness.* New York: Oxford University Press, 2008.

Hooker, B. "Does Moral Virtue Constitute a Benefit to the Agent?" In *How Should One Live?*, edited by Roger Crisp, 141–57. Oxford: Oxford University Press, 1996.

Hurka, Thomas. *Perfectionism.* New York: Oxford University Press, 1993.

Lyubomirsky, S., L. King, and E. Diener. "The Benefits of Frequent Positive Affect: Does Happiness Lead to Success?" *Psychological Bulletin* 131 (2005): 803–55.

Mill, J. S. *A System of Logic.* Honolulu: University Press of the Pacific, 2002.

Nozick, R. *Philosophical Explanations.* Cambridge, Mass.: Belknap Press, 1981.

Suikkanen, J. "An Improved Whole Life Satisfaction Theory of Happiness." *International Journal of Wellbeing* 1, no. 1 (2011): 149–66.

Sumner, L. W. "Two Theories of the Good." In *The Good Life and the Human Good*, edited by Ellen Frankel Paul, Fred D. Miller, Jr., and Jeffrey Paul, 1–15. New York: Cambridge University Press, 1992.

Sumner, L. W. *Welfare, Happiness, and Ethics.* Oxford: Clarendon Press, 1996.

Tatarkiewicz, W. *Analysis of Happiness.* Dordrecht: Kluwer Academic Publishers, 1976.

Telfer, E. *Happiness.* New York: St. Martin's Press, 1980.

Veenhoven, R. "Happiness in Nations: Subjective Appreciation of Life in 56 Nations 1946–1992." World Database of Happiness, Erasmus University Rotterdam, 1993.

Veenhoven, R. "Is Happiness Relative?" *Social Indicators Research* 24, no. 1 (1991): 1–34.

4

The Elements of the Good Life: It is a Very Big List

We've noted that it is almost platitudinous to say "I just want to be happy" or "I just want my children to be happy." From what we learned in the previous chapter, this translates into the desire to have positive moods and emotions along with sensory and attitudinal pleasure. Imagine translating these sentiments into policy: improvements upon our world are to be judged in terms of whether some alternate social arrangement yields greater positive moods along with sensory and attitudinal pleasure. Suppose we could send social scientists to investigate happiness in *Brave New World* through the Philosophers' Portal. No doubt they would report back that the citizens of *Brave New World* are much happier than we are. Between a carefully engineered society and *soma*, virtually every citizen is guaranteed far more positive moods and emotions along with greater sensory and attitudinal pleasure than their counterparts here. This reasoning suggests that we must conclude that those in *Brave New World* are much better off on average than we are. Given the distastefulness of this conclusion to most, we need to revisit the premises that allowed us to arrive at the conclusion.

An obvious move is to suggest that there must be more to the good life than happiness. This would allow us to say, although they may be happier in *Brave New World* than we are, they are not better off. Otherwise, it seems just pure pigheadedness to say we are better off than the denizens of *Brave New World*. The idea that there is more to the good life than happiness is something we will take seriously in this chapter. I will argue that, in

Happy-People-Pills For All, First Edition. Mark Walker.
© 2013 John Wiley & Sons, Inc. Published 2013 by John Wiley & Sons, Inc.

addition to happiness, the good life comprises a number of elements, including: athleticism, autonomy, beauty, creativity, desire satisfaction, friendship, health, knowledge, love, pleasure, truth, and wealth. This will open the door to a reply to the idea that those in *Brave New World* are better off: they may be happier but they lack many of the other items on this list. It is also suggestive of a criticism of those who "just want to be happy." Perhaps they aim far too low: it would be reasonable to want more for your children than just happiness.

4.1 Three Theories of the Good Life

As intimated in the previous chapter, in seeking an account of the good life we are looking for what philosophers sometimes term a theory of wellbeing, welfare or prudential good.[1] It will be useful to say a little bit more about the goal of this project, which is to inform us about how a life is going "for the individual whose life it is."[2] Welfare is sometimes said to be narrower than the "good life"[3] all considered, when lives are evaluated along moral or aesthetic dimensions.[4] Mother Teresa had a good life in the sense of a 'morally good life,' as exemplified in her work with the poor and diseased in India and other parts of the world. Her life was less exemplary from the point of view of prudential welfare: it seems she led a very hard life for many years and she struggled with doubts about her faith. The life of the consummate playboy may rate low in terms of the morally good life, but much higher in terms of prudential wellbeing. We will explore further the contrast between morality and prudential welfare in the next chapter. For the moment, the important point is that we are focusing on prudential welfare: the good life for the person whose life it is.

Philosophical theories of prudential value are often parsed according to a tripartite distinction: hedonism, desire satisfactionism, and objective list theories.[5] Hedonism says the good life comprises enjoyment or pleasure; desire satisfactionism suggests the good life is a life with satisfied desires. The last category is somewhat of a hodgepodge, but some preliminary understanding can be had simply by viewing it in relationship to its two competitors: wellbeing is more (or other) than simply pleasure or getting what you want.[6] Often, but not always, objective list theories are pluralistic: they suggest that wellbeing includes several values. It will simplify our discussion to assume that objective list theories are pluralistic.[7]

It may perhaps strike the reader as somewhat surprising that the idea that the good life is the happy life does not appear on this very common taxonomy. Those who say "I just want to be happy" seem to express a view about the good life that does not even appear within the usual philosophical catalogue. Part of the explanation for this is that philosophers have often thought that happiness might be reduced to one of the elements on this list. As we saw in the previous chapter, Fred Feldman attempt to reduce happiness to a form of hedonism, attitudinal hedonism.[8] J. S. Mill is another example of a philosopher who attempted to reduce happiness to pleasure.[9] Wayne Davis offers an analysis of happiness in terms of desire satisfaction.[10] So, it is not as if philosophers have neglected the common thought that happiness is intimately connected with wellbeing.

As is perhaps apparent, this chapter will defend the objective list theory. I will do so by showing the inadequacy of its two main competitors. One of the primary issues we will deal with is considerations of parsimony. It is often suggested that considerations of parsimony favor either hedonism or desire satisfaction accounts of wellbeing. The reason of course is that, unlike objective list theories, they appeal to a single value, and so they are simpler. To this point is added the claim that objective list theories have not met this challenge, in order to show that it is necessary to have multiple items.[11] So, objective list theories are to be rejected in favor of the more parsimonious alternatives. I will argue that any monistic theory is implausible.

We will also examine the criticism that objective list theories simply offer a capricious salmagundi of prudential goods.[12] We may think of this as 'inventory skepticism': there is no non-arbitrary way to establish the inventory of prudential items on the objective list. Richard Arneson summarizes the objection thus: "One criticism [of the objective list theory] consists in skeptical doubt that there is no uniquely rational way to determine what putative goods qualify as entries on the list. Skepticism here is a genuine worry, but not one this essay considers."[13] The skeptical worry seems borne out in practice. Surprisingly few of those who endorse an objective list theory attempt to provide a list.[14] On the relatively rare occasions when lists are delivered, they do not always have many common elements. Compare John Finis's list: knowledge, life, play, aesthetic experience, sociability (friendship), practical reasonableness, and religion and the pursuit of the ultimate questions of meaning,[15] with Bernard Gert's: consciousness, ability, freedom, and pleasure.[16] The fact that such radically different lists are proposed supports Arneson's contention that inventory skepticism is a serious challenge.

Both issues can be handled by using the method of difference from the previous chapter. Moreover, we shall see that the same methodology makes for a very powerful case for objective list theory. I argue that repeated application of the method of difference results in a very big objective list of prudential values, perhaps the most extensive list contemplated so far. The resulting theory I (imaginatively) term the "big objective list" theory of wellbeing. As noted, it includes the two main contemporary competitors to objective list theories – hedonism and desire satisfactionism – as proper parts, as well as athleticism, autonomy, beauty, creativity, friendship, happiness, health, knowledge, love, truth, and wealth.

4.2   The Method of Difference

In the previous chapter we used the method of difference to argue for the composite view of 'happiness.' In applying it to the question of prudential value, we are returning to its original provenance. The method harkens back to Plato's criticism of hedonism in the *Philebus*, and it has been discussed a number of times subsequently.[17] Applying it to the question of prudential value, the basic and purest form of the strategy is to imagine two different versions of a person's life that are identical in terms of non-disputed prudential value but differ in the disputed benefit (and whatever else is logically entailed by possession of the disputed value). If the version of the life with the putative value appears to be better, prudentially speaking, then there must be at least one other intrinsic prudential benefit. The same argument can be applied to groups of people, or indeed whole worlds: compare two worlds that are identical in every way except that one has the disputed value (and everything that is logically entailed by having, or having more of, the disputed value) while the other does not, and see if one world is better prudentially for its denizens. An impure version of the method of difference asks us to evaluate two versions of a life or lives identical in non-disputed benefits, but not identical in *relative amounts* of the disputed benefit, for example in how much health or knowledge a person has. The advantage of the impure strategy is that it may be hard to imagine lives completely lacking in some values, for example a life with "no health." Indeed, it is hard to know what a life with "no health" means, but it is easy to imagine persons being healthier or unhealthier. Similarly, it is hard to imagine a person lacking all knowledge, and much easier to imagine persons more or less knowledgeable.[18] So, the impure strategy would ask us to compare lives that are identical in the non-disputed prudential values, and then consider two versions of a person's life, one where they are healthier (or more knowledgeable) and one where they are less healthy (or less knowledgeable).

The method of difference is reminiscent of method of control group experimentation in science. Control and experimental groups are (ideally) as similar as possible except with respect to the variable under investigation. The experimental group in the method of difference is the individual or individuals who have (more of) some disputed value than the control group, but the two groups are otherwise as similar as possible. If, on reflection (the experiment), we judge the experimental group to have more prudential value, then the item in question has intrinsic prudential value.* If not, then we reject the assumption that the item in question has intrinsic prudential value.

4.3   Refutation of Hedonism

In this section we will apply the method of difference to hedonism. As noted, the hedonist's single intrinsic value or benefit is the experience or feeling of pleasure.† Hedonists have long realized that their view seems to fly in the face of our everyday understanding of prudential value. As Aristotle observed, "the common person" offers any number of candidates for what makes a life go well: " . . . pleasure, wealth, or honor; some say it is one thing and others another, and often the very same person identifies it with different things at different times: when he is sick he thinks it is health, and when he is poor he says it is wealth . . . "[19] It seems, at least on this score, not much has changed since Aristotle. However, hedonists have a ready answer: the value of these items can be accounted for in purely instrumental terms. Health, wealth, and so on are prudentially valuable only to the extent that they directly or indirectly promote the intrinsic value of pleasure.

Since the big objective list accepts pleasure as an intrinsic value, this is not under dispute with the hedonist. Rather, it is the hedonist's contention

---

*   Actually, this is not quite right, since the disputed item might have instrumental value for some further intrinsic value. See the discussion of knowledge and pleasure below for clarification of this point.

†   For the present, we will concentrate on sensory hedonism. See below for discussion of the difference between sensory and attitudinal hedonism. Also, for simplicity's sake, I ignore, for the most part, the harms associated with each of these theories of welfare: pain, unfulfilled desires, and so on. Also, I take the usual short-cut and assert that hedonism holds that there is a single intrinsic value, but as Feldman ("Basic Intrinsic Value") points out, this leads to the embarrassing consequence that lives or possible worlds cannot be intrinsically good.

that pleasure is the sole intrinsic value. To simplify matters at this stage, we will assume that knowledge is the only candidate other than pleasure for inclusion on an inventory of intrinsic prudential good. Other values on the big objective list could have served, but one reason for choosing knowledge is that it makes for a bright contrast with pleasure. At least since Plato, pleasure and knowledge have been taken as paradigmatic contrasts in terms of intrinsic prudential benefits.[20]

Taking J. S. Mill as our example, let us imagine two versions of his life identical in pleasure but different in knowledge. So, in one version of his life, he has high levels of pleasure in addition to high levels of knowledge (P+K+), while in the other he has high levels of pleasure and very low levels of knowledge (P+K−). Which life is better in terms of wellbeing? Which life should we wish for Mill, if we are wishing the best life for him? For the hedonist, the answer must be that the two lives are of equal value, for they are identical in terms of the hedonist's sole intrinsic value: pleasure. The hedonist must say that it is a matter of complete indifference, prudentially speaking, which life Mill leads. If coerced into making a decision, we might imagine a hedonist resorting to flipping a coin to decide between the two lives. The reasoning of course is that this would be as good a means as any to decide between the two lives, since they are identical in terms of wellbeing according to the hedonist.

While it may not be possible to convince the dyed-in-the-wool hedonist, for those of us who think the inventory question concerning intrinsic values is open this line of argument pretty convincingly shows that pleasure is not the sole intrinsic value: the life with knowledge (P+K+) is better for Mill, and so hedonism is wrong. The intuition that Mill's life is better with knowledge is widely shared.[‡] So this is one point in favor of the big objective list, for the big objective list has a very plausible explanation for why the (H+K+) life is better: both pleasure and knowledge are intrinsic values.

It may be thought that this example is implausible since it is difficult to see how Mill might have more knowledge and not find greater pleasure in this knowledge. Notice, however, that the method of difference requires us

---

[‡] I have asked literally thousands of students, and a good number of non-students, a version of the question of which life is better for Mill, and easily more than 90% say that the life with knowledge in addition to pleasure is better. Sometimes the answer is supported by remarks along the lines of: "if knowledge can be had for free – at no cost in terms of pleasure – then why wouldn't this life be better?" Many think the answer is so obvious that there must be some trick. I certainly can't say that my polling has been done with the rigor one might expect from a scientific study of the issue, but I have tried hard not to indicate my own view about the matter when doing the polling.

to imagine two versions of his life identical *in the amount of pleasure*. If Mill obtains happiness from pursuing knowledge in the (P+K+) version, we must imagine a corresponding loss of *some other source* of pleasure to keep the two versions of his life equal in pleasure. We can imagine a 'compensatory equalizer': while Mill gains pleasure from knowledge in the (P+K+) life, his overall pleasure is not higher because (let us imagine) he has less genetic propensity for pleasure. In other words, let us agree that the ledger sheet for the (P+K+) version of his life would require factoring in the instrumental value of knowledge: pleasure obtained through the pursuit and attainment of knowledge. In order to equalize the amount of pleasure, we must imagine subtracting pleasure somewhere else in his life. We imagine, for example, a genetic propensity to not experience quite as much pleasure from food in the (P+K+) life, so the pleasure gained from knowledge is offset by the loss of pleasure from dining. (Of course we can imagine any number of compensatory mechanisms: we might imagine Mill suffers an accident that makes it more difficult to experience pleasure in the (P+K+) version of his life, or that the (P+K+) world is much less benign: in general, one has to work harder in this world to obtain pleasure.)

For the objective list theorist, the method of difference is most helpful in combating the "instrumental strategy" – attempting to explain away some purported intrinsic value as merely instrumental.[21] I suspect this is the most common argumentative strategy employed by hedonists against pluralists: what pluralists allege are intrinsic prudential values are really only instrumental values. In the present case, we should imagine the hedonist trying to explain away the contention that knowledge has intrinsic value by suggesting that its value is merely instrumental in obtaining pleasure. The method of difference allows us to accept that knowledge may have instrumental value in promoting pleasure, but it also shows that its contribution to a life cannot be *completely explained away* in these terms. Anyone who has some reason to think that the (P+K+) version of Mill's life offers more prudential value cannot explain this in terms of additional pleasure, and so cannot appeal to the instrumental strategy.[22]

We assumed above that knowledge was the only other candidate for an intrinsic prudential value, but the argument against hedonism can actually jettison this assumption. Since the life with knowledge is prudentially better, this shows that there must be at least one intrinsic value other than pleasure. Either knowledge is an intrinsic value, as we assumed, or there is another intrinsic value, truth perhaps, in addition to pleasure, which knowledge is instrumental in obtaining. In either case, as long as we agree that the (P+K+) life contains more prudential value, the source of this additional value cannot be pleasure, so hedonism must be rejected.

4.4   Refutation of Perfectionism

Perfectionism is sometimes understood as a theory of prudential value.[23] According to Thomas Hurka, perfectionism accords pleasure no value.[24] Rather, perfectionists enjoin us to develop certain characteristics or capacities of human nature such as knowledge, friendship, and the accomplishment of complex tasks.[25] Since perfectionists see knowledge as something that ought to be perfected,[26] perfectionists have a ready answer to why Mill is better off in the (P+K+) life, namely, that he has more of the sole intrinsic value, perfection, and, in particular, knowledge. Mill's pleasure is irrelevant: it adds nothing in terms of prudential value. But we can reverse the thought experiment to show that pleasure is an intrinsic value.

Let us imagine that Mill experiences identically high levels of knowledge in the two versions of his life. However, in one version of his life he has, in addition, high levels of pleasure (K+P+), while in the other he has very low levels of pleasure (K+P−). The question then is which life is better in terms of prudential benefit: which life should we wish for Mill if we are wishing the best life for him? For the perfectionist the answer must be that the two lives are of equal value, for they are identical in terms of the perfectionist's sole intrinsic value: perfection. The perfectionist must say that it is a matter of indifference which life Mill leads. If coerced into making a decision, we might imagine a perfectionist resorting to flipping a coin to decide between the two lives. The reasoning of course is that this would be as good a means as any to decide between the two lives, since, according to the perfectionist, they are identical in terms of the one item of prudential good.[27]

The hedonist fails to explain why the (P+K+) life is better than the (P+K− life); and the perfectionist fails to explain why the (K+P+) life is better than the (K+P−) life. Thus, the hedonist and the perfectionist have merely partial views, while the big objective list provides the intuitively correct response in both cases.

4.5   A Very Big Objective List

Accepting the general line of argumentation seems to open the floodgates to a very big objective list of values. For instance, it seems that we can establish that friendship is an intrinsic value using the very same procedure. So, building on our previous result, where we said that Mill's life goes better in the version where he has pleasure and knowledge, we now apply the same procedure to the question of friendship. Thus, we must imagine two versions of Mill's life in which he enjoys exactly the same high level of knowledge and pleasure (K+P+); but in one version he lacks good friends (K+P+F−). In the other, he has a number of good friends (K+P+F+). If knowledge and pleasure are the only intrinsic prudential values, then there is no reason to prefer the life with friendship rather than the life without, at least for Mill's sake. Someone who thinks that knowledge and pleasure are the only intrinsic values might flip a coin to decide which life is better for Mill. But this is absurd. If Mill can have friends at no cost to the amount of pleasure he experiences and the amount of knowledge he obtains, then it seems that the life with many friends adds to his wellbeing.

The same argument might be used to establish that physical beauty is an intrinsic benefit. Consider two versions of Mill's life where he has exactly the same amount of happiness, with knowledge and friendship in each. In one permutation he lacks physical attractiveness and in the other he is extremely physically attractive. All else being equal, it seems that the life with physical beauty is better for Mill. Why not take good looks if he can get them for free?

It would take too much time to run through all of these, but I believe the same line of argument could be used to establish other items on our list, in addition to those that we have discussed: pleasure (P), knowledge (K) friendship (F), and beauty (B). Additional items include athleticism (At), autonomy (Au), creativity (C), positive moods and emotions (PM), health (HL), intelligence (I), love (L), truth (T), and wealth (W). Thus, we might say that one version of Mill's life, where he has a super-abundance of all these items, is better than any life where he has the identical amount of prudential pleasure less any one of these values. In other words, we can apply the method of difference to each value on our list as illustrated in Table 4.1. The left-hand column contains an abundance of all the items on our list; the right-hand column contains every item in abundance but one. The conclusion offered is that the left-hand

Table 4.1 Method of difference

Life with (or with more of) the disputed value	Disputed value	Life without (or with less of) the disputed value
At+, Au+, B+ C+, PM+, HL+ F+, K+, I+, L+, P+, T+, W+	At	**At−**, Au+, B+ C+, PM+, HL+ F+, K+, I+, L+, P+, T+ W+
At+, Au+, B+ C+, PM+, HL+ F+, K+, I+, L+, P+, T+, W+	Au	At+, **Au−**, B+ C+, PM+, HL+ F+, K+, I+, L+, P+, T+, W+
At+, Au+, B+ C+, PM+, HL+ F+, K+, I+, L+, P+, T+, W+	B	At−, Au+, **B−**, C+, PM+, HL+ F+, K+, I+, L+, P+, T+, W+
At+, Au+, B+ C+, PM+, HL+ F+, K+, I+, L+, P+, T+, W+	C	At−, Au+, B+ **C−**, PM+, HL+ F+, K+, I+, L+, P+, T+, W+
At+, Au+, B+ C+, PM+, HL+ F+, K+, I+, L+, P+, T+, W+	PM	At−, Au+, B+ C+, **PM−**, HL+ F+, K+, I+, L+, P+, T+, W+
At+, Au+, B+ C+, PM+, HL+ F+, K+, I+, L+, P+, T+, W+	HL	At−, Au+, B+ C+, PM+, **HL−** F+, K+, I+, L+, P+, T+, W+
At+, Au+, B+ C+, PM+, HL+ F+, K+, I+, L+, P+, T+, W+	F	At−, Au+, B+ C+, PM+, HL+ **F−**, K+, I+, L+, P+, T+, W+
At+, Au+, B+ C+, PM+, HL+ F+, K+, I+, L+, P+, T+, W+	K−	At−, Au+, B+ C+, PM+, HL+ F+, **K−**, I+, L+, P+, T+, W+
At+, Au+, B+ C+, PM+, HL+ F+, K+, I+, L+, P+, T+, W+	I	At−, Au+, B+ C+, PM+, HL+ F+, K+, **I−**, L+, P+, T+, W+
At+, Au+, B+ C+, PM+, HL+ F+, K+, I+, L+, P+, T+, W+	L	At−, Au+, B+ C+, PM+, HL+ F+, K+, I+, **L−**, P+, T+, W+
At+, Au+, B+ C+, PM+, HL+ F+, K+, I+, L+, P+, T+, W+	P	At−, Au+, B+ C+, PM+, HL+ F+, K+, I+, L+, **P−**, T+, W+
At+, Au+, B+ C+, PM+, HL+ F+, K+, I+, L+, P+, T+, W+	T	At−, Au+, B+ C+, PM+, HL+ F+, K+, I+, L+, P+, **T−**, W+
At+, Au+, B+ C+, PM+, HL+ F+, K+, I+, L+, P+, T+, W+	W	At−, Au+, B+ C+, PM+, HL+ F+, K+, I+, L+, P+, T+, **W−**

column always contains more prudential value than the same row in the right-hand column.

4.6   Desire Satisfaction and the Big Objective List

The argument for the big objective list is not quite complete, since there is still one competitor that we have not dealt with: desire satisfactionism. Pleasure has appeared on many objective lists, starting perhaps with Aristotle, but desire satisfactionism doesn't typically get the same billing.[28] The method of difference can show that desire satisfaction is an intrinsic benefit.

For the desire fulfillment theory, what counts for a life going well is the fulfillment of desires. Wellbeing consists of getting what you want.[29] Again, the desire fulfillment theory can attribute value to friendship and knowledge, but only to the extent that they are desired. Friendship, when friendship is not desired, has no prudential value. The sole intrinsic value on this view is the fulfillment of desires: to the extent that one's desires are satisfied, one's life goes better.[30] The theory typically takes on a number of refinements. For example, usually the theory is restricted to the satisfaction of intrinsic desires: my life goes better to the extent that my intrinsic desires are fulfilled. Also, some allowance is usually made for the importance of desires in terms of intensity and duration. Other qualifications sometimes considered include the ideas that desires are rational, self-regarding, autonomous, and authentic.[31] Our discussion will ignore these qualifications, since nothing turns on exploiting difficulties in specifying any of these refinements.

To establish that desire satisfaction should be on the list of prudential values, consider two versions of Mill's life exactly balanced in terms of our aforementioned intrinsic goods on the big objective list, but in one life he has more satisfied desires. Which life goes better for Mill? There seems to be something fundamentally right about the intuition that, other things being equal, the more our desires are satisfied, the better our lives go. If so, then satisfied desires have intrinsic value.

To secure this point, imagine trying to decide whether to surprise your friend on her birthday with a mushroom pizza or an onion pizza. You know that your friend desires mushrooms more than onions. Which should you bring if you know that the pizza decision will not affect the total quantity of the other intrinsic values? Surely the fact that she wants a mushroom pizza provides you with some reason to get a mushroom pizza and say that her life goes better for it. Conversely, if desire satisfaction is not part of the objective list, then there would be no reason to decide between a mushroom and an onion pizza – one might as well flip a coin, since the other values on the list are equally balanced.

It might be protested that this thought experiment assumes the implausible: bringing a mushroom pizza will bring your friend more pleasure; hence the increased pleasure is sufficient to decide the case, so desire satisfaction is not necessary. The reason she desires a mushroom pizza is that it will bring her more pleasure than an onion pizza. To skirt this objection we need to imagine some compensatory mechanism to balance out the total amount of pleasure. Suppose it is determined by your trusty magic crystal ball that your friend will eat more of the mushroom pizza than the onion pizza and so feel sleepy after dinner. This eventuates in your early exit, thus reducing the total amount of pleasure derived from your company. The increased pleasure from the mushroom pizza is exactly compensated for by the reduced time to experience other pleasures. Those who deny that desire satisfaction is an intrinsic value have no reason to prefer one version of events to the other. Since every item on the objective list (sans desire satisfaction) is identical between the two versions of your friend's life, a coin toss might as well determine the choice.

Such cases can be multiplied ad nauseam: simply look for desires that fall between the cracks of our big list. It is true that in the grand scheme of things, fulfilling one desire may not make much difference in terms of evaluating a whole life. Still, in this case, if this is the sole basis we have for choosing between two otherwise identical versions of a life, then the one with (more) satisfied desires is better. In other words, I maintain that unless there is a prior commitment to the falsity of desire satisfactionism, the explanation that you choose the mushroom pizza because your friend desires this more than an onion pizza, and this make her life (ever so slightly) better off, is entirely plausible. Conversely, frustrating the desire for mushroom pizza, when all other intrinsic prudential values remain the same, takes away a little something from your friend's life. This suggests that we need to add desire satisfaction to our list.

We have just argued that one advantage of desire satisfactionism is its breadth: it can account for items that appear valuable but must be dismissed as merely *de minimis* to objective lists that do not include desire satisfaction. But the breadth of desire satisfactionism also seems to pose an imminent threat to the big objective list: it may seem that the desire satisfaction theorist can simply annex every item on the objective list in a similar manner, that is, for each of the items on the objective list it seems it may be said by the desire theorist that it is valuable because it is desired. However, the method of difference can be applied to defeat this line of argument.

George has just finished high school and is trying to decide his next move. He has narrowed it down to taking a full scholarship to Cambridge or taking up a life as a shepherd. The attraction of the former is to continue his high school chemistry project (which won him the scholarship) investigating a novel way of sequestering carbon dioxide to reduce global warming. The attraction of the shepherd's life is to give him ample opportunity to sodomize and torture animals.[32] George is aware that these two lives are quite incompatible. A life of sodomizing and torturing animals is sure to attract attention in an academic setting (even in Cambridge). It would be stupid to put the work into an academic career and then risk it by indulging in these depraved proclivities. He really must make a choice. And George's dilemma is that his desire for each life is exactly equal. He can see the advantages of each for himself, but can find no way to decide between them simply by consulting his desires. If it is objected that if George gets caught performing acts of bestiality or torture, many of his desires will be frustrated, so he should take the chemistry life, then let us imagine that we consult our trusty crystal ball and each version of George's life has as many, and as important, desires satisfied and unsatisfied.

For the desire satisfactionist, there is no choosing between the two lives: George may as well flip a coin to decide between the two lives. The big objective list has a ready answer as to why the life of a chemist is better. In this life George will obtain more knowledge and friendship (being a shepherd can be a lonely business). Of course the big objective list cannot explain why this life is better in terms of desires for knowledge and friendship, since his desires are exactly balanced by the desires to torture and engage in bestiality. Rather, the big objective list says that knowledge and friendship, other things being equal, are of benefit to a person whether they desire them more or not. Since they have intrinsic value, they add value to George's life, and so this life offers more prudential value.

To account for the previous case it might be thought that the desire satisfactionist might amend the theory by attributing greater value to worthy desires.[33] The life of chemistry is better because the object of the desire is more worthy than the object of desire in the life of bestiality. This amounts to some concession by the desire satisfactionist theory, since now desire satisfaction is no longer sufficient for determining intrinsic prudential value. However, it may not be thought a complete capitulation, since desire may still be thought necessary. Derek Parfit explores this sort of hybrid view: "What is of value, or is good for someone, is to have both: to be engaged in these activities," for example the pursuit of knowledge, "and to be strongly wanting to be so engaged."[34] In other words, on the hybrid view knowledge is only good for someone if he wants it.

Even the weakened hybrid or "organic unity" view can be shown to be inadequate using the method of difference. George has had a religious epiphany of Pascalian proportions. He finds his previous desires to pursue chemistry or bestiality repugnant. His new and strong desire is to join the church. Unfortunately, the Galactic Overlords forbid him his new desire, and further insist that we decide for him which of the two previous lives he should pursue. Using the resources of desire satisfactionism we are stuck, for in consulting his desires we see that he no longer desires to pursue chemistry or bestiality – he considers either pursuit an anathema to his true mission. Despite this lack of preference, we should choose the life of chemistry as the one with greater prudential value. This decision is based on the intrinsic value of knowledge over bestiality. Obviously, even modified desire satisfactionist theory has no resources for explaining the difference: he has no desire for these lives, and an equal aversion to both, so one of hybridism's necessary conditions for intrinsic prudential value is missing. That is, even if the chemistry life is more worthy, the hybrid account attributes it no prudential value unless it is desired. The hybrid desire satisfactionist might as well flip a coin to decide the issue – but this is absurd. The big objective list may concede that both lives might be bad for George, perhaps so bad that even death is preferable, because he has no desire for either. All that the big objective list is committed to is the claim that the life of bestiality is worse, if only ever so slightly.

4.7   Objections to the Big Objective List

I have argued that the method of difference leads to the big objective list. In this section we shall consider objections to the big objective list, and in the following section objections to the method of difference. The following quote from Feldman nicely summarizes a frequent criticism[35] of objective list theories in general:

> Suppose some pluralist tells me that knowledge and virtue will make my life better. Suppose I dutifully go about obtaining knowledge and virtue. After a tedious and exhausting period of training, I become knowledgeable. I behave virtuously. I find the whole thing utterly unsatisfying. The pluralist tells me

my life is going well for me. I dispute it. I think that I might be better off *intellectually*, and *morally*, but my welfare is, if anything, going downhill. Surely a man might have lots of knowledge and virtue and yet have a life that is not good in itself for him.[36]

The argument is such an obvious straw person it is a wonder that it is so frequently made. If Feldman and other hedonists are correct that pleasure is a necessary component of the good life, then at best we can conclude from his example that pleasure ought to be on an objective list, and objective lists that do not include pleasure ought to be rejected. What does not follow is that all objective list theories are untenable. As noted, others have made this same criticism but the straw person seems particularly egregious in Feldman's case. In the paragraph before the one cited above, Feldman discusses Ross's objective list, which includes virtue, pleasure, knowledge, and justice. Since Ross thinks that pleasure is a necessary feature, it is surprising that Feldman uncharitably drops pleasure from the list in order to make his criticism.

Perhaps it may be thought that Feldman's point can be made even if pleasure is part of the objective list. We can imagine a person's life not going well because in the pursuit of other values on the objective list, for example knowledge and virtue, he must forgo a certain amount of pleasure, or experience a certain amount of pain, which he would not have had to do otherwise. But if this is what Feldman has in mind, it is clear that it does not tell against objective list theories in general.

To see why, we should distinguish between the inventory and indexing questions of prudential value. The former is the one we have been pursuing: what items are intrinsically prudentially valuable? The latter asks: how much weight should be assigned to the various intrinsic prudential values? These two questions are independent: two people may have the same list of intrinsic prudential values but disagree on their relative worth. Thus, one could agree with Ross's inventory: knowledge, pleasure, virtue, and justice are intrinsic prudential values; but disagree with his indexing, which makes knowledge more important than pleasure.[37] Thus, depending on how the indexing question is answered, an objective list theorist can agree that one ought not to pursue knowledge and virtue if the opportunity cost is something more valuable, namely, pleasure. So, again, Feldman's example does not work against all forms of objective list theories.

Still, it may be thought that a somewhat analogous point might be made against the big objective list: it sets the standard for the good life too high. Consider the consummate hedonist: Hugh Hefner, the publisher of *Playboy*, who for decades has enjoyed the proverbial sex, drugs, and rock and roll lifestyle. Let us suppose, whether this is true of the real Hefner or not, that he has little in the way of knowledge. Although it may not be the life we would choose, it seems like a good life for Hefner. This runs counter to the big objective list, so the objection goes, which says that there is something lacking in his life, namely, more knowledge.

However, the big objective list need not deny that Hefner is having a good life. The reason is that the connection between the questions of what are intrinsic prudential values and whether a life meets the threshold for a good life is indirect, at best. To see why, it will help to think about different conceptions of the 'good life' using the distinctions between 'threshold' and 'superlative' discussed in the previous chapter.

The lowest standard of wellbeing commonly applied is that which asks whether the wellbeing in a life is sufficient to make the life worth living. For example, sometimes the question is broached as to whether it is in the interests of a severely disabled child to be born, that is, the issue is whether existence is better than non-existence for that child. As many have argued, the standard here might be surprisingly low, but this is because often the alternative is to not exist at all.[38] At the other extreme is the idea of 'superlative wellbeing' or 'ideal wellbeing': the highest standard of the good life. The idealized aspect asks us to factor out all contingent impediments to wellbeing when we ask, "What is the best possible life for those whose life it is?" The point of ideal wellbeing is to factor out the inevitable tradeoffs that human life typically imposes. The fact that such tradeoffs often must be made does not show that ideally one would not be better off to have high levels of both.

Finally there is what we think of as 'threshold wellbeing' or 'satisfactory wellbeing,' meaning something less than ideal wellbeing. It is quite possible to say: "John is doing very well" or "John had a good life" without thereby implying that his life could not have been better. Although it is not always easy to tell, it seems this standard is often in play in discussions of wellbeing: a standard where we might appraise a life as having gone well while admitting room for further prudential value.[39]

Applying these distinctions, we can see that the big objective list can consistently hold the position that pleasure is sufficient for threshold or satisfactory wellbeing, but not the ideally good life. The big objective list might even concede that Hefner had the best life of anyone in history. For the big objective list can still maintain that we can imagine a better life: a life with all the bacchanalian pleasures of Hefner's life, but with the addition of other elements of the big objective list. The big objective list is committed to saying that the ideal life – one where the usual tradeoffs between different values do not happen – will have all the elements of the big objective list. When we move away from ideal wellbeing, nothing directly follows from the big objective list about the standards of a minimally or satisfactorily good life. To think otherwise is to conflate the inventory and the indexing questions. So one can consistently endorse the big objective list and claim that Hefner's is a good life, so long as pleasure (or perhaps desire satisfaction) is accorded sufficient weight.

4.8　Objections to the Method of Difference

It may be thought that the method of difference is trivial, since any item can be added to the list by the same reasoning. To this it may be responded that there are two sorts of item that fail the test: those with negative intrinsic prudential value and those with neutral intrinsic prudential value. As an example of the former, consider the two versions of Mill's life: they are otherwise equal in the prudential values of the big objective list, but one version has lots of pain and one has little pain. A life with lots of pain is worse for Mill, not better, so not everything passes the method of difference. While we won't explore this further, the suggestion is that the method of difference can also be used to delineate intrinsic harms.

A plausible case where a change of characteristic does not add or subtract from the prudential value of a life is hair color. Being a blond, brunette or redhead seems to make no difference to prudential value, other things being equal. This is not to say that hair color may not have some instrumental value, e.g., if the cliché that blonds have more fun is true, then hair color may be instrumentally valuable in promoting fun (and fun may be instrumentally valuable in promoting pleasure).[40] The point is that if other values are held constant, if hair color is stripped of any instrumental value by the method of difference, then there seems to be no reason to prefer one hair color over another. Hair color is intrinsically prudentially neutral.

The final objection we shall consider is one that directly confronts the intuitive judgment that the method of difference leverages to construct the big objective list. Thus, with reference to our first example, the hedonist might use the skeptical strategy to argue that the (P+K+) and (P+K−) lives are indeed equivalent in terms of welfare – there is no choosing between them. The idea is to be skeptical about the intuitive judgments about these two versions of Mill's life. But the skeptical strategy, as we shall understand it, is not merely digging in one's heels and claiming that the intuitive judgments of others are wrong, but rather it offers some explanation of why so many are so often mistaken in their intuitive judgments.

To be effective, the skeptical strategy must be deployed with some delicacy; in particular, it must meet at least two conditions. First, the skepticism cannot be a global doubt about the ability to ascertain prudential value. Such skepticism would not favor monists like hedonists and desire satisfactionists because of its generality: it undermines the cognitive resources necessary to decide the issue. A second condition is that the monist's preferred intrinsic value must itself be immune from the skepticism.

Roger Crisp offers a fine example of the skeptical strategy in his defense of hedonism:

> Those who achieved more in the field – who brought back more meat, or more fungi and fruit – would have been rewarded by their fellows, partly with a larger share of the available goods, but also with esteem and status within the group. Now this story is of course not on its own sufficient to debunk the claim of accomplishment to independent non-hedonic value for individuals. But it does, I suggest, throw that claim into some doubt. Could it not be that our valuing of accomplishment is an example of a kind of collective bad faith, with its roots in the spontaneous and largely unreflective social practices of our distant ancestors?[41]

Crisp's argument seems to meet the first condition. He offers a reason to think that we might be deceived about achievement in particular, not about all prudential value. Crisp's argument, however, fails to meet the second condition. The same skeptical strategy, it seems, could just as easily be deployed against pleasure as achievement. Crisp, as far as I can tell, is suggesting that cultural or perhaps evolutionary forces cause us to mistake the instrumental value of achievement for intrinsic value. But this puts a lot of pressure on Crisp's explanation to be empirically plausible. Not only does Crisp provide no evidence (assuming we do not count the rhetorical question at the end of the quote above as adding any evidential weight), but psychologists inform us that the arrow of causation is bidirectional: feeling good can lead to achievement, and vice versa.[42] So, we could just as easily say that our ancestors had reason to encourage people to enjoy themselves to promote better physical excellence and knowledge in hunting and fungi-gathering expeditions. After all, given that feeling good leads to doing more, the model predicts that persons would better secure these perfectionist goods. We might offer the alternative explanation that through collective bad faith people began to think that enjoyment has intrinsic value, confusing its instrumental value with intrinsic value. In other words, the skeptical strategy Crisp invokes can just as easily be deployed against pleasure as against achievement. So, we have little reason to suppose that Crisp's version of skepticism about achievement is any more plausible than a similar skepticism mounted against pleasure using the same strategy.

Moreover, even if Crisp's skepticism *explains* why we might be mistaken about non-hedonic values, this does not show that such skepticism is *justified*. No independent reason is offered to suppose that he is right in his most general claim that people might be suffering some kind of collective bad faith whereby they confuse instrumental and intrinsic values, rather than supposing that people are not so confused. To think that reasoning using this distinction misfires only when it comes to achievement seems to me to be in danger of arguing *from* rather than *to* hedonism, that is, begging the question.

The fact that Crisp's argument is not particularly convincing does not show that all attempts at the skeptical strategy must fail. It does, however, serve to highlight one of the attractive features about using the method of difference to establish pluralism: the evidential basis is fairly narrow and uncontroversial. The primary assumption is that our intuitive judgments about the prudential value of various lives (real and imaginary) are reasonably reliable. To successfully deploy the skeptical strategy, monists must deny this assumption without undermining their own position – a tough row to hoe.

It is worth making another remark about the method of difference. Obviously it relies crucially on describing cases and asking the fair-minded reader to make judgments about wellbeing. In this respect it is no different from what one will find in all sophisticated philosophical discussions of wellbeing. I can't think of a single case where an author does not employ the argumentative strategy to describe various lives and to ask the fair-minded reader whether he or she judges the life to be one high or low in wellbeing. Certainly this is the case for some of the best-known and most widely discussed recent contributions to the debate.[43] This is not an argument ad populum, but merely to point out that the method of difference hardly distinguishes itself in asking readers to make judgments about cases, and using these as data. Judgments about cases are used as data because the exercise is supposed to be one of arguing *to* rather than *from* a theory of wellbeing. By this I mean that the exercise in making judgments about cases is supposed to go like this: we consider a number of cases and make pre-theoretical judgments about the degree of wellbeing. Theory X nicely explains these judgments, while theories Y and Z fail to, so we have reason to adopt theory X. This would be arguing *to* theory X. Arguing *from* theory X would say something like this: Theory X is correct, so we ought to make such and such judgments about the intuitive cases. Nothing about the method of difference is inconsistent with arguing to a big objective list. Nor do we need to assume that our judgments about cases are always reliable. Indeed, the method of difference takes seriously the charge by hedonists and desire satisfactionists that people can easily confuse instrumental and intrinsic value. Proponents of the method of difference may agree that this is a significant worry, and indeed, this is precisely what the method of difference seeks to control for.

To summarize, critics of the method of difference should ask themselves whether they are global or local skeptics. They are global skeptics if they doubt our ability to establish much by asking fair-minded readers to make judgments about the degree of wellbeing of adequately described cases. I have no general answer to this skepticism, but then again such skepticism impugns all theories of wellbeing. More local worries, like those expressed by Crisp, must be adequately motivated. It is not enough to say that we could be mistaken in our intuitive judgments about such cases. Of course we could. I could also jump over the moon with the cow and the spoon. The point is only relevant if we have good reason to suppose that our intuitive judgments are mistaken.

Finally, we can ask "what" and "why" of a theory of welfare. The big objective list, as presented here, is a theory about what wellbeing consists of. Life goes better for the person whose life it is, other things being equal, the more that life has of each of the items on the big objective list. The parallel for hedonism is the claim that wellbeing comprises pleasure. We could also ask a hedonist why wellbeing comprises pleasure. Here the hedonist might say such things as: "because evolution made us that way," "because God intended it that way," or "there is no deeper reason than that pleasure provides the best theoretical unity to our intuitive judgments about what makes for a good life." These same answers, *mutatis mutandis*, as to why wellbeing comprises the items on the big objective list are available to the big objective list theorist. Of course, our concern here is the what-question, not the why-question, and so in this respect it is incomplete. However, in this respect it is in good company: most contemporary discussions of welfare are focused exclusively on the what-question. Sumner and Feldman, for example, in their book-length treatment of wellbeing, realize there is a why-question, but never seek to answer it.[44]

4.9　Inventory and Indexing

The method of difference shows that there is a very strong case that the inventory question should be resolved in favor of the big objective list. However, I have not claimed that the big objective list, as presented above, is complete or fully specified. By 'complete' I mean that every intrinsic prudential value appears on the list; for example, we should ask, as we shall in the next chapter, whether virtue should be included on a complete big objective list. It may be too that some of the items on the list are redundant, that some reductionist arguments might be plausible. There is the question, going back to Plato's discussion in the *Meno*, about whether knowledge adds anything of value over and above true belief.[45] Another example is whether wealth might be reduced to some aspect of autonomy. Often autonomy is thought of as a threshold concept: is the patient autonomous or not? If we think of it as a variable concept – one which persons can have more or less of – and we analyze wealth in terms of social power, then the possibility is open that we might say that wealth increases one's autonomy, suggesting that wealth could be reduced to a dimension of autonomy. Ross thought that friendship could be reduced to other things like knowledge, pleasure, and virtue. Clearly it is well beyond the scope of this work to explore such matters; but I will say this much: such matters can be accommodated as disagreements *within* the big objective list; they are not in themselves objections *to* the big objective list. For these disputes are about the nature of the proper parts of the big objective list, not about the big objective list itself. The big objective list can hardly be blamed, for example, if we have not resolved the *Meno* question.

　　Nor have I claimed that the method is capable of deciding all inventory questions. It is possible, for example, that a putative intrinsic value may be so slight that our intuitions may not be self-consistent or consistent with others. I have a colleague who seems generally sympathetic to the line of argument suggested by the paper, but rejects the claim that the method of difference reveals that physical beauty has intrinsic value. I disagree (and he is ugly), but the method of difference does not need to be accepted only on the condition that it solves all such disputes. The fact that we agree on the intrinsic prudential value of pleasure, autonomy, knowledge, friendship, desire satisfaction, etc. is sufficient to put us both in the big objective list camp.

Although there is much latitude in how the big objective list might be developed, saying that the big objective list is correct is not without content: if the big objective list is correct, then the list of intrinsic prudential values is much longer than the typical objective list theory.

Perhaps the most significant limitation of the argument is that it says nothing about the indexing question; for example, nothing has been said about the relative prudential worth of pleasure and knowledge. So, admittedly, much of the dispute formally associated with the inventory problem merely reappears in a slightly altered form with the indexing problem. Imagine, for example, that a hedonist and a perfectionist accept the line of argument suggested by the method of difference and reform their views. The reformed hedonist is now a pluralist, but insists that pleasure is the most important intrinsic benefit and so is lexically prior to everything else on the objective list. Conversely, the perfectionist is now a pluralist but thinks that knowledge is the most important intrinsic benefit, and so argues that knowledge is lexically prior to every other value, including pleasure. It is of course not quite the old battle, since they both agree about what counts as an intrinsic benefit. Still, these two different versions of the big objective list could give diametrically opposed recommendations about the good life in many cases.

The indexing question may not be easy to answer, but, fortunately for us, we do not need to answer it. As we shall see, starting in Chapter 6, for most people there is no need to choose between being happier and achieving more. This is because happiness causes achievement. As expounded above, the big objective list does not tell us how to decide between happiness and achievement, if we really must choose between them. It does tell us that if the choice is the status quo or more happiness *and* achievement, then we should go for more happiness and achievement. As noted, this is precisely what will be argued.

Notes

1. Griffin, *Well-Being*, 3–4.
2. Sumner, *Welfare, Happiness, and Ethics*, 20. Further clarification can be found in Arneson, "Human Flourishing Versus Desire Satisfaction" and Zimmerman, "Understanding What is Good for Us."
3. Feldman, *Pleasure and the Good Life.*

4. Julia Annas (*The Morality of Happiness*) argues that most of the Ancient Greeks rejected (or did not even consider) the idea that there are additional dimensions upon which to evaluate a human life. Getting clear on how wellbeing differs from these other dimensions is no easy task. It is partly for this reason that I avoid talking about virtue as an intrinsic prudential benefit until the next chapter.

5. Parfit, *Reasons and Persons*; Griffin, *Well-Being*.

6. Arneson, "Human Flourishing Versus Desire Satisfaction."

7. As Brad Hooker notes, one could view perfectionism as an objective list theory with a single entry: perfection ("Does Moral Virtue Constitute a Benefit to the Agent?").

8. Feldman, *What Is This Thing Called Happiness?*

9. Mill, *Utilitarianism*.

10. Davis, "A Theory of Happiness."

11. Sumner, *Welfare, Happiness, and Ethics*; Mill, *Utilitarianism*.

12. See Sumner, *Welfare, Happiness, and Ethics*, 45–6, Crisp, "Well-being", and Arneson ("Human Flourishing Versus Desire Satisfaction").

13. Arneson, "Human Flourishing Versus Desire Satisfaction."

14. Keller, "Welfare as Success"; Wolf, "Happiness and Meaning"; Brink, *Moral Realism and the Foundations of Ethics*.

15. J. Finnis, *Natural Law and Natural Rights*, 86–90.

16. Gert, *Morality*, 94.

17. Plato, *Plato's Philebus*; Ross, *The Right and the Good*; Hooker, "Does Moral Virtue Constitute a Benefit to the Agent?"; Feldman, *Pleasure and the Good Life*; Mendola, "Intuitive Hedonism."

18. Even the determined skeptic will have a hard time showing that we do not know at least some truths, e.g., the minimal principle of non-contradiction: not every statement is true and false. Putnam, "There is At Least One A Priori Truth."

19. Aristotle, *Nichomachean Ethics*, 24–5.

20. See Plato, *Plato's Philebus*, Hurka, *Virtue, Vice, and Value*, and Sumner, "Two Theories of the Good."

21. See Sumner, *Welfare, Happiness, and Ethics*, for a sophisticated version of this argument.

22. It may be thought that Mill's doctrine of higher and lower pleasures might be of some avail here. The cogency of this doctrine is a matter of some dispute (Feldman, "Mill, Moore, and the Consistency of Qualified Hedonism"; Ryberg, "Higher and Lower Pleasures"; Rabinowicz, "Ryberg's Doubts About Higher and Lower Pleasures – Put to Rest?"; Schmidt-Petri, "Mill on Quality and Quantity"). We can side-step the issue simply by assuming that Mill does not get any pleasure from knowledge: the Galactic Overlords stop him from experiencing pleasure when he gains knowledge. Since he does not get any

pleasure from the knowledge, the explanation for the difference here cannot be in terms of the greater worth of higher pleasures.

23. See Griffin, *Well-Being*; Sumner, *Welfare, Happiness, and Ethics*; and Hooker, "Does Moral Virtue Constitute a Benefit to the Agent?" Hurka (*Perfectionism*) does not understand it as a theory of prudential value. In terms of our tripartite distinction above, perfectionism is often classified as a particular form of objective list theory (for discussion see Hooker, "Does Moral Virtue Constitute a Benefit to the Agent?").

24. Hurka (*Perfectionism*, 27), at this point in his discussion, seems to use 'pleasure' and 'satisfaction' interchangeably. I'm not sure why pure perfectionism rejects pleasure; certainly there is little in Hurka's masterful presentation of perfectionism to suggest why this is the case. After all, if perfectionism (at least in some forms) enjoins us to develop certain aspects of human nature, then why is pleasure not one of the excellences to be developed? A historical answer might be that hedonism and perfectionism have traditionally been at loggerheads (ibid.). The only remotely plausible argument I can think of is that pleasure is passive, whereas perfectionism enjoins us to develop excellence. However, Aristotle long ago questioned this line of reasoning: pleasures can be cultivated. So, I am simply following suit here, rather than endorsing this contrast.

25. Hurka (*Perfectionism*, 5). I am using 'perfectionism' in the narrow sense defined by Hurka, which ties it to human nature (p. 4).

26. Hurka's list of perfectionists includes: Plato, Aristotle, Aquinas, Leibniz, Spinoza, Kant, Hegel, Marx, Bradley, Green, and Bosanquet (ibid., p. 3). A possible exception is Nietzsche, at least as Hurka ("Nietzsche: Perfectionist") understands him. My own view is that Hurka is correct that Nietzsche is a perfectionist about power, but he overlooks the fact that Nietzsche may have held a reductionist view: knowledge is power.

27. We are ignoring other possible aspects of Mill's perfection that might be of interest to the perfectionist, e.g., athleticism, friendship or health (Hurka, *Perfectionism*).

28. Assuming, of course, that Aristotle is correctly described as an objective list theorist. Whether this assumption is correct is of little concern at present. Sen ("Plural Utility") considers desire satisfaction to be part of a plural conception of the good. Arneson ("Human Flourishing Versus Desire Satisfaction," 124) cogitates on the possibility of adding desire satisfaction to an objective list, but takes no definitive stand on the issue.

29. See Brandt, *A Theory of the Good and the Right*, Ch. 6. Desire satisfactionism is often understood as a formal theory. Very, very crudely: some object O is good for person X just in case X desires O, and that desire is satisfied. O, then, is the thing that is intrinsically good. I tend to think that it is more charitable to understand it as a substantive theory: desire satisfaction is an intrinsic

prudential good. Nothing of substance turns on this for present purposes: see the following footnote.

30. Whether desire satisfactionism is a monistic theory clearly depends on how one counts intrinsic benefits; e.g., Hooker, "Does Moral Virtue Constitute a Benefit to the Agent?," 144, seems to deny that it is monistic. The formal understanding of the theory, where each object that is desired is intrinsically good for the desiring agent, seems to suggest a potentially infinite set of intrinsic prudential goods, since there are potentially an infinite number of objects that we might desire. For present purposes, absolutely nothing interesting hangs on whether we say that desire satisfaction holds that there is only one intrinsic value (the satisfaction of desires), or a potentially infinite number of intrinsic values (the objects of desire). In what follows, I will talk as if desire satisfaction is a monistic theory, but this should be understood as meaning that either desire satisfaction is the single prudential good, or desire satisfaction is the single criterion of a potentially infinite number of intrinsic prudential goods. Both views are challenged by the counterexample offered below: items that are good for an agent even when the agent does not desire the item.

31. Bykvist, "What Are Desires Good For?," 290.

32. Moore asks us to imagine that "the greatest possible pleasure could be obtained by a perpetual indulgence in bestiality" (*Principia Ethica*, section 56). I defer to his authority on this point.

33. Griffin, *Well-Being*.

34. Parfit, *Reasons and Persons*, 502. Although Parfit considers a hybrid between hedonism and an objective list, he seems to slip between hedonism and desire satisfactionism in his discussion of hybridism. Variants of hybridism can be found in Darwall, *Welfare and Rational Care*, Ch. 4; Dworkin, "Foundations of Liberal Equality"; Brandt, "Overvold on Self-Interest and Self-Sacrifice"; Adams, *Finite and Infinite Goods*; Feldman, *Pleasure and the Good Life*; Kraut, *What Is Good and Why*. Feldman does not acknowledge the hybrid character, but as Serena Olsaretti argues, it is difficult to see on what basis this hybridism might be denied ("The Limits of Hedonism"). As Guy Fletcher points out, it is not clear how committed Kraut is to ubiquitous hybridism as a general theory ("Review of *What Is Good and Why*").

35. Griffin, *Well-Being*; Sumner, "Two Theories of the Good"; Arneson, "Human Flourishing Versus Desire Satisfaction"; Kagan, "Well-being as Enjoying the Good."

36. Feldman, *Pleasure and the Good Life*, 19.

37. Ross, *The Right and the Good*, 149–50.

38. See for instance, Glover, *Choosing Children*.

39. It may be that something like this distinction is at work in Plato's discussions of pleasure and virtue in *The Republic* where he gives what seem to be competing

accounts in Books IV and IX. The problem, in a nutshell, is whether virtue is sufficient for wellbeing, a view Aristotle lampoons (*Nichomachean Ethics*, 1096a). The view may not be quite so ridiculous (even if not plausible) if we think of Plato suggesting that a life of virtue is sufficient for a satisfactorily good life while maintaining that it could be made better by the addition of pleasure, as he seems to suggest in Book IX.

40. There is some evidence that red hair may be correlated with increased levels of pain for a given stimulus (Mogil, Ritchie, and Smith, "Melanocortin-1 Receptor Gene Variants Affect Pain and Mu-opioid Analgesia in Mice and Humans"). This would suggest that red hair is instrumentally detrimental in this regard; however, the method of difference controls for this by stipulating that the levels of pain are identical between all hair colors.

41. Crisp, "Hedonism Reconsidered," 638–9. See also Crisp, *Reasons and the Good*, 121–2.

42. As noted, we will discuss in Chapter 6 the large meta-study by Lyubomirsky, King, and Diener, "The Benefits of Frequent Positive Affect," which shows that positive affect can lead to achievement and vice versa.

43. Parfit, *Reasons and Persons*; Griffin, *Well-Being*; Sumner, *Welfare, Happiness, and Ethics*; Feldman, *Pleasure and the Good Life*.

44. Sumner, *Welfare, Happiness, and Ethics*; Feldman, *Pleasure and the Good Life*.

45. David, "Truth as the Primary Epistemic Goal."

References

Adams, R. M. *Finite and Infinite Goods: A Framework for Ethics*. New York: Oxford University Press, 1999.

Annas, J. *The Morality of Happiness*. New York: Oxford University Press, 1993.

Aristotle. *Nichomachean Ethics*. New York: Macmillan, 1962.

Arneson, Richard. "Human Flourishing Versus Desire Satisfaction." *Social Philosophy and Policy* 16, no. 1 (1999): 113–42.

Brandt, R. B. "Overvold on Self-Interest and Self-Sacrifice." *Journal of Philosophical Research*, no. 16 (1991): 353–63.

Brandt, R. B. *A Theory of the Good and the Right*. Oxford: Clarendon Press, 1979.

Brink, D. O. *Moral Realism and the Foundations of Ethics*. Cambridge: Cambridge University Press, 1989.

Bykvist, K. "What Are Desires Good For? Towards a Coherent Endorsement Theory." *Ratio* 19, no. 3 (2006): 286–304.

Crisp, R. "Hedonism Reconsidered." *Philosophy and Phenomenological Research* 73, no. 3 (2006): 619–45.

Crisp, R. *Reasons and the Good*. New York: Oxford University Press, 2006.

Crisp, R. "Well-being." In *The Stanford Encyclopedia of Philosophy* (Fall 2008 edn.), edited by Edward N. Zalta. http://plato.stanford.edu/archives/win2008/entries/well-being/.

Darwall, S. *Welfare and Rational Care*. Princeton, N.J.: Princeton University Press, 2002.

David, M. "Truth as the Primary Epistemic Goal: A Working Hypothesis." In *Contemporary Debates in Epistemology*, edited by E. Sosa and M. Steup, 296–312. Oxford: Blackwell, 2005.

Davis, Wayne A. "A Theory of Happiness." *American Philosophical Quarterly* 18, no. 2 (1981): 111–20.

Dworkin, R. "Foundations of Liberal Equality." In *The Tanner Lectures on Human Values*, II: 1–119. Salt Lake City: University of Utah Press, 1990.

Feldman, F. "Mill, Moore, and the Consistency of Qualified Hedonism." *Midwest Studies in Philosophy* 20, no. 1 (1995): 318–31.

Feldman, F. *Pleasure and the Good Life: Concerning the Nature, Varieties, and Plausibility of Hedonism*. Oxford: Clarendon Press, 2004.

Feldman, F. *What Is This Thing Called Happiness?* New York: Oxford University Press, 2010.

Finnis, J. *Natural Law and Natural Rights*. Oxford: Oxford University Press, 1980.

Fletcher, G. "Review of *What Is Good and Why*." *Analysis* 69, no. 3 (2009): 576–8.

Gert, B. *Morality: Its Nature and Justification*. New York: Oxford University Press, 1998.

Glover, J. *Choosing Children: Genes, Disability, and Design*. Oxford: Oxford University Press, 2006.

Griffin, J. *Well-Being: Its Meaning, Measurement, and Moral Importance*. Oxford: Clarendon Press, 1986.

Hooker, B. "Does Moral Virtue Constitute a Benefit to the Agent?" In *How Should One Live?*, edited by Roger Crisp, 141–57. Oxford: Oxford University Press, 1996.

Hurka, Thomas. "Nietzsche: Perfectionist." In *Nietzsche and Morality*, edited by Brian Leiter and Neil Sinhababu, 9–31. Oxford: Clarendon Press, 2007.

Hurka, Thomas. *Perfectionism*. New York: Oxford University Press, 1993.

Hurka, Thomas. *Virtue, Vice, and Value*. New York: Oxford University Press, 2001.

Kagan, S. "Well-being as Enjoying the Good." *Philosophical Perspectives* 23, no. 1 (2009): 253–72.

Keller, S. "Welfare as Success." *Noûs* 43, no. 4 (2009): 656–83.

Kraut, R. *What Is Good and Why: The Ethics of Well-Being*. Cambridge, Mass.: Harvard University Press, 2007.

Lyubomirsky, S., L. King, and E. Diener. "The Benefits of Frequent Positive Affect: Does Happiness Lead to Success?" *Psychological Bulletin* 131 (2005): 803–55.

Mendola, Joseph. "Intuitive Hedonism." *Philosophical Studies* 128 (2006): 441–77.

Mill, J. S. *Utilitarianism*. Chicago, Ill.: University of Chicago Press, 1906.

Moore, G. E. *Principia Ethica*. Cambridge: Cambridge University Press, 1903.

Mogil, J. S., J. Ritchie, and S. Smith. "Melanocortin-1 Receptor Gene Variants Affect Pain and Mu-opioid Analgesia in Mice and Humans." *Journal of Medical Genetics* 42, no. 7 (July 2005): 583–7.

Olsaretti, S. "The Limits of Hedonism: Feldman on the Value of Attitudinal Pleasure." *Philosophical Studies* 136 (2007): 409–15.

Parfit, D. *Reasons and Persons*. Oxford: Oxford University Press, 1987.

Plato. *Plato's Philebus*, trans. R. Hackforth. Cambridge: At the University Press, 1972.

Plato. *The Republic*. Indianapolis, Ind.: Hackett, 2004.

Putnam, H. "There is At Least One A Priori Truth." *Erkenntnis* 13, no. 1 (1978): 153–70.

Rabinowicz, W. "Ryberg's Doubts About Higher and Lower Pleasures – Put to Rest?" *Ethical Theory and Moral Practice* 6, no. 2 (2003): 231–7.

Ross, W. D. *The Right and the Good*. Indianapolis, Ind.: Hackett, 1988.

Ryberg, J. "Higher and Lower Pleasures: Doubts on Justification." *Ethical Theory and Moral Practice* 5, no. 4 (2002): 415–29.

Schmidt-Petri, C. "Mill on Quality and Quantity." *Philosophical Quarterly* 53, no. 210 (2003): 102–4.

Sen, A. "Plural Utility." *Proceedings of the Aristotelian Society*, 81 (1980): 193–215.

Sumner, L. W. "Two Theories of the Good." In *The Good Life and the Human Good*, edited by Ellen Frankel Paul, Fred D. Miller, Jr., and Jeffrey Paul, 1–15. New York: Cambridge University Press, 1992.

Sumner, L. W. *Welfare, Happiness, and Ethics*. Oxford: Clarendon Press, 1996.

Wolf, S. "Happiness and Meaning: Two Aspects of the Good Life." *Social Philosophy and Policy* 14, no. 1 (1997): 207–25.

Zimmerman, M. "Understanding What is Good for Us." *Ethical Theory and Moral Practice* 12 (2009): 429–39.

5

Wellbeing and Virtue

In this chapter we will argue that virtue is a component of wellbeing. This will set the stage for subsequent chapters wherein it will be argued that happiness causes virtue.

In thinking about the role of virtue in wellbeing it will help to consider again John the Savage's cost argument: "*'But I don't want comfort. I want God, I want poetry, I want real danger, I want freedom, I want goodness. I want sin.'*" We have yet to deal with John's claim that he wants sin. It is not entirely clear from the novel what John's complaint about a lack of opportunity for sin amounts to. The most obvious interpretation is that John thinks *Brave New World* lacks a moral dimension. The reason for the hesitancy in understanding John in this way is that it seems obviously false. It is true that the lower classes are so intellectually stunted, and so heavily conditioned, that arguably they have no moral dimension to their lives – no more so than a well-trained dog. However, even the Beta class might be said to have at least some moral dimension to their lives.

Early in the novel there is a discussion between Lenina and her friend Fanny about Lenina's involvement with the dashing Henry Foster. Basically, Fanny takes Lenina to task for not following the norms of having multiple sexual partners. Lenina's "sin" is one of desiring a monogamous relationship. Now, we may disagree with the norm, and no doubt John the Savage does (John is smitten with Lenina, yet repulsed by her sexual promiscuity), but the discussion certainly appears to have a moral dimension to it: Fanny is morally admonishing Lenina for not following a norm

Happy-People-Pills For All, First Edition. Mark Walker.
© 2013 John Wiley & Sons, Inc. Published 2013 by John Wiley & Sons, Inc.

that is generally recognized as good for society. In effect, Fanny argues that Lenina must sacrifice some of her own personal welfare, specifically, her desire to be only with Henry, for she has a duty to have sexual relations with other men. I take it that this is a very recognizable form of moral argument. Interestingly, the moral admonishment by Fanny is pivotal for the plot development. Lenina was vacillating as to whether to agree to Bernard's request to go to the Savage Reservation, and this conversation with its moral admonishing may have turned the tide in favor of her accompanying Bernard.

Another clear case of moral reasoning is the Controller's reply to the question of why he did not move to an island to pursue his love of science:

> "I was given the choice; to be sent to an island, where I could have got on with my pure science, or to be taken on to the Controllers' Council with the prospect of succeeding in due course to an actual Controllership. I chose this and let the science go." After a little silence, "Sometimes," he added, "I rather regret the science. Happiness is a hard master – particularly other people's happiness. A much harder master, if one isn't conditioned to accept it unquestioningly, than truth." He sighed, fell silent again, then continued in a brisker tone. "Well, duty's duty. One can't consult one's own preferences."[1]

The idea that the Controller has a duty to serve the happiness of others, rather than merely consult his predilections, has a distinctly moral tone. Immanuel Kant or J. S. Mill could not have said it better.

However, whether *Brave New World*ers are capable of moral action is not ultimately our concern; rather, what we want to pursue is the idea that moral goodness confers a prudential benefit. At least one understanding of John's argument is that he thinks his life (and the lives of others) is diminished by not having the possibility of moral action. Understood in this way the question is whether moral action enriches the lives of moral agents, rather than the recipients. Consider a trite example: you help the proverbial old lady across the street. Most agree that the old lady benefits from the action, but did you, as moral agent, benefit? Some argue that you did as well. This is the "virtue is its own reward" school of thought. Others suggest that the moral actor (typically) does not benefit (at least directly) through moral action, so moral action does not contribute to your wellbeing. It is this question we want to pursue here. We will argue on the "virtue is its own reward" side; specifically, the claim is that moral virtue is an intrinsic prudential benefit.

5.1 Gyges' Ring

The myth of Gyges' Ring might be used to further locate our topic. Plato, in the *Republic*,[2] tells the story of a simple shepherd who discovers a magic ring that has the power of conferring invisibility. Gyges uses the ring's power to kill the king and sleep with his wife. Given the power of the ring, and the fact that Gyges wants to be king and sleep with the queen, it seems that Gyges' actions are perfectly reasonable in terms of promoting his own wellbeing. To the objection that he is not acting in a just manner – it is a grave injustice to kill the king – it seems that Gyges might say that he has little need for justice once he has the power of the ring. So the challenge is made in Plato's dialogue to show that Gyges should act justly even if he has the power to escape punishment when he acts unjustly.

So, how can this challenge be met? Modern ethical theory, for the most part, says the challenge cannot be met, that is, being moral is not in Gyges' prudential interest. This is not to say that modern moral theory recommends that Gyges ought to go ahead and commit the crimes. Rather, modern moral theory says that Gyges ought to heed the governor of morality. That is, while it may be in Gyges' prudential interest to kill the king and sleep with the queen, to do so would be to act in an immoral manner. For example, utilitarians might explain the impermissibility of the action in terms of failing to promote the greatest amount of happiness for all. The moral error Gyges falls into here is to weight his happiness more than that of others. (This is not to say that utilitarians think that Gyges should not factor in his own happiness, only that it should not count for more than that of others.) Kant would explain Gyges' error here in terms of violation of the categorical imperative. Gyges treats the king as a mere means to Gyges' ambitions – he does not treat the king with the dignity and respect due to persons. Thus, the indictment would be that Gyges puts the principle of self-love before the principle of moral duty. So, while they may explain the moral error here in different terms, nevertheless they agree that morality requires restraining prudential interest in such a case. The challenge Plato takes up is to show that it is not in Gyges' prudential interest to kill the king and sleep with the queen. His life, prudentially considered, will be worse. So, the Modern versus the Ancient way of meeting this challenge is quite different.

The views do, however, share a common problem. Both must account for the "common" conception of the prudential view of one's life. The common conception here says that given that Gyges wants the riches, the power, and the wife of the king, and he can obtain these with little cost to himself thanks to the power of the ring, his life will be better. Modern theories, in general, do not ask us to rethink the common view of what is in our prudential interest; rather, they suggest that this is not the only view of your life you must take. You must also think of your life from a moral point of view, and, when you do, this will constrain the prudential view. In this case the moral view constrains Gyges' prudential interest in becoming king. The difficulty for modern conceptions is how to explain the source of the moral point of view, and why we should think it has any claim on us. Gyges might claim that he is more than happy to forgo any good feelings that arise from doing what the moral point of view requires in exchange for a kingdom. Again, the Ancients do not have this motivational problem, since they do not appeal to the moral point of view over and above the prudential view. But where at least some of the Ancients find difficulty is in their disagreement with the common view about the nature of the prudential conception of wellbeing. For example, Plato and Aristotle would say that, in fact, Gyges is actually worse off becoming king. The trouble is to show how this can be the case – how can we think that this is even remotely plausible? If Gyges desperately wants to become king and sleep with the queen, how can it be that he is worse off? Plato's reasoning, which we will not explore here, is that killing the king will require Gyges to act in a vicious (i.e., not in accordance with virtue) manner, and such viciousness means his soul will be "out of harmony." Our conclusion is a little more optimistic than the prototypical modern theory, which says that moral action is not in our prudential interest, and less ambitious than Plato's view, which says that it is necessary and sufficient for the good life.[3] It will be argued that virtue is necessary for an ideally good life.

5.2 Moral Virtue

Virtues are often classified as 'self-regarding' and 'other-regarding' depending on whether the primary benefit of the virtues accrues to the virtuous agent, or some other.[4] So, the virtue of 'industry' is sometimes said to be self-regarding because the primary benefit accrues to the person who is industrious. Those who are industrious, so the thought goes, will often accrue benefits such as material prosperity. Others in society may benefit, at least indirectly, from the productivity of the industrious, but in the typical case the greatest benefit goes to the industrious person.[5] In the case of an other-regarding virtue like justice,[6] the primary benefit is conferred upon those who are affected by the agent exhibiting the virtue of justice; for example, someone who is involved with a just person in some sort of distribution of goods, such as selling property, may benefit by being treated fairly in the exchange. I shall assume that caring, justice, and honesty are other-regarding virtues, or what we shall term 'moral virtues'. Assuming, as we shall, that others are the primary beneficiaries of moral virtues, still it makes sense to ask: does moral virtue provide a benefit for the morally virtuous?[7]

I believe that most will grant that, at least in some cases, the answer to this question is "yes." For instance, being (or at least appearing to be) morally virtuous may well prove a benefit to someone in securing positive letters of recommendation when applying to medical school. Note that even if we accept this example of how being morally virtuous may confer a benefit on the agent, it seems we will have shown only the instrumental benefit of moral virtue. We have explained its benefit in terms of a means to realizing some other benefit for the agent, namely, the benefit of getting into medical school. Our question is whether moral virtue constitutes an intrinsic benefit to the agent; that is, does it confer some benefit on the agent irrespective of any means it has in realizing some other benefit?

We will say more about this below, but even if our argument is successful, it does not provide an argument against the immoralist: it still may be that Gyges acts against his prudential interest in killing the king and sleeping with the queen. If Gyges takes much pleasure in these activities, then the benefit of this pleasure may outweigh the benefit of acting virtuously; that is, the prudential value of that greater pleasure outweighs the prudential value of being just. What would follow is that there is at least some prudential cost to acting immorally.

5.3   The Method of Difference

Applying the method of difference argument that we examined in the previous chapters shows that moral virtue is a benefit to the agent. First we imagine two versions of a person's life balanced in terms of non-disputed intrinsic benefits. In thinking about any disputed intrinsic benefits, it is best to imagine an expansive list of non-disputed intrinsic benefits. The reason the expansive list is an advantage here is that it may help us avoid confusing instrumental benefit with intrinsic benefit. Thus, suppose we did not have pleasure on our list of intrinsic benefits, when in fact it is an intrinsic benefit. We might be more inclined to think that moral virtue is a benefit when we think about the pleasure it evokes. If we reasoned in this way, of course, we would be confusing the instrumental benefit of moral virtue with the intrinsic benefit of pleasure. The confusion in this case is attributable to our not including pleasure as an intrinsic benefit. In other words, the more items on the list, the greater the possibility of explaining any benefit of moral virtue in instrumental terms. An expansive list, then, is to the argumentative advantage of those who think that moral virtue is not an intrinsic benefit.

To apply the method of difference, let us imagine two versions of Serena's life: each has an identical amount of our big objective list (BOL) of prudential values: athleticism, autonomy, beauty, creativity, desire satisfaction, friendship, health, knowledge, love, pleasure, positive moods and emotions, truth and wealth. In one life (BOLV+) Serena has moral virtue (V+); in the other (BOLV−) she is almost completely lacking moral virtue (V−). Now we ask, prudentially speaking, which life is better for Serena? The (BOLV+) version, I want to suggest, is the better life. Remember, in (BOLV+) Serena is not required to sacrifice other intrinsic benefits. In (BOLV+) she has as much athleticism, autonomy, beauty, creativity, desire satisfaction, friendship, health, knowledge, love, pleasure, positive moods and emotions, truth, and wealth as in (BOLV−), so moral virtue does not require any sacrifice in terms of non-disputed intrinsic benefits.

Intuitively it seems that Serena's life goes better in (BOLV+), and I have difficulty seeing how (BOLV−) could be said to be better, or equivalent. However, it is unlikely that everyone will agree that (BOLV+) is better than (BOLV−). Part of the reason for this is that even when asked about knowledge or pleasure in seemingly paradigmatic cases of intrinsic benefit,[8] a small percentage of people (less than 10 percent)[9] think that knowledge or pleasure adds nothing of intrinsic benefit. With a more contentious item like moral virtue, it is foreseeable that there will be even less agreement about this.[10] Still, I think – at least for those of us for whom the question of the prudential value of virtue is an open question – the argument as it stands is fairly convincing.

It can be bolstered by considering what else might be said of virtue. If one thinks it is not a intrinsic benefit then there are only two other options: either it is intrinsically prudentially harmful or intrinsically neutral. To say it is intrinsically harmful would be to make virtue analogous to paradigmatic harms such as pain. That is, with pain, we tend to think lives that have less of it, other things being equal, go better, and those with more of it worse.

So on this view, the (BOLV−) life is actually better for Serena than the (BOLV+). Sometimes the thought that the (BOLV−) life is better is based on confused reasoning. For instance, sometimes it is suggested that the (BOLV−) life is better, because if one gets the same long list of non-virtue prudential goods in both lives, the (BOLV−) life is better because it does not require the hard effort or sacrifice of the (BOLV+). But of course this is to explain why (BOLV−) is better in terms of less pain – the pain of effort. Since pain is a prudential harm, this violates the requirement that other prudential values are kept equal. In any event, in order to make the case for (BOLV−) being better, the objector will have to assume that an equal amount of effort is required. True, being virtuous typically requires more effort on occasion than being non-virtuous, but we can imagine that Serena has to work harder to obtain other prudential goods in the (BOLV−) version of her life, so that effort balances out. (For example, if Serena is non-virtuous it may be harder for her to obtain friends. Or perhaps she is not as naturally gifted in the (BOLV−) version, so she has to work harder to obtain knowledge.) Once we balance out the non-disputed intrinsic prudential benefits (as required by the method of difference), the view that virtue is a harm does not look the least bit plausible.

Much more common is the idea that moral virtue is neither an intrinsic benefit nor a harm: it is a matter of indifference to prudential wellbeing which life Serena lives. So long as other things are equal, her life goes equally well in the (BOLV+) and the (BOLV−) versions. An uncontroversial example of something that is intrinsically prudentially neutral is whether one has an odd or an even number of hairs on one's head. There is no intrinsic benefit to having either an even or an odd number of hairs.

I have no knock-down argument that virtue is not prudentially neutral but will suggest that those who hold that virtue is prudentially neutral owe us some account about how something that is so causally productive in our lives can be completely intrinsically neutral. By 'causally productive in our lives,' I mean having a great influence on how our lives unfold. It is easy to tell a story about why having an odd or an even number of hairs is not causally productive in our lives. It is not something we know or are aware of: I don't know anyone who knows whether they have an even or an odd number of hairs. It is not likely that it will make a difference to how aerodynamically efficient we are, and so on. The effect on our lives of having an odd or an even number of hairs really makes no appreciable difference. (Having more or less hair may, but one can move from odd to even by adding or subtracting a single hair.) Contrast that with the case of moral virtue, which does seem causally productive in our lives. If we are honest, caring, and just, our lives will likely unfold quite differently than if we are dishonest, uncaring, and unjust. Notice that I am not saying here that they will unfold for the better or for the worse, I am simply saying it will have an appreciable effect on how our lives will unfold. Even the immoralist will agree that being virtuous or vicious makes a difference in our lives. With a slight touch of hyperbole I would suggest that it would be a matter of cosmic coincidence that virtue has not even the slightest intrinsic benefit or harm given how causally productive it is in our lives. It is difficult to think of any other item in our lives that is so causally productive and yet is entirely intrinsically prudentially neutral. Pain, pleasure, happiness, unhappiness, knowledge, ignorance, friendship, isolation, health, illness, etc. are also things that are causally productive in our lives, and yet they are all prudential benefits or harms. It seems a minor miracle that virtue could land exactly in the middle of the scale and be neither a harm nor a benefit. I am not saying this is not possible, but it would help to make this position more plausible if some explanation could be provided.

5.4 The Sympathy Test

A different means of assessing whether moral virtue ought to be included on our objective list has recently been suggested by Brad Hooker.[11] The sympathy test starts with the thought that "how sorry we feel for someone is influenced by how badly from the point of view of his own good we think that person's life has gone, that is, by whether we think his life has lacked important prudential goods."[12] This, combined with the method of difference, is the sympathy test.[13] For example, one application of the sympathy test is this: " . . . if two people's lives contained the same amounts of pleasure, knowledge, and autonomy, but one has contained significantly more achievement than the other, we feel sorrier for the person whose life contained less achievement."[14]

Hooker applies the sympathy test to the question of whether moral virtue is a benefit to the agent:

> Consider two people who lead sad and wretched lives. Suppose that one of these two people is morally virtuous, and that the other is not. Let us use the name 'Upright' for the one who is morally virtuous, and the name 'Unscrupulous' for the one who is not. We would *not* feel *sorrier* for Unscrupulous. This suggests that we do not really believe that moral virtue has the same status on the list as pleasure, knowledge, achievement, and friendship.[15]

This looks like a fairly persuasive case that moral virtue is not an intrinsic benefit. For it does seem that when we apply the sympathy test to other possible items on our objective list, such as pleasure, knowledge, and friendship, we do feel sorrier for those who lack these items in their lives; yet, we do not feel sorrier for Unscrupulous, so it is difficult to see how moral virtue can be an intrinsic benefit to the agent if we do not feel sorrier for those who lack moral virtue.

I propose to argue against Hooker's conclusion on two fronts. First, there are limitations to the sympathy test: specifically, the test seems to track matters other than wellbeing, and our becoming aware of these tends to undermine the idea that sympathy reliably tracks wellbeing. Second, I believe that a better application of the sympathy test will reveal that moral virtue is an intrinsic benefit.

One of the limitations of the sympathy test is that whether we feel sympathy for someone seems to be affected by whether the agent is at fault for the lack of prudential goodness in their lives. So, consider Eddy and Freddy: their lives are equal in terms of prudential benefits such as pleasure, knowledge, autonomy, and friendship. If Eddy does not have friends because he passed up overtures of friendship from others, we may feel less sympathy for him than for Freddy, who had no opportunities for friendship. Even though they have exactly the same amount of prudential benefit in their lives, it is difficult to feel as much sympathy for Eddy. The difference here seems to be that Eddy is at fault for his lack of friends. Hooker considers this a possible objection to why we don't feel sorrier for Unscrupulous if moral virtue really is an intrinsic benefit, namely, that Unscrupulous is responsible for this lack of benefit.[16]

Hooker says there are two good responses to this argument. We will consider the first response in this section, and the second in the next section. Regarding the first reason, Hooker says that someone's failure to obtain some prudential good through their own fault does not in itself preclude us being sympathetic. We might think that someone may be suffering from lung cancer as a result of years of smoking, yet we may feel sympathy for her even though we assign fault for the lung cancer in terms of smoking. This seems a sound point. From this Hooker concludes, " . . . we should demand some explanation of why sympathy is absent in the case of our reactions to Unscrupulous."[17]

But there is something terribly wrong with Hooker's use of this example. When Hooker asked about Upright and Unscrupulous, the question was whom we feel *sorrier* for, not whether we feel any sympathy at all. Recall that both "lead sad and wretched lives," so I think it is quite possible that we might feel sorry for both of them. And yet the conclusion that Hooker draws is that "We would *not* feel *sorrier* for Unscrupulous." In other words, his conclusion is a comparative point about who we will feel *sorrier for*, not whether we will *feel any sympathy at all*. To make his point, Hooker needs to show that fault cannot explain the comparative difference in sympathy. In effect, Hooker has confused the comparative and threshold senses we distinguished in Chapter 3. Both Scrupulous and Unscrupulous may meet the threshold for evoking sympathy without being identical in terms of receiving our sympathy.

We can modify Hooker's example to elicit such a comparative judgment. Suppose Matt and Pat have lives identical in terms of all the prudential values we can think of: pleasure, knowledge, friendship, autonomy, health, etc. Unfortunately, both have just been diagnosed with lung cancer. Matt has lung cancer because he was a heavy smoker; while Pat has lung cancer because, unbeknownst to everyone, there were high levels of carcinogens in his workplace. We can agree with Hooker in feeling sympathy for the smoker, but I take it that most of us feel more sympathy for Pat. If the sympathy test tracks wellbeing, and only wellbeing, then we ought to feel equally sorry for Matt and Pat. Both are facing a terrible disease, and both have the same level of wellbeing up to that point in their lives. The fact that Pat is less responsible for the cancer should not affect the judgment about the levels of wellbeing they actually have.[18] Since their past, present, and future levels of wellbeing are similar, we should feel equal sympathy for the wellbeing that they in fact have. Since responsibility clearly does make a difference to our unreflective judgments of sympathy in this case, it calls into question the idea that the sympathy test tracks wellbeing and only wellbeing.

There is a second confounding variable in our judgment of sympathy, in addition to responsibility, that Hooker does not acknowledge: the agent's effects on the lives of others may affect our sympathy. Consider Fred, Ned, and Ted. Their lives, up to the fatal evening in question, were identical in prudential good: each had the same amount of knowledge, friendship, autonomy, pleasure, and so on. As it happens, they were born on the same day in three different towns and each is out celebrating his twenty-first birthday with a group of friends. Fred's twenty-first birthday evening was great. Although he lost the toss to see who would be the designated driver, he ended up having a very long and pleasant conversation with a friend he hadn't seen since high school. As Fred drove his friends home they were all killed in a head-on collision with a drunk driver. The police report says that the other driver swerved into Fred's lane at the last second and so Fred was entirely blameless. Ned had a less pleasant evening than Fred. Ned found himself trapped in a club that played awful music and so he drank to dull his displeasure. Inebriated, Ned drove into a telephone pole that killed him and his friends instantly. Ted had the least pleasant evening of the three. It was agreed before they got to the bar that Ted would be the designated driver. After a fight with his friends over the relative merits of a local sports team, Ted left them for several hours and returned (unbeknownst to them) inebriated. Not letting on that he was no longer fit to drive, Ted crashed into a telephone pole and died along with his friends, instantly. Thirty seconds after the initial impact the telephone pole crashed onto a school bus that just happened to be turning a corner at that moment. The crash and ensuing fire killed fifty children and fifty puppies on board the bus.

In asking whom we feel greater sympathy for, it is perhaps best to think about their lives up to the instant of their deaths, so as to avoid any controversial assumptions about postmortem effects on wellbeing. Thus, up to the instant of their deaths, whom do we feel most sympathy for, Fred, Ned or Ted? When asked, the most common (untutored) response is that we feel the greatest sympathy for Fred, followed by Ned and then Ted. But, as in the case of Matt and Pat, the sympathy test gets the answer to the question of wellbeing wrong. As Hooker presents it, the sympathy test is supposed to track an individual's level of wellbeing, not whether persons deserve their level of wellbeing. Yet, as the case is described, they have equal amounts of wellbeing up to their fatal nights out; furthermore, Fred has more prudential value that evening than Ned, and Ned more than Ted. So, if the sympathy test tracked prudential value rather than our judgments about whether they deserved that value, then we should feel sorriest for Ted, followed by Ned and finally Fred. After all, Ted had a slightly less good life overall, since their lives were identical up to that evening, and his evening was worse than the other two. Likewise, Ned's night was not as good as Fred's so overall his life was not quite as good as Fred's.* So, if we use our untutored sympathy responses to determine wellbeing, we get the ordering precisely backwards.

---

* Obviously the differences in total wellbeing here are pretty small, but even if we think they are not enough to make a difference in overall wellbeing, we should have equal sympathy for the three.

Notice too that responsibility cannot fully explain the difference in sympathy for Ned and Ted. Both Ned and Ted are responsible for their own loss of future wellbeing, so both equally deserve (or don't deserve) their fate. What distinguishes the two cases? The effects on others: Ted killed fifty children. So, the effects on others seem to be independent of how much responsibility we assign to the agent for his or her own wellbeing. Even though Ted's wellbeing is less than Ned's, we feel less sympathy for someone who caused so much suffering to others.

In sum, the sympathy test does not always track only wellbeing. If we are to use sympathy to assess wellbeing, then we must be aware of the aforementioned confounding influences. If this is so, then we have a good explanation for Hooker's original question of why we don't feel more sympathy for Unscrupulous, namely, that his loss of prudential value is his own fault, and his loss of prudential value in all likelihood negatively affected the prudential value of others. This does not show that virtue is a prudential value, or that it passes the sympathy test, but it does show that Hooker needs to address the reliability of the sympathy test to track wellbeing and only wellbeing.

5.5 Upright, Unscrupulous, and Non-virtuous

The second argument that Hooker considers in response to the idea that an agent's fault may affect our sympathy is as follows. Suppose Unscrupulous was raised in an environment where there was no possibility for him to develop moral virtue. Imagine there were no morally good role models, and so anyone raised in this environment would not develop moral virtue. In this case, it can hardly be said to be Unscrupulous's fault that he turned out as he did. "And if Unscrupulous's turning out to lack moral virtues is not his fault, our not feeling sorry for Unscrupulous cannot be explained by reference to the matter of fault."[19] So, this emendation to our understanding of Unscrupulous is designed to address the possible confounding influence of responsibility.

Incredibly, Hooker does not consider the possibility that our judgment about the sympathy for Unscrupulous might change if we know that it is not his fault that he does not have moral virtue. By this I mean that there is no argument whatsoever in Hooker's paper that the assumption that Unscrupulous is not at fault does not change how sympathetic we are to him. This is a serious omission, because, in my experience, knowing this changes how sympathetic people feel towards Unscrupulous.

One way to see this is to consider three persons who have equivalent amounts of the undisputed prudential values of knowledge, autonomy, pleasure, achievement, and friendship. Both Upright and Unscrupulous are raised in environments where moral education is available. Upright, of course, used his moral education to become morally virtuous, whereas Unscrupulous did not. Non-virtuous is not morally virtuous, but through no fault of her own: she was raised in an environment where there was not the requisite moral education. In other words, what we have done is disambiguated Hooker's original 'Unscrupulous'. We have assigned responsibility to 'Unscrupulous' for not being morally virtuous, and absolved 'Non-virtuous' of all responsibility for not being morally virtuous.

I have surveyed a fair number of people on this thought experiment (mostly students and colleagues). But it might be useful for the reader to take one version of the survey for him- or herself before discussing the results. One version of the survey asks three questions.

1. Do you have greater sympathy for Upright or Unscrupulous (or neither)?
2. Do you have greater sympathy for Upright or Non-virtuous (or neither)?
3. Do you have greater sympathy for Unscrupulous or Non-virtuous (or neither)?

Although there is some variation in answers to each of these questions, the most consistent response is to questions 1 and 3: most feel more sympathy for Upright than for Unscrupulous, and to the third question most feel more sympathy for Non-virtuous than for Unscrupulous. In my experience, with respect to question 2, people have greater sympathy for Upright than for Non-virtuous, but the response here is not quite as consistent as the response to questions 1 and 3.

These responses seem to support Hooker's assessment that the sympathy test does not support the idea that virtue is an intrinsic benefit. However, there are two arguments against this conclusion. First, the explanations of how people make the sympathy rankings invariably involves considerations that are extraneous to judgments of wellbeing.

The following is an explanation by one participant in the survey:

My gut reaction says that Upright in #1 should get my sympathy because he has the hardship of trying to do what's best.... Upright in #2 also gets my sympathy, because he is constrained by rules that Non-virtuous doesn't have, and that makes me feel bad for him. In #3 I feel more sympathy for Non-virtuous because she never got to learn that there are other ways to live. (Non-Virtuous didn't win out in #2 because the hardship of being selfless for the sake of morality seemed to win out over the hardship of lack of education.) I don't seem to like Unscrupulous very much, and I seem to feel very bad for virtuous people![20]

Notice how the justification for the sympathy rankings is not made exclusively in terms of actual wellbeing, but considerations of desert are also present. The underlying thought running throughout is that being virtuous requires some sacrifice in prudential goods and so when the virtuous have only as much prudential good as the vicious we feel sorrier for the virtuous because we feel they deserve to do better than the vicious. But this means that such judgments about sympathy are useless for the purposes of assessing whether virtue is an intrinsic benefit. Recall that the thought behind the sympathy test was that we could use it to track prudential value by assessing sympathy. But the test will work only if sympathy tracks actual wellbeing exclusively, that is, is not influenced by considerations of how much wellbeing we think the individual deserves. But in this response we see that sympathy is so influenced. It is worth pointing out that I chose the above response because it articulates well what seems to me to be the most common response to the sympathy test.

The second point invokes considerations of logical consistency to suggest people include in their ranking factors other than wellbeing. To see our way to this point, consider first what sort of judgment consistency demands. As we noted above, with respect to virtue there are three, and only three, options for the prudential value of virtue: it is prudentially neutral, an intrinsic harm, or it is an intrinsic benefit. If virtue is intrinsically prudentially neutral, then we should feel equal sympathy for all three: their lives are otherwise equal in prudential value and virtue neither adds nor subtracts anything. If virtue is an intrinsic benefit, then we ought to have equal sympathy for both Unscrupulous and Non-virtuous, since they both lack this benefit, and we ought to have less sympathy for Upright, who enjoys the benefit. If virtue is an intrinsic harm, then we should have more sympathy for Upright and equally less for Unscrupulous and Non-virtuous. However, almost no one gives one of these assessments without considerable tutoring. If people are attempting to assess actual wellbeing, they are being incredibly inconsistent. True, people make logical errors all the time, but I, for one, am reluctant to attribute this much inconsistency to people. The point is perhaps easiest to appreciate with respect to the comparison between Unscrupulous and Non-virtuous. No matter whether virtue is a benefit, a harm or neutral, we should have equal sympathy for them. As noted, almost no one arrives at this conclusion.

If the sympathy test works at all, I think it does support the view that virtue is an intrinsic benefit. To see this we need to focus on sympathy judgments based just on their actual wellbeing and not on their deserved wellbeing. Thus focused, we know that we should feel equal sympathy for them if we put aside the question of virtue. So, the question of sympathy resolves to whether we should feel some sympathy for Unscrupulous and Non-virtuous because they lack something in their lives, namely virtue. I believe the answer here is yes. If they could be virtuous "for free," with no cost to any other prudential value, then indeed they would be better off. So, we should feel sympathy that they did not get virtue for free. Turning the question around, do we feel sympathy for Upright and Non-virtuous because they lack viciousness in their lives? I think the answer here is no. Nothing would be added to their lives even if they could get viciousness "for free." Indeed, we should think they are worse off.

Although this is a better application of the sympathy test, I have my doubts about how independent it is of the method of difference argument. The way the argument is made in the previous paragraph, we seem to have the explanatory order reversed from what Hooker imagines. Hooker says we can read off prudential value from our assessments of sympathy. One may wonder whether in the previous paragraph we are basing our judgment of sympathy on how we should judge. If so, this gets things precisely backwards: the sympathy test is supposed to base judgments of prudential value on sympathy. I think this is a significant worry, so I think the conclusion we can draw is conditional only: If the sympathy test works for assessing prudential value, then virtue is an intrinsic benefit.

5.6   The Immoralist Challenge

It will help to situate the view advocated here, that virtue is an intrinsic benefit, by reference again to the immoralist's challenge. Recall the challenge put to Socrates that Gyges is better off being just a shepherd than being an unjust king. Our argument is not sufficient to answer this challenge. At best it would show that, other things being equal, Gyges is better off being morally virtuous. Of course the entire challenge of Gyges' ring is based on things not being equal: the point is that the life of a king looks much more attractive, prudentially speaking. But having admitted this, our argument is not entirely powerless against a weaker challenge by the immoralist. To illustrate, consider the following remarks by Daniel Haybron:

> The successful Southern slaveholder who enjoys the approbation of his community and a comfortable existence with a loving family has obvious moral shortcomings, yet it is hard to see in what sense his life must be "impoverished." Why must he be in *any* way worse off than he would be were he more enlightened about human equality? Why must he be worse off than a morally better counterpart who enjoys as much wealth, comfort, success, love, and reputation, but without ever wronging anyone?[21]

The last sentence reads like a rhetorical question, that is, as an assertion that the counterpart is not any better off. But if this is the case the entire issue has been begged. It is not enough to simply assert that the two lives are equally good: some reason must be provided. Perhaps a more generous interpretation suggests that Haybron takes this to be an open question. But consider how Haybron follows up:

> This point arises with greater force in the case of a brutal warlord like Genghis Khan, who directed the slaughter of tens of millions. He appears to have done so largely with the blessing of his culture's moral code. It is not hard to imagine that his relatively long life, which appeared to be rather successful on his terms, went very well for him indeed. And while his idea of happiness or well-being is not exactly yours or mine, it is difficult to see the grounds for gainsaying it (as a conception of well-being!). Is humanitarian concern for strangers really necessary for a full, rich, or characteristically human life? History offers little reason for optimism on this count.[22]

But notice that the Genghis Khan example does not support the previous claim that the Southern slaveholder would not be better off living a more virtuous life. For the question in the Genghis Khan example is whether one can have a full and rich life without moral virtue. Suppose we answer in the affirmative to this. This in no way implies that, other things being equal, a life is better if it is one of virtue rather than one of vice.

The point can be reinforced by reference to the distinction between ideal and satisfactory wellbeing expounded in Chapter 4. Satisfactory wellbeing means that a certain amount of wellbeing has been obtained in a life. Ideal wellbeing asks us how a life would go best. It is not entirely clear whether Haybron means 'satisfactory wellbeing' or 'ideal wellbeing,' so we will examine both possibilities before settling with the former.

If Haybron means satisfactory wellbeing, then it is clear that the argument is missing a crucial step. What is required is a premise that says that if a satisfactory life can be had without X, then X is not an intrinsic value. In other words, what is required is some argument that everything that is an intrinsic benefit must be part of our conception of a satisfactory life. No argument is offered for this premise, and indeed it looks independently implausible. Consider a scientist who is an extreme loner: she spends almost every waking moment in her lab and has no friends. She seems and claims to be very happy, and so excels at her work that she wins the Nobel Prize in physics. When asked about winning the prize she says that yes, that made her happy, but it does not compare to the joys of investigating nature's secrets that she gets every day when she is in her lab. Her life seems perfectly satisfactory, even though it does not include friendship. But this does not show that her life would not have been better if she could have achieved as much happiness and scientific success while squeezing in some time for friendship. Notice too that it is not enough to show that some intrinsic benefits are necessary for satisfactory wellbeing. Perhaps no life counts as satisfactory without at least some happiness, for instance. For this still leaves open the possibility that some items are intrinsic benefits, but are not necessary for satisfactory wellbeing.

As we noted in the previous chapter, ideal wellbeing seems the more appropriate notion for attempting to ascertain whether something is an intrinsic benefit. But if Haybron has in mind ideal wellbeing, then it is clear from his discussion that he is not asking the relevant question as to whether virtue is an intrinsic benefit. What needs to be asked is this: if the Southern plantation owner and Genghis Khan could have achieved the same level of non-virtuous prudential goods while leading a virtuous life, then would they have been better off? Of course, the social realities in which the two lived may have made obtaining the non-virtuous prudential goods as well as living virtuously impossible. For example, it may well be that Khan's reputation for viciousness helped him achieve much of his military success. But it is at least logically possible that he might have achieved as much while being virtuous. The fact that he does not explore this line of reasoning suggests that Haybron has in mind satisfactory wellbeing.

The modest position here is consistent with Haybron's claim that one can have a perfectly satisfactory "full, rich, or characteristically human life" without virtue. It is also consistent with a capitulation to the immoralists' position with respect to the challenge of Gyges' ring: Gyges may have reasoned correctly in acting viciously to obtain more prudential benefit. However, the modest position does not capitulate to the immoralist who says that virtue is merely instrumentally valuable. If Gyges, the plantation owner, and Genghis Khan could have achieved the same non-virtuous prudential benefits while being virtuous, then their lives would have more prudential value.

We noted above that it is questionable whether morality and virtue are entirely absent in *Brave New World*, as John alleges. Without deciding the issue, our response can be put conditionally: if virtue is absent in *Brave New World*, then John is correct that this is one of the costs of *Brave New World*. Our modest position does not help us decide whether this cost is worth it: Does the increase in happiness outweigh the loss in virtue? But John is at least right in that the loss of virtue is, other things being equal, a loss in prudential value. As we shall see below, this point is enough for the argument we shall make: happy-people-pills do not always require us to choose between intrinsic benefits. Often, we can have it all.

Notes

1. Huxley, *Brave New World and Brave New World Revisited*, 214.
2. Plato, *The Republic*, 359a–360d.
3. Annas, *The Morality of Happiness*, "Should Virtue Make You Happy?"
4. Taylor and Wolfram, "The Self-Regarding and Other-Regarding Virtues."
5. It is not clear that even a good Marxian must disagree here. If I earn a whopping four dollars an hour for my industriousness at the factory, the capitalist may earn only an average profit of one dollar an hour on my labor. Where capitalists do well is in the fact that they can make a similar profit on any number of workers. The Marxian need not deny the relative split in the benefit of my industriousness, but will take issue with the capitalist receiving any benefit from my industriousness.
6. I am of course speaking here of "individual justice." See Slote, "Justice as a Virtue."
7. It may be objected that if putative moral virtuousness turns out to be a benefit to the putatively morally virtuous then they are not truly morally virtuous, because they are not properly altruistic. This is not the place to answer this question, but may mark some difference between Ancient and Modern conceptions of ethics. It is worth noting that it is a caricature of Kant to think that he believes we cannot receive benefit from moral acts (Wood, *Kant's Ethical Thought*).
8. Hurka, *Virtue, Vice, and Value*.

9.   This is based on my unscientific polling. I welcome investigation of this phenomenon by so-called 'experimental philosophers.'

10. A second reason is that the method of difference argument seems open to this objection: in thinking about the two possible lives of Serena, we may not be clearly distinguishing between a benefit for Serena and a benefit for others. The thought then is that if there is no cost to Serena in terms of intrinsic benefits then (BOLV+) is better, because others will benefit, but not because Serena's life is better. The question then is whether we are muddling the benefit to others and the benefit to Serena. This seems a utilitarian/consequentialist way of putting the point. The Kantian way of putting it is: a good will has a kind of value (dignity) that is independent of its prudential value to self *or* others. So the difference between ethical and prudential value (for the Kantian) does not correspond to the distinction between what's good for others and what's good for oneself. Certainly we cannot conclude from the fact that opting for (BOLV+) does not require any sacrifice from Serena, prudentially speaking, that moral virtue is in fact a benefit to Serena. For obviously, even when something does not cost us in terms of prudential value, it does not follow that the item in question is prudentially valuable. After all, it could be prudentially neutral (see below).

11. Hooker, "Does Moral Virtue Constitute a Benefit to the Agent?" credits Amartya Sen for antecedents of this test.

12. Hooker, "Does Moral Virtue Constitute a Benefit to the Agent?," 149.

13. I will not explore this difference here, but roughly the sympathy test seems to engage our emotional responses more than the method of difference test.

14. Hooker, "Does Moral Virtue Constitute a Benefit to the Agent?," 148.

15. Ibid., 149–50.

16. Ibid., 153.

17. Ibid.

18. Here and below I take it that agents do not necessarily benefit by having the level of wellbeing they deserve. A serial killer like Charles Manson deserves the low level of wellbeing that he has in jail, but I don't think he benefits from it. (Even Kant would say that Manson's dignity is supported by punishment, but Manson's wellbeing is not promoted.)

19. Hooker, "Does Moral Virtue Constitute a Benefit to the Agent?," 153.

20. Sarah Cashmore, July, 2009, personal communication.

21. Haybron, *The Pursuit of Unhappiness*, 159.

22. Ibid.

References

Annas, J. *The Morality of Happiness*. New York: Oxford University Press, 1993.

Annas, J. "Should Virtue Make You Happy?" *Apeiron* 35, no. 4 (2002): 1–19.

Haybron, D. *The Pursuit of Unhappiness*. New York: Oxford University Press, 2008.

Hooker, B. "Does Moral Virtue Constitute a Benefit to the Agent?" In *How Should One Live?*, edited by Roger Crisp, 141–57. Oxford: Oxford University Press, 1996.

Hurka, Thomas. *Virtue, Vice, and Value*. New York: Oxford University Press, 2001.

Huxley, A. *Brave New World and Brave New World Revisited*. Toronto: Vintage Books, 2007.

Plato. *The Republic*. Indianapolis, Ind.: Hackett, 2004.

Slote, M. "Justice as a Virtue." In *The Stanford Encyclopedia of Philosophy* (Fall 2010 edn.), edited by Edward N. Zalta. http://plato.stanford.edu/archives/fall2010/entries/justice-virtue/.

Taylor, G. and S. Wolfram. "The Self-Regarding and Other-Regarding Virtues." *Philosophical Quarterly* 18, no. 72 (1968): 238–48.

Wood, A. W. *Kant's Ethical Thought*. New York: Cambridge University Press, 1999.

6

Happiness Promotes Perfection

The main purpose of this chapter is to examine some of the social science data concerning the relationship between happiness and achievement. However, in this introduction I will briefly review the conclusions of Chapters 3, 4, and 5 for those who have chosen to proceed directly here. Those who have read these chapters may want to skip ahead to the next section.

The primary purpose of Chapter 3 is to offer an analysis of happiness. It was argued that happiness has a cognitive and an affective component. The cognitive component involves being pleased or delighted by things. Prototypical instances of this aspect of happiness are the following: "I am pleased by the rain," "I am delighted by the course of my life." So the things that one might be pleased about include relatively small matters, for example rain, and larger matters, the course of one's life. Anything of the form "I am pleased by _____," where the blank is filled in by a phrase that describes such large or small matters, counts towards the happiness of the subject. The affect component includes both positive moods and sensations of pleasure. So, moods or emotions such as joy, excitement, and contentment count towards a subject's happiness, as do experiences of pleasure such as an ice-cream cone on a hot summer's day. The chapter does not say how much of either component is necessary to be happy. The argument is simply that, other things being equal, the more a person has the cognitive component or the affective component, the happier they are. It was noted that inhabitants of the *Brave New World* seem happier than

Happy-People-Pills For All, First Edition. Mark Walker.
© 2013 John Wiley & Sons, Inc. Published 2013 by John Wiley & Sons, Inc.

the inhabitants of our world, for they more often are in positive moods, experience sensory pleasure, and are pleased with things more than we are.

Chapter 4 investigates the question of the prudentially good life or wellbeing. A 'prudentially good life' means a good life for the one whose life it is; it does not mean a 'morally good life.' A pirate may have a morally depraved life, but a prudentially good life. The chapter considers the obvious thought that to have a prudentially good life one needs only happiness. This view, happinessism, is refuted. It is argued that there are a large number of items that make up an ideal prudentially good life: athleticism, autonomy, beauty, creativity, desire satisfaction, friendship, health, knowledge, love, pleasure, truth, and wealth. The argument is *not* that happiness is not part of a prudentially good life, only that there are other components to a good life. This opens up a potential criticism of *Brave New World*: they may be happier than we are, but they may not be better off. The reason of course is that they lack so many items of prudential value: love, knowledge, beauty, autonomy, and so on. The chapter does not in fact argue that the inhabitants of *Brave New World* are worse off. Rather, the more modest claim is made: it does not follow that those in Huxley's world are better off simply because they are happier. A corollary is this: we can imagine a world better than our own, one where we are happier and obtain more of the non-happiness components of the good life, in other words, a world that combines the greater happiness of *Brave New World* with more of the "higher" aspects of humanity we enjoy in this world.

Chapter 5 argues that moral virtues, for example the virtues of beneficence and justice, are prudentially valuable. Again, the claim is rather modest. I do not claim that a pirate could not have a great life simply because he lacks virtue. Rather, the claim is that, other things being equal, a life goes better if it is a virtuous life.

6.1 Huxley's Dilemma

This is a good time to take stock of where we are going, especially since the overall direction of the argument to this point may seem a bit counterintuitive. After all, if the goal is to support the use of happy-people-pills, the account of wellbeing we have developed does not look particularly well suited to this argument. Thus, it might be thought that the most natural argument to make would be for happinessism – again, the view that happiness is all there is to wellbeing – for this position seems a natural ally for happy-people-pills. There are two reasons for not attempting to argue for happinessism (besides the obvious reason of intellectual honesty).

First, such an argument would have things precisely backwards. The goal is not to find a theory of wellbeing that fits happy-people-pills, but to see whether happy-people-pills fits a plausible theory of wellbeing. In other words, we want to know what it is for our lives to go well and then see if happy-people-pills will serve this goal. Secondly, there is a certain dialectical advantage in arguing from a broader conception of wellbeing of the sort outlined here. Many critics of happy-people-pills have criticized bioprogressives for having a narrow understanding of wellbeing. As we shall see below, this is a root complaint by critics of happy-people-pills like Kass, Fukuyama, and Elliott. I won't comment on whether their criticism hits the mark with respect to other happy-people-pills progressivists, but it definitely does not apply to the present argument. That is, the argument here shares with many critics a broad conception of wellbeing, and so on this fundamental issue we are agreed.

As we noted in Chapter 2, Huxley's dilemma is the tragic choice between the happiness that might be achieved in a society organized like *Brave New World*, and a society like our own where we have reduced happiness, but a greater portion of the "higher" aspects of human life: knowledge, autonomy, virtue, etc., aspects of life that we may lump under the terms 'perfection' or 'achievement.' Indeed, as we have said, if we were to compare the two worlds on the single value of happiness, then *Brave New World* wins hands down. But if we compare the two worlds in terms of perfectionist goods, such as friendship, marriage, work success, and virtue, *Brave New World* is seriously lacking. For instance, relations between individuals in *Brave New World* are, by and large, shallow and transitory, since *Brave New World* is socially engineered to exclude marriage and deep lasting friendships. The workplace is carefully managed to keep people occupied rather than to foster any achievement, and the population for the most part seems relatively oblivious to the suffering of individuals. This leads to the classic dilemma Huxley forces on his readers: either we choose our world where there is the possibility of serious achievement but considerable unhappiness; or, we use technology to make ourselves happy with *soma* (or *soma* analogues), but forgo serious pursuit of achievement, that is, excellence in intellectual, cultural, interpersonal, and social goals.

For the bioprogressivists, there are three, and only three, ways to deal with this dilemma. First, bioprogressivists could deny that achievement has any intrinsic value. For example, this strategy is available to the bioprogressivist who endorsed happinessism. The argument then would be that happy-people-pills do a better job of promoting happiness than achievement does, so achievement may be done away with. We rejected this line of argument in the last two chapters, based as it is on a narrow theory of wellbeing, so this strategy is foreclosed to us.

The second means to tackle the dilemma is to acknowledge the intrinsic value of achievement, but claim that happy-people-pills offer more overall value, even if it means renouncing some achievement. This, in effect, is the argument of the Controller in *Brave New World*. The cost associated with the increased happiness of *Brave New World* is decreased achievement. But the increase in happiness gained in *Brave New World*, according to the Controller, is more than worth it in terms of loss of achievement. Nothing we have said directly contradicts the Controller's argument. We have argued for the intrinsic value of perfectionist goods, but we have not said anything about the relative weightings of any of the elements of the good life that we have identified. On the one hand, our big objective list is compatible with someone saying that achievement is much more valuable than happiness, even though both are valuable; on the other hand, nothing in our argument contradicts the Controller's position that happiness is much more valuable than achievement. Of course, if the bioprogressivist were to side with the Controller, then we would need to come up with an argument stating that happiness is more important than achievement. I do not know of any convincing argument to this end, but fortunately, it is not one that we need to consider. We will take the third option.

The third option is to reject the dilemma itself. What if, in addition to the two alternatives offered by Huxley, there is the possibility of a world with both greater happiness and greater achievement than our own world? Consider again *Mark's Braver New World*, where people are significantly *happier and achieve more* than in our world. Added to the mix it would leave us with a trilemma: our world, the *Brave New World* or *Mark's Braver New World*. The last is (other things being equal) the obvious choice. In fact, the proposed sequel to Huxley's novel would be terribly boring because, unlike *Brave New World*, the third possibility here does not ask how much we would be willing to sacrifice for happiness. Rather, it offers us even more of both sides of Huxley's dilemma: more happiness and more achievement. Our argument will be that using happy-people-pills will promote happiness and achievement.

I think most people are not likely to take the third possibility seriously because of the common assumption about the arrow of causality between happiness and achievement. Specifically, it is a common assumption both in "folk psychology" and among professional researchers on happiness that achievement causes happiness.[1] The thought here is that, for example, winning an award at work, getting married or developing friendships often causes us to be happier. Conversely, being unhappy or dissatisfied with our lives is the spur to action: if we were happy, then we would have no reason to achieve at work, get married or develop friendships. It is certainly true that recent success can cause us to be happier: it may boost our moods and most will take attitudinal enjoyment in the success. So, winning an award at work, getting married or meeting new friends can cause at least a temporary spike in our happiness. But this tells us only about one direction of causality. The fact that X causes Y does not preclude Y causing X. Thus, being healthy makes it easier to exercise, and exercising often leads to better health. So, our question is this: does happiness cause achievement or does unhappiness cause achievement? We will look at both "common sense" arguments and social science research for the answer to this question. Our argument will be that in both instances a good case can be made that happiness causes achievement. If this defense can be made, then we have good reason to reject Huxley's dilemma. If we develop an appropriate technological means to increase average happiness, then we should also thereby boost average achievement. In a slogan: to achieve more, first get happier. So, given this arrow of causality, there is no reason to suppose that happy-people-pills would force us to choose between happiness and achievement. Huxley offers us a false dichotomy: making people happier will make them achieve more, not less.

6.2   Happiness Causes Achievement: the Common-Sense Case

In this section I want to explore further the idea that there are causal links between happiness and achievement, focusing on what common sense has to say about these matters.

Consider four hypotheses:

1. Happiness causes less achievement.
2. Happiness causes more achievement.
3. Unhappiness causes less achievement.
4. Unhappiness causes more achievement.

The common-sense case against the thesis that happiness causes achieve-ment endorses 1 and 4 and rejects 2 and 3. The reasoning goes something like this: suppose you are happy. If you are happy, then you are pleased with how things are going. If you are pleased with how things are going, then there is little need to change anything, so there is little need to achieve anything. Thus, we should believe that 1 is true and 2 is false. Conversely, if you are unhappy it means you are not pleased with the way things are, so you will seek to rectify this through some achievement. So, 3 is false and 4 is true. In short, the untutored common-sense view sees unhappiness as the spur in our sides which causes us to achieve: without the spur of unhappiness prodding us in the side there will be less achievement. We can see how the 'spur of unhappiness' argument nicely dovetails with the Huxley dilemma: if we have more happiness, we will have less achievement; and if we want more achievement, then we will have to have less happiness.

The above line of reasoning is often the first thing that comes to people's minds, but careful consideration, "reflective common sense," shows that the case is not as open and shut as it may first appear. Consider, for instance, if it is true that unhappiness causes achievement, then one might suppose that the clinically depressed would be the greatest achievers. But this is hardly the case. One of the symptoms of depression for some people is that they withdraw from many of their regular activities, and so achieve less, not more. The severely or even moderately depressed are not likely out saving whales, making new friends, getting married or finding a cure for cancer; they are more likely to be huddled in their rooms with the blinds drawn. The depressed, then, are doubly unfortunate: they are unhappy and lacking in achievement.

Perhaps it may be remonstrated that the intuitive model is supposed to apply only to those in the "healthy" range of happiness. Again common sense suggests that this might not be the case. Imagine Clayton who is just barely in the healthy range of happiness. If Clayton were just a bit unhappier, he would be diagnosed with a mild form of depression, but he does not quite fit the category. Should we predict that Clayton achieves more than his peers who are much happier, but who are otherwise similarly situated? I think common sense tells us that a figure as dour as Clayton is not as likely to achieve as much as others. He may not be in his room with the curtains drawn, but his negative mood propensity seems more likely to interfere with than to promote achievement. It seems implausible to suppose that being unhappy in this way is going to cause people to save whales, make new friends, get married or find a cure for cancer more than their more upbeat peers. This example does not show that happiness causes achievement, but it should shake a little of the confidence that the connection between unhappiness and achievement is straightforward.

Here is an example that invites reflection on your own psychology.

History 1: *It is March 21st, the light streams through the window, waking you at 6:42 on the first morning of spring. You are in a bad mood. You turn over to rest, perchance to go back to sleep, but the chirping of the damn birds makes this impossible. You drag yourself downstairs and make some coffee. Thinking that this has been a terrible start to your weekend, you mull over your options, which you quickly reduce to two. You could spend the morning reading the newspaper and watch the ballgame that starts at 11:00 am. The game ends at about 3 pm, and then you can work out what to do from there. The other choice is to take advantage of the fact that this is the first day of the year that the Canadian weather will permit you to start on the large landscaping project you have been secretly planning all winter. The idea is to install a large koi pond along with some significant landscaping renovations. The thought of getting out there in the backyard messing around in the muck, having to go shopping and deal with sales clerks simply to procure a few supplies to even get started seems like a big drag.*

History 2: *It is March 21st, the light streams through the window, waking you at 6:42 on the first morning of spring. You are in a great mood. You turn over to rest, to take in the beautiful sound of the birds chirping in celebration of the day. With a spring in your step, you bound downstairs and make some coffee. Thinking that this has been a great start to your weekend, you mull over your options, which you quickly reduce to two. You could spend the morning reading the newspaper, and watch the ballgame that starts at 11:00 am. The game ends at about 3 pm, and then you can work out what to do from there. The other choice is to take advantage of the fact that this is the first day of the year that the Canadian weather will permit you to start on the large landscaping project you have been secretly planning all winter. The idea is to install a large koi pond along with some significant landscaping renovations. The thought of getting out there in the backyard messing around in the muck brings back memories of fun times playing in the mud as a child, and the chance to go shopping and get your hands on some supplies will make the project seem that much more real.*

Question: in which of these two alternate histories do you think you are more likely to actually start the project? I think the answer for most of us is the second case. This is meant simply as an average. Perhaps some days waking up in a particularly good mood you might indulge yourself and lounge around and watch the game. Why not? You deserve it. Other times you might suck it up and go out and face the world despite your foul mood. Still, I suspect that most of us will be more inclined to start something like this when we find ourselves in the mood described in the second scenario.

Notice too that there is a sense in which you are equally unhappy about something in both cases. You are unhappy *about* the landscaping in your backyard; you are attitudinally displeased about the state of your backyard. In our two histories we must imagine that you hold the same cognitive attitude to the state of your landscaping: it is a source of attitudinal displeasure. Of course, if you took enormous attitudinal pleasure in the present landscaping, then it is hard to imagine why you would undertake such a landscaping project. (Let us put aside trivial counterexamples where you are happy with the landscaping but your spouse is not, so you want to start on such a project.) It seems then that the best spur to action is where our moods are positive and where we have attitudinal displeasure about some state of affairs. Indeed, I suspect some of the reason for thinking that unhappiness is the spur to action turns on confusing these two senses of happiness. Being happy in terms of positive mood may actually spur us to action and so to do something that we are attitudinally displeased about.

To summarize, reflective common-sense psychology supports the proposition that those who experience positive moods may be more likely to get out and achieve; and those who are less positive may be less likely to do so. None of this is to deny that achieving may also promote positive moods. A good start on the koi pond may turn a foul mood positive, or help sustain a good mood. So, reflective common sense supports a bidirectional model of causation: good moods often cause achievement and achievement often causes good moods.

6.3 Happiness Causes Achievement: Social Science Research

We have just argued that reflective folk psychology provides some support for the idea that the causal relationship between happiness and achievement is bidirectional. Social scientists, until relatively recently, by and large held the same view as unreflective common sense: achievement causes happiness. That some causal relationship between happiness and achievement is likely is suggested by the long-established correlation between happiness and achievement noted by social science researchers. Thus, as Sonja Lyubomirsky, Laura King, and Ed Diener point out, researchers have found considerable evidence that happiness correlates with marriage, income, better mental health, and longer life.[2] Lyubomirsky, King, and Diener comment on these correlations:

> Such associations between desirable life outcomes and happiness have led most investigators to assume that success makes people happy. This assumption can be found throughout the literature in this area. For example, Diener, Suh, Lucas, and Smith (1999) reviewed the correlations between happiness and a variety of resources, desirable characteristics, and favorable life circumstances. Although the authors recognized that the causality can be bidirectional, they frequently used wording implying that cause flows from the resource to happiness. For example, they suggested that marriage might have "greater benefits for men than for women" (p. 290), apparently overlooking the possibility that sex differences in marital patterns could be due to differential selection into marriage based on well-being. Similarly, after reviewing links between money and well-being, Diener and his colleagues pointed out that "even when extremely wealthy individuals are examined, the *effects* [italics added] of income are small" (p. 287), again assuming a causal direction from income to happiness. We use quotes from one of us to avoid pointing fingers at others, but such examples could be garnered from the majority of scientific publications in this area. The quotes underscore the pervasiveness of the assumption among well-being investigators that successful outcomes foster happiness.[3]

However, the massive meta-study by these authors makes a powerful case that happiness can cause achievement. The authors do not challenge the assumption that achievement causes happiness, rather, they suggest in line with our previous argument that the arrow of causation is bidirectional: it is not simply that achievement causes happiness, but happiness may also cause achievement. We will review and comment on their findings in this section. In general, we can say that our confidence in the study turns on its comprehensiveness: the authors looked at 225 papers by hundreds of different researchers.[4] A proper meta-study, of course, does not simply review the literature that reports evidence that is favorable to the hypothesis of the meta-study, but looks for independent measures in its literature search. Thus, they looked for as many studies as could be found that relate happiness to achievement. Their search resulted in 225 papers with 293 samples comprising over 275,000 participants.[5] In short, they had a huge amount of data with which to test their hypothesis.

6.4   Measuring Happiness

The authors understand "happiness" in terms of the experience of frequent positive moods and emotions. That is, individuals who are happy are "those who experience frequent positive emotions, such as joy, interest, and pride, and infrequent (though not absent) negative emotions, such as sadness, anxiety, and anger."[6] A few words about this definition are perhaps in order. First, they understand 'positive affect' to refer to both positive moods and emotions, in part because the distinction between moods and emotions is rarely made in the happiness literature of the study.[7] There is considerable debate as to how to distinguish moods and emotions outside of happiness research. For example, it is sometimes suggested that emotions are typically shorter- and moods longer-lasting, that emotions have an intentional object: some stimulus or event, while moods typically lack an intentional object, and that emotions are more foregrounded in consciousness whereas moods are more in the background. The authors seem correct that since there is little distinction in the literature, there is little point in defining happiness exclusively in terms of emotions and moods, even supposing that such a distinction can be clearly made.

Second, there is the obvious question: why this definition of happiness? Their answer is elegant and straightforward: because this definition of happiness is correlated with the areas of achievement that they wish to investigate:

> Although many definitions of happiness have been used in the literature, ranging from life satisfaction and an appreciation of life to momentary feelings of pleasure, we define happiness here as a shorthand way of referring to the frequent experience of positive emotions. In our theoretical framework, it is the experience of positive emotions that leads to the behavioral outcomes we review, and "happiness" describes people who experience such emotions a large percentage of the time (Diener, Sandvik, & Pavot, 1991).[8]

So, the authors use part of the affective sense of happiness we delineated in Chapter 3. One of the typical problems in a meta-study is to get a heterogeneous set of measurements to "speak a common language." For example, suppose one is doing a meta-study on whether rising unemployment leads to increased crime. One of the problems researchers will typically face is that there are different ways of defining 'unemployment' and 'crime.' One study might use figures from unemployment insurance schemes and another might use telephone surveys. Both have obvious limitations. The former, for instance, does not track those who are unemployed but are no longer eligible for unemployment benefits, and the latter may be skewed if more of the unemployed do not have phones. Meta-surveys invariably have to contend with the fact that the constructs they investigate are not always defined and measured in the same way. This is an inherent limitation of any meta-study. The research by Lyubomirsky, King, and Diener is no exception. For example, some of the studies included in the meta-study defined happiness in terms of life satisfaction, and so being happy in this sense would be evidenced by scoring high on a life satisfaction survey. As we noted in Chapter 3, these are quite different conceptions of happiness, so it is a good question as to why Lyubomirsky, King, and Diener included life-satisfaction studies as part of their data. In part the justification for including such studies is the fact that

> they frequently represent the only available evidence in an area. Furthermore, life satisfaction and positive affect have been found to correlate at around .40 to .50 in undergraduates (Lucas, Diener, & Suh, 1996) and .52 in business students (Staw & Barsade, 1993). In addition, of people who say they are above neutral in satisfaction with their lives, 85% have been found to report that they feel happy at least half of the time (Lucas et al., 1996). Thus, life satisfaction is a defensible proxy for chronic happiness, in cases in which no studies exist using more direct measures of happiness . . . [9]

So, the authors are aware of the limitations and add that " . . . we eagerly await the day when a full set of findings based on measures of positive affect, as well as related concepts, is available."[10]

We noted in Chapter 3 that many measurements of happiness, either life satisfaction or positive affect, rely on subjective reports. The General Social Science Survey (GSS) question is: "Taken all together, how would you say things are these days? Would you say that you are very happy, pretty happy, or not too happy?" A similar question is asked in the World Value Survey: "All things considered, how satisfied are you with your life as a whole these days?" The World Value Survey offers interesting cross-cultural data on happiness as it tracks respondents in over 180 countries.[11] These and similar questions ask respondents to make global retrospective judgments. This raises at least two worries: whether there are potential biases in making a global judgment, and whether subjects can accurately access and assess the appropriate information. For instance, a potential bias exists in responding according to cultural norms: one may feel they ought to be happy because they have it all: a nice car, 1.9 children, and a beautiful house in the suburbs, even if they are not. As for memory, the data on lapses in human memory are well established. Of particular relevance here is the phenomenon for most people to remember things as more positive than they were actually experienced at the time.

There is an extensive literature on the reliability of subjective reports on happiness. Some of it is quite shocking. Consider the following experiment. Schwarz had subjects photocopy a piece of paper before filling out a life satisfaction survey. Half the subjects "found" a dime on the photocopier – of course the dime was placed there as part of the experiment. Reported life satisfaction was substantially higher in those who found the dime.[12] Asking respondents to complete a life satisfaction survey on a sunny day can also raise scores.[13] The obvious disturbing aspect of such studies is that it is hard to believe that one's life as a whole goes that much better because of finding a dime or because it happens to be sunny.

I will make two points in response to skepticism about subjective reports being inherently unreliable. The first point is that social scientists have long sought to collect alternate data to assess the reliability and validity of global retrospective subjective reports. One method is what is sometimes described as "beeper studies." One investigation had 228 subjects report their happiness every 20 minutes with the prompting of their beeper. Beeper studies are designed to mitigate potential memory biases in subjective reports. Happiness researchers also look to independent measures of happiness to assess the reliability of subjective evaluations, including reports from informants (friends, family, and colleagues), interviews by trained clinicians, observations of non-verbal behavior and physiological assessments, and so on. All such independent assessments support the judgment that self-reports of happiness are reasonably reliable.[14]

The second point is that data is only ever good or bad relative to some purpose. A simple example may illustrate the point. Suppose you are looking to see if height is correlated with income and your measuring tape is off by two inches. Unbeknownst to you, everyone you measure is actually two inches shorter. Suppose too that everyone exaggerates their income by 5,000 dollars. Although your records will have false data for each individual – everyone makes less and is shorter than your records indicate – your investigation is not undermined: if there is a correlation, it should still show up in your inflated figures. This is important for us because we are not attempting to use subjective reports of happiness to assess individual happiness, but to see if there is a causal relationship between happiness and achievement. Just like in the height and income study, *systematic* overestimations of happiness will not affect the result. Nor should influences like the weather matter in a large statistical sample. At least on a population level, which is our primary interest here, such influences should all come out in the statistical wash.

None of this is to say that it would not be nice to have more measures of happiness that did not rely so much on subjective reports. Of course this is just to assert the banality that, as with all science, it is better to have more independent measures of a given phenomenon.

Not only do social scientists often use the positive moods and emotions formulation of 'happiness,' but so too do researchers interested in the pharmacology of happiness. This is readily apparent in research into depression, where 'happy' is often understood as the antipode to 'depressed.' Depression is typically understood by such researchers as a "mood disorder," which again suggests that happiness is to be understood in terms of positive moods. According to the analysis of Chapter 3, strictly speaking we are forced to say that scientists who identify happiness with positive moods and emotions are wrong, since positive moods and emotions are only a part of happiness. Despite the fact that this is technically incorrect, in what follows we shall often follow suit and think of 'happiness' in terms of positive moods and emotions. The reader should understand this as a short-cut and that, strictly speaking, it would be more accurate to say "the positive mood and emotion component of happiness" in reference to many scientific findings. One reason for the short-cut is that it would obviously get tiring pretty quickly to replace every reference to 'happiness' with "the positive mood and emotion component of happiness." Furthermore, there are good reasons to suppose that the cognitive component of happiness – attitudinal hedonism – will often have a similar valence to moods and emotions.[15] To illustrate: the attitudinal hedonism component of happiness will say that someone who sees the proverbial glass as half full is happier in this respect than the person who sees the glass as half empty. Common-sense psychology suggests that positive moods are more likely to generate judgments that the glass is half full, and judgments that the glass is half full are more likely to engender positive moods. So, the two will often go hand in hand. Furthermore, readers of Chapter 3 will recall that there is a large overlap in certain instruments for assessing life satisfaction and attitudinal hedonism. This means that the correlation noted above between positive moods and emotions and life satisfaction ratings should spill over into assessments of the positive mental states valued by attitudinal hedonism. All this should be tempered with a nod to the obvious: the degree to which positive moods and emotions are correlated with the other aspects of happiness is an empirical matter. Since attitudinal hedonism, to the best of my knowledge, has not been investigated by social scientists, what I have said is speculative. I think it is a good bet that the two will prove to be highly correlated, and hopefully future research will confirm this bet.[16]

6.5   Effect Size

Before we look at the studies in support of the claim that happiness promotes achievement, it is worth pausing here to consider the notion of 'effect size': a concept often invoked in meta-studies, in contrast to the usual statistical measure of statistical significance. A statistically significant difference is one in which the relationship between the variables is not likely to have occurred by chance. The difference in heights of girls aged 13 years and 6 months and those who are one month older are likely to be found to be statistically significant. That is, if one had a huge sample to study, and one measured the heights of all those aged 13 and 6 months and compared them with the heights of those aged 13 and 7 months, the difference in height between the two groups would not be explained by chance. This tells us that there is a statistically significant relationship between height and these two ages. Notice however, that the difference in height will be extremely small even though statistically significant. Statistical significance tells us only that there is a difference that is probably not due to chance, not the strength or degree of the difference.

Effect size tells us the strength or degree of difference. Jacob Cohen offers the classic illustration of the concept where he (somewhat reluctantly) defined effect size as small=0.2, medium=0.5, and large=0.8. [17] Cohen used the following illustration. The heights of 15- and 16-year-old girls in the US represent a small effect size. One may not be able to tell with the naked eye the small difference in height. The difference in height between 14- and 18-year-old girls represents a medium effect size and the difference between the heights of 13- and 18-year-old girls is a large effect size. Another illustration of a large effect size according to Cohen is the difference in IQ between the average college freshman and the average person with a PhD. As we shall see, many of the studies suggest a medium effect size of happiness on achievement. So, as a somewhat crude analogy, if we equate achievement with height, the effect of happiness on achievement is similar to the effect of age on the heights of 14- and 18-year-old girls.

6.6 Correlation Studies

Part of the case authors Lyubomirsky, King, and Diener make is based on correlation studies between happiness and achievement. The authors are well aware that correlation is not sufficient to establish a causal relation, but it is a necessary condition. So, for example, if someone says drinking milk causes little Jimmy's stomachaches and we find no correlation between his stomachaches and his drinking milk, then the causal claim has been disproven. Conversely, a correlation between Jimmy's drinking milk and his stomachaches does not mean that the one causes the other. Perhaps he drinks milk only when washing down hallucinogenic magic mushrooms and the mushrooms cause his stomach problems, or perhaps he drinks milk when he is nervous, and nervousness is the cause. So, the presence of correlation does not show causation, but the absence of a correlation shows an absence of causation.*

In examining the correlation evidence, Lyubomirsky, King, and Diener look at success in three domains: work, relationships, and health. In terms of work, happier people succeed along many dimensions. For example, they note that Staw and Barasade had observers rate managers on such abilities as information mastery and leadership and found that those high in positive affect were likely to be rated higher.[18] A study by Wright and Cropanzano found a correlation between a supervisor's judgment that a worker's job performance is superior and that worker's happiness.[19] A correlation was found between desirable jobs and happiness in research conducted by Staw, Sutton, and Pelled; specifically, happier people tended to have jobs that were rated higher in terms of autonomy, meaning and variety as rated by trained observers.[20] As well, they found that happier people were more likely to have a higher annual salary.

Their 'work' category summarizes some other interesting studies. For example, happiness has been found to correlate with the batting average of professional cricket players.[21] Another interesting linkage is between happiness and what business researchers sometimes term 'organizational citizenship,' which refers to supererogatory (going above and beyond the

---

* At least in the typical situation. This purposely ignores third variables that might explain the lack of correlation.

call of duty) acts in the workplace, such as spreading goodwill and assisting coworkers.[22]

The second category examined by Lyubomirsky, King, and Diener is social relations, which included many of the strongest correlations. In terms of friendships, happy people tend to have more friends, social support and companionship. Conversely, loneliness is negatively correlated with happiness[23] and positively correlated with depression.[24] Happiness is also correlated with marriage: married people are happier than individuals who are single, divorced or widowed.[25] The correlation between happiness and marriage holds up across a vast number of countries and cultures.[26]

The third and final category is health. Research shows that happy people have superior mental and physical health. In terms of mental health, the happiest people tend to have fewer psychiatric ailments such as depression, hypochondria, schizophrenia, anxiety and social phobia.[27] Happiness is correlated with better physical health outcomes in cancer treatment and sickle cell disease[28] as well as allergic reactions.[29] Happiness is inversely correlated with cortisol levels, with a 32.1 percent difference between the levels of the happiest people and the least happy.[30] The relevance to health is that higher cortisol levels are linked with hypertension, obesity and autoimmune disease.

Lyubomirsky, King, and Diener summarize the correlation evidence thus: "happy people appear to be more successful than their less happy peers in the three primary life domains: work (mean $r = .27$), relationships (mean $r = .27$), and health (mean $r = .32$)."[31]

In a section dedicated to "behaviors paralleling success" Lyubomirsky, King, and Diener consider several issues, two of which are particularly germane for our discussion. The first is altruistic or what social scientists sometimes refer to as "prosocial behavior." Lyubomirsky, King, and Diener summarize the empirical literature that indicates a correlation between happiness and prosocial behavior as follows: " . . . happy people are inclined to be kind and charitable people."[32] The fact that the data were collected from diverse samples, such as high school students, male twins and psychology undergraduates, provides additional confidence in the robustness of the conclusion.[33] The studies tended to operationalize prosocial behavior in different ways, but were recognizable forms of what most of us would understand as 'helping others.'[34] In terms of the virtues, such activity might be best described as exhibiting the virtue of beneficence.

The other issue is creativity. There is a well-known stereotype of the brooding artist. In fact we exploited this stereotype in Chapter 3 when we discussed Harriet the depressed artist. However, empirical research on the matter suggests the contrary is more often the case. Happy children and adults with high positive affect score higher on tests of creativity.[35]

6.7   Longitudinal and Laboratory Studies

We have cited evidence that happiness is correlated with achievement. As noted above, this does not in itself prove causation, and indeed is open to the obvious rebuttal that of course happiness and achievement are correlated, because achievement causes happiness. Workplace success, good health, marriage, and good friends are all conducive to making people happier. While no one denies that achievement often causes positive affect, the question of whether positive affect causes achievement can be addressed by two sorts of studies. One type is longitudinal studies; the other is laboratory studies. We will look at these in turn.

Longitudinal studies, as the name suggests, typically sample a population over time. If we have two correlated variables X and Y, and we are not sure which is the cause and which is the effect, we look to see whether one precedes the other in time. If X causes Y, then X should be present earlier than Y; conversely, if Y causes X, then Y should be apparent earlier than X. To illustrate, consider a study by Diener and his colleagues.[36] The study assessed the cheerfulness of college freshman and their income 19 years later. The group assessed as more cheerful in college earned more than their less cheerful cohorts 19 years later. The evidence here is suggestive that happiness causes increased earnings. As with any attribution of causality, there are significant worries about confounding variables. In this case, an obvious one is parental income. It does not seem out of the realm of possibility that freshmen whose parents earn more may be happier, and higher parental income may explain why their children are able to earn more. To sort out possible confounding influences, researchers "control" for such variables. Thus, in this study, when parental income was "high," defined as above $50,000, the most cheerful college students made a whopping $25,000 more than their less cheerful counterparts. In this case, parental income cannot be used to explain the difference in income because they all come from similarly high-income families.

In their review of longitudinal evidence, Lyubomirsky, King, and Diener found that "study after study shows that happiness precedes important outcomes and indicators of thriving, including fulfilling and productive work (mean $r = .24$), satisfying relationships (mean $r = .21$), and superior mental and physical health and longevity (mean $r = .18$)."[37] They also noted the relative paucity of studies in this area compared with correlation studies. By definition, longitudinal studies require a passage of time, and so often require foresight and patience – but not always. Sometimes the data has been collected by others, such as in the GSS database, and simply needs to be mined and analyzed. Sometimes researchers find novel sources of data. For example, Harker and Keltner found a correlation between the happiness and the marital satisfaction of women 31 years later.[38] To measure happiness, they assessed in terms of "appearing happy" the college yearbook photos taken when the women were 21.

The second type of evidence is from laboratory studies. Here the basic protocol is to induce an emotion in a test group and compare the result against controls, and then observe the result. Thus one experiment tested the reasoning of practicing physicians.[39] The test group were given a small bag of candy to induce a positive mood and then the physicians were asked to reason out loud about their diagnosis of a patient with liver cancer. Those with the induced mood were found to faster and better integrate the case study information. One of the obvious advantages of laboratory experiments is that they make it possible to minimize confounding influences, insuring that the test and control groups are as identical as possible except for the test condition. One limitation of just about all laboratory experiments is whether the artificial conditions of the laboratory translate into the "real world." A second, and for us more important, point is that laboratory experiments, at least the ones conducted so far, focus on short-term induction of moods. In these experiments, relatively minor things or events induce mood. In addition to candy, positive-mood inducers include a small gift, and seeing a humorous video clip and false positive information. The limitation here is that we are focusing on chronic positive affect: frequent positive moods. The inference that needs to be made in the case of laboratory studies is that the effects of short-term mood induction are parallel to the effects of chronic positive affect. In the above study of physicians, for example, we need to suppose that physicians who are higher in chronic positive affect are more likely to faster and better integrate the case study information. While the inference seems plausible enough – there is nothing to suggest it is not correct – there is an obvious need for "bridge" studies that test the relationship between short-term inducement of positive affect and chronic positive affect.

Lyubomirsky, King, and Diener summarize the experimental evidence thus:

> Our review of the relevant experimental literature reveals compelling evidence that positive affect fosters the following resources, skills, and behaviors: sociability and activity (mean r = .51), altruism (mean r = .43), liking of self and others (mean r = .36), strong bodies and immune systems (mean r = .38), and effective conflict resolution skills (mean r = .33). The evidence is weaker, but still consistent, that pleasant moods promote original thinking (mean r = .25).[40,41]

6.8   A Causal Model: Broaden and Build

Correlation, longitudinal, and experimental studies converge to show that positive moods and emotions cause achievement. Still, it may be wondered how they do so. That is, what is the mechanism that connects positive moods with achievement? The authors of the meta-study, along with many others in the positive psychology movement, accept the 'broaden-and-build theory' proposed by Barbara Fredrickson.[42] Fredrickson notes that positive emotions look puzzling if observed through the same lens as negative emotions such as anger, fear, and disgust. The evolutionary adaptations of negative emotions to challenges faced by our ancestors seem obvious. Anger evokes the desire to fight, fear the desire for flight, and disgust the desire to expel. As a response to threats, the easily recognizable facial, behavioral, and physiological changes evoked by these negative emotions appear to be very adaptive, as evolutionary theorists going back to Darwin have long realized. The trouble is that positive emotions do not appear to fit neatly into the framework: their existence cannot be explained in terms of an adaption to a specific evolutionarily important activity; for example, the experience of joy does not lead to (say) procreation in the way that fear leads to fleeing. Frederickson offers the following explanation for this asymmetry:

> Instead of solving problems of immediate survival, positive emotions solve problems concerning personal growth and development. Experiencing a positive emotion leads to states of mind and to modes of behavior that indirectly prepare an individual for later hard times. In my broaden-and-build theory, I propose that the positive emotions broaden an individual's momentary mindset, and by doing so help to build enduring personal resources.[43]

So, the broaden-and-build theory says that positive emotions differ from negative emotions along two dimensions. First, negative emotions are geared for the short term: fear and anger evolved as responses to immediate problems in the environment. Positive emotions are geared for the long term. Broadening and building is about building up resources for the long-term future. Second, the desires associated with positive emotions are less object-specific than negative emotions. A fear response, for instance, is typically about some immediate threat. With positive emotions the desire is more likely to be directed to some more abstract or diffuse goal. The "open mindset" suggests that people are more open to developing preexisting skills or attempting to develop new ones. The evolutionary payoff is that in hard times individuals will have more resources to fall back on. Persons who develop their social resources will have more allies to call upon in hard times, persons with greater hunting and gathering acumen will be better prepared for times of food scarcity, and so on.

It may help to visual the difference in positive and negative emotions by reflecting on an example adapted from Frederickson.[44] Imagine two children at a park. One is sitting alone, the other playing ball with several other children. It is pretty obvious, if one had to bet, which child is in a positive mood and which is in a negative mood, where to lay one's wager. It is also obvious which child is more likely developing resources, like social skills, hand−eye coordination, and cardiovascular fitness. Lyubomirsky, King, and Diener summarize the theoretical model thus:

> Positive emotions produce the tendency to approach rather than to avoid and to prepare the individual to seek out and undertake new goals. Thus, we propose that the success of happy people rests on two main factors. First, because happy people experience frequent positive moods, they have a greater likelihood of working actively toward new goals while experiencing those moods. Second, happy people are in possession of past skills and resources, which they have built over time during previous pleasant moods.[45]

So the broaden-and-build theory has an explanation for why happiness leads to achievement: those who are more frequently in positive moods will develop the resources to achieve more. Although the broaden-and-build explanation supports the idea that happiness can cause achievement, nothing in this work crucially depends on this being the correct explanation. What is crucial is the fact that happiness causes achievement, not what mechanism explains the causal relation. It is often the case that we know that A causes B without knowing the mechanism of action. For example, it has been known for over a century by Western science that aspirin causes pain to subside, but it was only in the 1970s that the mechanism of action was explained: the active ingredient in aspirin, acetylsalicylic acid, binds an enzyme which reduces prostaglandins, which are instrumental in sending pain messages to the brain. Suppose science is wrong about the mechanism of action: it turns out that ingesting aspirin releases tiny angels who soothe souls who are in pain. If this or some other mechanism turns out to be doing the work, it still won't change the fact that aspirin causes pain relief. Similarly, if the broaden-and-build hypothesis is replaced by a neurological model, it won't change the fact that happiness causes achievement.

6.9   Why Don't People in the *Brave New World* Achieve More?

Despite the wealth of empirical evidence that happiness causes achievement, many find the causal connection counterintuitive. Some may even find *Brave New World* itself a good counterexample to the thesis. Specifically, if happiness causes achievement, then we ought to predict (so the objection goes) that *Brave New World*ers will achieve more than we do, since they are so much happier. Since they don't achieve more than us, there must be something wrong with the putative causal link between happiness and achievement.

There are a number of good responses to this objection, not the least of which is that the novel is, well, a piece of fiction. Recall that my great unwritten novel, *Mark's Braver New World*, depicts an imaginary future where everyone is happier and achieves more. But so what? Obviously we should take this criticism seriously only if we think we can read off empirical psychology simply from what we glean from fiction writers. Very few of us think that fiction is likely to be a more reliable guide to predicting human behavior than empirical psychology. While this may seem all too obvious, it seems to be missed by many critics of happy-people-pills who seem to think that Huxley's novel illuminates the connection between happiness and achievement. (We will meet some of these critics again in Chapter 9.)

Second, to say that A causes B is not to say that A inevitably causes B. Obvious cases where this is not so are where there are confounding causal influences. We can't disprove the claim that aspirin causes pain relief by giving someone an aspirin for a mild headache and then triumphantly claiming it does not work when the person screams in pain as we torture them. In this case, being tortured is a confounding causal influence. In *Brave New World* Huxley introduces a number of confounding influences, including indoctrination and the other types of social manipulation we documented above, that are carefully deployed to suppress most kinds of achievement.

Third, it is worth noting an alternate reading of the connection between happiness and achievement in *Brave New World*. The Alpha class, of course, is most like people of our world: they are the least indoctrinated and not intellectually dulled with alcohol during gestation. Of the three Alpha class members readers have the most acquaintance with, Bernard, Helmholtz, and Mustapha, two show some predilection for achievement. Helmholtz has nascent poetic urges and Mustapha waxes wistful about his promising career as a scientist cut short by the previous generation of controllers. This impulse for achievement, despite it being officially frowned upon by society and government officials, is noteworthy. Furthermore, Bernard is clearly the least happy of the three and also shows the least inclination to achieve. Of course, *Brave New World* is just a piece of fiction, so there is no point in trying to make much of this. Still, there is a certain irony in the fact that the text can just as easily be read in support of the idea that happiness causes achievement.

6.10   Can We Be Too Happy?

Our preliminary conclusion of this chapter is this: Social science research suggests that those who are happier than average will be doubly blessed: they are happier and, on average, they will achieve more. But is more happiness always better? Can we be too happy?

The answer is a definite yes: clearly it is possible to be too happy. We can easily imagine a bad science fiction movie where an alien predatory species, the Happerions (sensitive to elevated neurochemical levels associated with happiness, let's say), eat the happiest people. When the Happerions land it would be best to stay unhappy. On the other hand, if one does not care to survive in a world dominated by Happerions, then you can't be too happy: being extremely happy may serve the goal of getting the Happerions to eat you. The example is purposely fanciful in the extreme, but it does tell us that in asking whether it is possible to be too happy we are asking whether a certain level of happiness thwarts some goal.

There is very little that addresses, in a systematic fashion, the question of whether it is possible to be too happy.[46] One of the most comprehensive studies is by Oishi, Diener, and Lucas, who argue that "although happiness has positive consequences in general, being happier is not always better. Once a moderate level of happiness is achieved, further increases can sometimes be detrimental."[47] As we have just seen, we should ask: detrimental to what goal? The answer seems to be suggested by the title of their paper: "The Optimum Level of Well-Being: Can People Be Too Happy?" Their basic idea is that happiness promotes wellbeing to a certain extent, but has diminishing and even negative returns, at least for some persons, as they reach the hyperthymic end of the scale.

One of the interesting things about their study is that the "too much happiness is detrimental for some" hypothesis seems to apply to only certain domains:

> The optimal level of happiness in the domains of volunteer work and relationships is the highest possible level of happiness. In contrast, the optimal level of happiness for achievement outcomes including income and education is a moderate (but still high) level of happiness.[48]

The upshot of this research sounds like a tragic choice: if we want to excel in terms of volunteer work and personal relationships, then we ought to strive to realize the highest level of happiness. If we seek to attain the highest level of education and income, then we should not try to be so happy.

The study is exactly the sort of empirical research we need to get a more nuanced understanding of the effects of happiness on achievement. It is worth noticing how this study is consistent with but different from the study by Lyubomirsky, King, and Diener. In the latter, to see whether happiness causes achievement subjects are typically divided into two groups in terms of their happiness ranking. The top half is the 'happy group' and the lower half the 'unhappy group': they use a version of the threshold sense of 'happiness' discussed in Chapter 3. What the Lyubomirsky, King, and Diener study found is that being in the top half causes more achievement. Notice that from this it does not follow that being happier always causes more achievement. As an analogy, imagine dividing students into two groups according to how much time they spend studying for a test the night before. Half the students spend two hours or less studying and half spend more than two hours studying. Let us suppose our research confirms what seems obvious: the group that studies more receives a higher score on the test. Obviously this does not imply that studying more always leads to a better exam result. Some students in the more-study-time group may study too long: imagine they are up most of the night studying and consequently are too tired to perform well on the test. We might find that studying for four hours leads to the best results. Finding a drop-off in performance is consistent with the original finding that those in the plus-two-hours-of-study group perform better on average than those in the two-hours-or-less-study group. By parallel reasoning we can see that research that confirms that being in the happiest half of the population leads to greater achievement does not show that more happiness always leads to more achievement. The study by Oishi, Diener, and Lucas addresses a question not systematically addressed in the Lyubomirsky, King, and Diener study.

One shortcoming of the Oishi, Diener, and Lucas study has to do with the explanation provided for the non-linear relationship between happiness on the one hand and income and educational achievement on the other. Suppose the relationship was positive and linear; then we would expect to see something like Figure 6.1. If the relationship was negative and linear we would expect something like Figure 6.2. The trouble is that the relationship is not linear but slightly curved, as in Figure 6.3, from Oishi, Diener, and

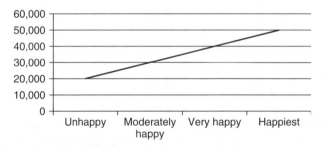

Figure 6.1   Happiness causes higher income.

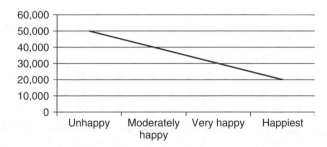

Figure 6.2   Unhappiness causes higher income.

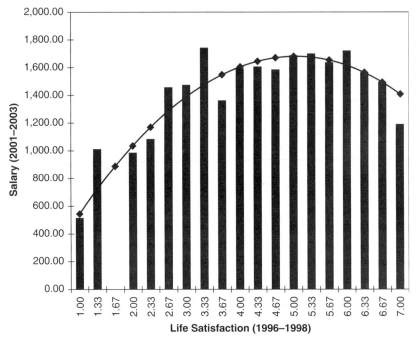

Figure 6.3   Life satisfaction and salary in the British Household Panel Study. Bars reflect average income at the listed life satisfaction level. The line reflects the estimated quadratic effect of life satisfaction on salary. From Oishi, Diener, and Lucas, "The Optimum Level of Well-being."

Lucas. In other words, happiness is positively correlated with income up to a certain point, and then negatively curved. The curve is shaped somewhat like the arm of someone making a basketball wrist shot.

The explanation the authors offer for the wrist-shot curve is somewhat baffling. They say, "individuals who consistently experience positive affect and never experience dissatisfaction might be less likely to make a change to improve their life circumstances. Thus, a very high level of satisfaction might lead individuals to fail to attain their full potential."[49] The trouble with this explanation is that it does not really explain the shape of the curve. If unhappiness is the spur to action, then any happiness seems an impediment to achieving more. This suggests the negative linear association depicted in Figure 6.2. In other words, their explanation does not tell us why happiness is positively correlated up to a certain point, and then negatively correlated. So, it is not clear, at present, why there is a non-linear curve.[50]

A simple explanation that may explain at least some of the wrist-shot curve is the "crowding-out" hypothesis: extremely high levels of happiness do not directly result in lower education or income attainment; rather, achievement in these areas is reduced as a consequence of success in other areas. A simple example can be seen from data that Oishi, Diener, and Lucas present concerning college students. The unhappiest students in their survey spent about a half-hour each week dating, while the happiest spent close to five hours each week dating. Students spend about 13 hours a week studying on average,[51] so imagine the unhappiest studied while the happiest were out dating. Over the course of a typical semester, the unhappiest would devote one workday equivalent in time (eight hours) to dating, while the happiest would devote about two weeks of workday equivalent in time to dating. I'm not saying that this is *the* explanation, only that it is a possible explanation. The general thought would be that the happier one is, the more one achieves, and the more one achieves, the more the demands on one's time (other things being equal of course). It would be interesting to study time allocation in relation to different levels of happiness. In any event, the important point here for us is that the authors of the study have not ruled out the possibility that the highest levels of happiness are only an indirect cause of lower income and education. It may well be that happiness causes us to be more social, more altruistic, and so on, and being more successful in these areas cause us to be less successful in other areas. Even the hyperthymic might have to deal with the fact that there are only 24 hours in a day.

Another problem with the study is that it is not clear how some of the measured indices relate to wellbeing; for example, it is not clear that having a higher income correlates with more wellbeing. This may sound like a minor quibble, since most of us believe that, other things being equal, a higher-paying job is better than a lower-paying job. Two points can be made in response. First, higher-paying jobs do not necessarily promote individual wellbeing. Riskier jobs, jobs with a longer commute, jobs that require one to be away for extended times from friends and family, and jobs with less social prestige tend to pay more, other things being equal. Some jobs pay more but require the sacrifice of our dignity and humanity: I would be earning a lot more if I had chosen to go into law with my father. Every year different lists of the "best jobs" are published, and, to the best of my knowledge, none of them names income as the sole criterion of what makes for a good job. It would be interesting to see whether happiness correlates in a more linear fashion with the quality of the job, which would

Table 6.1   19-year longitudinal study of cheerfulness
and income

Cheerfulness in 1976	Income in 1995
1 (lowest 10%)	$54,318
2 (below average)	$61,664
3 (average)	$63,509
4 (above average)	$66,144
5 (highest 10%)	$62,681

Source: Oishi, Diener, and Lucas. "The Optimum Level of Well-being"

look at aspects of a good job other than income: security, shorter hours, meaningful and safe work, etc.

Second, we should keep the tailing off of income in perspective. As noted, the moderately happy earn the most. Consider data from a 19-year-long panel study (Table 6.1).[52] The happiness of a group was measured in 1976 and correlated with their income in 1996. For the happiest group to earn as much as the moderately happy, they need a 5.5% pay increase. In comparison, the unhappiest require a 21.8% pay increase to match the moderately happy. The point then is that the effect size of being too happy is not that large. This point also reinforces the first: it is not hard to imagine at least some of the 5.5% income difference explained in terms of other aspects of work that make a job desirable. A similar unspectacular drop-off in scholastic achievement for college students is evidenced.[53] The moderately happy have the highest grade point average of 4.1 (on a 5-point scale), the happiest group have a grade point average of 3.8, and the unhappiest have a grade point average of 3.2. So, while there is some difference between the grade point averages of the moderately happy and the happiest group, it is not nearly as large as the difference between the unhappiest group and the moderately happy. It is a relatively small tail-off.

Even if we accept the data presented as unproblematic, there is still a large gap to show that the highest levels of happiness are not correlated with wellbeing. In the terms we have developed here, wellbeing is pluralistic: it contains a number of components. Assuming that the research shows that some components of wellbeing, like income and educational attainment,[†]

[†]   We do not need to assume that they are intrinsic benefits; for present purposes it does not matter whether they are only instrumentally beneficial.

fail to show a linear positive correlation, this still does not show that being in the happiest group is suboptimal for wellbeing. One way to close the gap in the reasoning would be to assume that "incomism" – all that matters for wellbeing is income – is true. If incomism is true, then clearly the data support the idea that too much happiness can thwart wellbeing: the happiest suffer a loss of wellbeing because their income is lower than the moderately happy. But obviously incomism is entirely implausible. Incomism does not take into account other aspects of wellbeing. Once we figure in other aspects of wellbeing it is clear that we need to ask whether the loss of income and educational attainment at the highest level of happiness is compensated for by gains in other aspects of wellbeing, in other words to make the argument a premise along the lines that income and educational attainment are of such great importance to wellbeing that the magnitude of the loss from the moderate to the happiest group means a reduction of wellbeing.

Our argument in Chapters 3 to 5 did not commit to the relative values of the intrinsic benefits, so it is consistent with what we said – that there is a loss of wellbeing. Still, it is perhaps apparent how implausible this position is. Imagine Mephistopheles offers a 5.5 percent pay raise to the happiest group in the 19-year panel study mentioned above. This would mean they would earn as much as their less happy peers, the moderately happy. The catch? They have to forgo the other benefits that come with being in the happiest group. If they accept the bargain, then they will be less happy, and have fewer friends, poorer relationships, and less virtue.[‡] Or imagine Mephistopheles makes the happiest students mentioned in the study above this offer: they can have their grade point raised 0.3 on average and be more contentious in exchange for a decrease in their average number of close friends, self-confidence, energy, time spent dating and happiness.[54] It is hard to imagine many taking up either of Mephistopheles' offers. The loss in certain aspects of wellbeing would not be compensated for by the gains. So the study does not show that happiness is not linearly correlated with wellbeing, that the happiest are not better off in terms of wellbeing.

It is worth noting too that even if the previous criticisms are incorrect, this still does not spell disaster for happy-people-pills progressivism. It claims that at least some persons who are not depressed, persons in the "normal range of happiness," will benefit from taking happy-people-pills. If it turns out that too much happiness reduces wellbeing, then this still leaves a large number of people who might benefit. For instance, in the grade

---

[‡] Using volunteering as a proxy for virtue.

point average study, those in the second-highest happiness group achieved the highest grade point average; 65 percent of students were not in the two highest happiness groups (126 out of 193). In an income study,[55] happiness is positively correlated with income in 9 out of 10 happiness categories, with a negative correlation only with the highest level of happiness. This means that persons in the lower eight categories of happiness could benefit from happy-people-pills. This amounts to 76 percent of the population study (38,266 out of 50,292 surveyed).

Finally, the research may suggest that there could be advantages to being slightly less happy at crucial junctures in one's life. Perhaps, in college, in an attempt to get the highest grade point average, students should only take half their weekly happy-people-pills rather than a full dose. Similarly, if there are strategic windows for moving up the corporate ladder, then perhaps a reduced dose of happy-people-pills would be in order. The point of course is that we need not say that happy is always better in all points in our lives.

To summarize this, if the only goal were to maximize earnings, even taking the data at face value most people would benefit from taking happy-people-pills to boost their happiness to moderately high levels. Very roughly, most people will benefit because most are not in the top 35 percent. Thus, even if we take everything written at face value, the news for happy-people-pills is not all bad. It would suggest that perhaps 50–60 percent of the population would benefit from taking happy-people-pills by increasing their chances of a higher income. If the goal were to increase stable relationships or to be altruistic, then everyone might benefit.

Notes

1. Lyubomirsky, King, and Diener, "The Benefits of Frequent Positive Affect."
2. Ibid., 803.
3. Ibid. The italics are added by the authors of the extract.
4. Ibid., 806.
5. Ibid.
6. Ibid., 816.
7. Ibid., 843.
8. Ibid., 816, 820.
9. Ibid., 822.
10. Ibid.
11. World Values Study Group, "World Values Survey, 1981–1984 and 1990–1993."

12. Schwarz, *Stimmung als Information*. Cited in Kahneman and Krueger, "Developments in the Measurement of Subjective Well-being."

13. Schwarz and Clore, "Mood, Misattribution, and Judgments of Well-being."

14. For review see Diener, "Assessing Subjective Well-being" and Schneider and Schimmack, "Self-informant Agreement in Well-being Ratings."

15. It seems likely that the other affective component of happiness, sensory hedonism, will also often be in lockstep with moods and emotions. As with attitudinal hedonism, I take this to be an empirical conjecture that has not yet been investigated in detail by social scientists.

16. What if it turns out there are two different mechanisms at work in happiness, one underlying the cognitive component and one the affective component? As noted, this would go against much of our best science, but still it is worth speculating on for a moment. My answer here would be simply to parse out the happy-people-pills-for-all project accordingly. That is, we would look to see to what extent these two happiness mechanisms are heritable, and then seek to put into pill form what the cognitive hyperthymic and the affective hyperthymic have thanks to the genetic lottery.

17. Cohen, *Statistical Power Analysis for the Behavioral Sciences*.

18. Staw and Barsade, "Affect and Managerial Performance." Most of the studies published before 2005 mentioned in this chapter are discussed in Lyubomirsky, King, and Diener, "The Benefits of Frequent Positive Affect."

19. Wright and Cropanzano, "Psychological Well-being and Job Satisfaction as Predictors of Job Performance."

20. Staw, Sutton, and Pelled, "Employee Positive Emotion and Favorable Outcomes at the Workplace."

21. Totterdell, "Catching Moods and Hitting Runs."

22. George and Brief, "Feeling Good–Doing Good"; Organ, *Organizational Citizenship Behavior*.

23. Lee and Ishii-Kuntz, "Social Interaction, Loneliness, and Emotional Well-being Among the Elderly."

24. Peplau and Perlman, *Loneliness*; Seligman, *Learned Optimism*.

25. Diener et al., "Subjective Well-being."

26. Mastekaasa, "Marital Status, Distress and Well-being"; Diener et al., "Similarity of the Relations Between Marital Status and Subjective Well-being Across Cultures"; Kozma and Stones, "Predictors of Happiness"; Lee, Seccombe, and Shehan, "Marital Status and Personal Happiness"; Marks and Fleming, "Influences and Consequences of Well-being Among Australian Young People"; Stack and Eshleman, "Marital Status and Happiness."

27. Diener and Seligman, "Very Happy People"; Chang and Farrehi, "Optimism/Pessimism and Information-Processing Styles"; Phillips, "Mental Health Status, Social Participation, and Happiness"; Kashdan and Roberts, "Trait and State Curiosity in the Genesis of Intimacy."

28. Collins et al., "Sense of Coherence Over Time in Cancer Patients"; Gil et al., "Daily Mood and Stress Predict Pain, Health Care Use, and Work Activity in African American Adults with Sickle-Cell Disease."

29. Laidlaw, Booth, and Large, "Reduction in Skin Reactions to Histamine After a Hypnotic Procedure."

30. Steptoe, Wardle, and Marmot, "Positive Affect and Health-Related Neuroendocrine, Cardiovascular, and Inflammatory Processes."

31. Lyubomirsky, King, and Diener, "The Benefits of Frequent Positive Affect," 825.

32. Ibid., 828.

33. Magen and Aharoni, "Adolescents' Contributing Toward Others"; Krueger, Hicks, and McGue, "Altruism and Antisocial Behavior"; Feingold, "Happiness, Unselfishness, and Popularity."

34. Feingold, "Happiness, Unselfishness, and Popularity"; Magen and Aharoni, "Adolescents' Contributing Toward Others."

35. Cacha, "Figural Creativity, Personality, and Peer Nominations of Preadolescents"; Schuldberg, "Schizotypal and Hypomanic Traits, Creativity, and Psychological Health."

36. Diener et al., "Dispositional Affect and Job Outcomes."

37. Lyubomirsky, King, and Diener, "The Benefits of Frequent Positive Affect," 834.

38. Harker and Keltner, "Expressions of Positive Emotion in Women's College Yearbook Pictures and Their Relationship to Personality and Life Outcomes Across Adulthood."

39. Estrada, Isen, and Young, "Positive Affect Facilitates Integration of Information and Decreases Anchoring in Reasoning Among Physicians."

40. Lyubomirsky, King, and Diener, "The Benefits of Frequent Positive Affect," 840.

41. Some recent research (Tan and Forgas, "When Happiness Makes Us Selfish, but Sadness Makes Us Fair") would tend to pull down the effect size of altruism. Their research suggests that happiness leads to selfishness. Their research has too many methodological problems to merit serious concern. To cite a single example: Tan and Forgas had subjects take a cognitive test, and good or bad moods were induced by providing either positive or negative feedback on the test. The feedback was randomly assigned; actual test scores were not used. Subjects were given raffle tickets for a $20 prize and asked to decide, after receiving the feedback, how many to keep for themselves and how many to give to others. Students provided with positive feedback tended to give away fewer raffle tickets than students who were provided with negative feedback. An obvious difficulty here is that praise for performance is a potential confounding variable. There may well be an expectation on

the part of subjects that one is more deserving of a prize if one has done well on a performance test. It would be interesting to see the results of the study done with a more traditional good-mood inducement such as luck, for example where the experimenters arrange that some subjects "just happen to find some money" or something else of value. The point, of course, is that one has to be careful teasing out whether the cause of the good mood is being tested, or the good mood itself. This is not to suggest that luck itself may not be a confounding variable, only that a different result would suggest that at least one of the inducements was a confounding variable.

42. Fredrickson, "What Good Are Positive Emotions?," "The Role of Positive Emotions in Positive Psychology," and "The Value of Positive Emotions."
43. Fredrickson, "The Value of Positive Emotions," 332.
44. Adapted from Frederickson, ibid., 333.
45. Lyubomirsky, King, and Diener, "The Benefits of Frequent Positive Affect," 804.
46. Oishi, Diener, and Lucas, "The Optimum Level of Well-being."
47. Ibid., 346.
48. Ibid., 356.
49. Ibid., 348.
50. It should be noted that the authors are upfront about the tentativeness of their explanation.
51. Babcock and Marks, *The Falling Time Cost of College*.
52. Oishi, Diener, and Lucas, "The Optimum Level of Well-being," 353.
53. Ibid., 352.
54. The study also measured number of classes missed, and event balance (ratio of positive to negative experience), neither of which is particularly relevant to our conception of wellbeing.
55. Oishi, Diener, and Lucas, "The Optimum Level of Well-being," 351.

References

Babcock, P. S. and M. Marks. *The Falling Time Cost of College: Evidence from Half a Century of Time Use Data*. Cambridge, Mass.: National Bureau of Economic Research, 2010.

Cacha, F. B. "Figural Creativity, Personality, and Peer Nominations of Pre-adolescents." *Gifted Child Quarterly* 20, no. 2 (1976): 187–95.

Chang, E. C. and A. S. Farrehi. "Optimism/Pessimism and Information-processing Styles: Can Their Influences Be Distinguished in Predicting Psychological Adjustment?" *Personality and Individual Differences* 31, no. 4 (2001): 555–62.

Cohen, J. *Statistical Power Analysis for the Behavioral Sciences*. Hillsdale, N.J.: Lawrence Erlbaum Associates; 1988.

Collins, J. F., K. Hanson, M. Mulhern, and R. M. Padberg. "Sense of Coherence Over Time in Cancer Patients: A Preliminary Report." *Medical Psychotherapy: An International Journal* 5 (1992): 73–82.

Diener, E. "Assessing Subjective Well-being: Progress and Opportunities." *Social Indicators Research* 31, no. 2 (1994): 103–57.

Diener, E., C. L. Gohm, E. Suh, and S. Oishi. "Similarity of the Relations Between Marital Status and Subjective Well-being Across Cultures." *Journal of Cross-Cultural Psychology* 31, no. 4 (2000): 419–36.

Diener, E., C. Nickerson, R. E. Lucas, and E. Sandvik. "Dispositional Affect and Job Outcomes." *Social Indicators Research* 59, no. 3 (2002): 229–59.

Diener, E. and M. E. P. Seligman. "Very Happy People." *Psychological Science* 13, no. 1 (2002): 81–4.

Diener, E., E. M. Suh, R. E. Lucas, and H. L. Smith. "Subjective Well-being: Three Decades of Progress." *Psychological Bulletin* 125, no. 2 (1999): 276–302.

Estrada, C. A., A. M. Isen, and M. J. Young. "Positive Affect Facilitates Integration of Information and Decreases Anchoring in Reasoning Among Physicians." *Organizational Behavior and Human Decision Processes* 72, no. 1 (1997): 117–35.

Feingold, A. "Happiness, Unselfishness, and Popularity." *Journal of Psychology* 115, no. 1 (1983): 3–5.

Fredrickson, B. L. "The Role of Positive Emotions in Positive Psychology: The Broaden-and-Build Theory of Positive Emotions." *American Psychologist* 56, no. 3 (2001): 218–26.

Fredrickson, B. L. "The Value of Positive Emotions: The Emerging Science of Positive Psychology is Coming to Understand Why It's Good to Feel Good." *American Scientist* 91, no. 4 (2003): 330–5.

Fredrickson, B. L. "What Good Are Positive Emotions?" *Review of General Psychology* 2, no. 3 (1998): 300–19.

George, J. M. and A. P. Brief. "Feeling Good–Doing Good: a Conceptual Analysis of the Mood at Work–Organizational Spontaneity Relationship." *Psychological Bulletin* 112, no. 2 (1992): 310–29.

Gil, K. M., J. W. Carson, L. S. Porter, C. Scipio, S. M. Bediako, and E. Orringer. "Daily Mood and Stress Predict Pain, Health Care Use, and Work Activity in African American Adults with Sickle-Cell Disease." *Health Psychology* 23, no. 3 (2004): 267–74.

Harker, L. A. and D. Keltner. "Expressions of Positive Emotion in Women's College Yearbook Pictures and Their Relationship to Personality and Life Outcomes Across Adulthood." *Journal of Personality and Social Psychology* 80, no. 1 (2001): 112–24.

Kahneman, D. and A. B. Krueger. "Developments in the Measurement of Subjective Well-being." *Journal of Economic Perspectives* 20, no. 1 (2006): 3–24.

Kashdan, T. B. and J. E. Roberts. "Trait and State Curiosity in the Genesis of Intimacy: Differentiation from Related Constructs." *Journal of Social and Clinical Psychology* 23, no. 6 (2004): 792–816.

Kozma, A. and M. J. Stones. "Predictors of Happiness." *Journal of Gerontology* 38, no. 5 (1983): 626–8.

Krueger, R. F., B. M. Hicks, and M. McGue. "Altruism and Antisocial Behavior: Independent Tendencies, Unique Personality Correlates, Distinct Etiologies." *Psychological Science* 12, no. 5 (2001): 397–402.

Laidlaw, T. M., R. J. Booth, and R. G. Large. "Reduction in Skin Reactions to Histamine After a Hypnotic Procedure." *Psychosomatic Medicine* 58, no. 3 (1996): 242–8.

Lee, G. R. and M. Ishii-Kuntz. "Social Interaction, Loneliness, and Emotional Well-being Among the Elderly." *Research on Aging* 9, no. 4 (1987): 459–82.

Lee, G. R., K. Seccombe, and C. L. Shehan. "Marital Status and Personal Happiness: An Analysis of Trend Data." *Journal of Marriage and the Family* 53, no. 4 (1991): 839–44.

Lyubomirsky, S., L. King, and E. Diener. "The Benefits of Frequent Positive Affect: Does Happiness Lead to Success?" *Psychological Bulletin* 131 (2005): 803–55.

Magen, Z. and R. Aharoni. "Adolescents' Contributing Toward Others." *Journal of Humanistic Psychology* 31, no. 2 (1991): 126–43.

Marks, G. N. and N. Fleming. "Influences and Consequences of Well-being Among Australian Young People: 1980–1995." *Social Indicators Research* 46, no. 3 (1999): 301–23.

Mastekaasa, A. "Marital Status, Distress and Well-being: An International Comparison." *Journal of Comparative Family Studies* 25, no. 2 (1994): 183–206.

Oishi, S., E. Diener, and R. E. Lucas. "The Optimum Level of Well-being: Can People Be Too Happy?" *Perspectives on Psychological Science* 2, no. 4 (2007): 346–60.

Organ, D. *Organizational Citizenship Behavior: The Good Soldier Syndrome.* Lexington, Mass.: Lexington Books, 1988.

Peplau, L. A. and D. Perlman. *Loneliness: A Sourcebook of Current Theory, Research, and Therapy.* Vol. 36. New York: Wiley, 1982.

Phillips, D. L. "Mental Health Status, Social Participation, and Happiness." *Journal of Health and Social Behavior* (1967): 285–91.

Schneider, L. and U. Schimmack. "Self-informant Agreement in Well-being Ratings: A Meta-analysis." *Social Indicators Research* 94, no. 3 (2009): 363–76.

Schuldberg, D. "Schizotypal and Hypomanic Traits, Creativity, and Psychological Health." *Creativity Research Journal* 3, no. 3 (1990): 218–30.

Schwarz, N. *Stimmung als Information: Untersuchungen zum Einfluß von Stimmungen auf die Bewertung des eigenen Lebens.* Heidelberg: Springer-Verlag, 1987.

Schwarz, N. and G. L. Clore. "Mood, Misattribution, and Judgments of Well-being: Informative and Directive Functions of Affective States." *Journal of Personality and Social Psychology* 45, no. 3 (1983): 513–23.

Seligman, M. *Learned Optimism*. New York: Knopf, 1991.

Stack, S. and J. R. Eshleman. "Marital Status and Happiness: A 17-Nation Study." *Journal of Marriage and the Family* 60 (1998): 527–36.

Staw, B. M. and S. G. Barsade. "Affect and Managerial Performance: A Test of the Sadder-but- Wiser vs. Happier-and-Smarter Hypotheses." *Administrative Science Quarterly* 38, no. 2 (1993): 304–31.

Staw, B. M., R. I. Sutton, and L. H. Pelled. "Employee Positive Emotion and Favorable Outcomes at the Workplace." *Organization Science* 5, no. 1 (1994): 51–71.

Steptoe, A., J. Wardle, and M. Marmot. "Positive Affect and Health-Related Neuroendocrine, Cardiovascular, and Inflammatory Processes." *Proceedings of the National Academy of Sciences of the United States of America* 102, no. 18 (2005): 6508–12.

Tan, H. B. and J. P. Forgas. "When Happiness Makes Us Selfish, but Sadness Makes Us Fair: Affective Influences on Interpersonal Strategies in the Dictator Game." *Journal of Experimental Social Psychology* 46, no. 3 (2010): 571–6.

Totterdell, P. "Catching Moods and Hitting Runs: Mood Linkage and Subjective Performance in Professional Sport Teams." *Journal of Applied Psychology* 85, no. 6 (2000): 848–59.

World Values Study Group, and others. "World Values Survey, 1981–1984 and 1990–1993." ICPSR, University of Michigan, 1994.

Wright, T. A. and R. Cropanzano. "Psychological Well-being and Job Satisfaction as Predictors of Job Performance." *Journal of Occupational Health Psychology* 5, no. 1 (2000): 84–94.

7

Happy Pharmacology

In the previous chapter we reviewed evidence from the social sciences that suggests that happy people are doubly blessed: they are happier and they achieve more. In this chapter we explore the question of what makes people happy, and how we might make people happier. As intimated previously, a good part of the explanation for differences in happiness has to do with genetics: some have won the proverbial "genetic lottery" and so are happier on average. Others have lost and are below the average range for positive affect. We will review the scientific data relevant to a heritable component to happiness, and the prospects for using current and future technologies to alter or "compensate" those who have not won the genetic lottery.

7.1 Heritability Measures

Of all the surprising results discovered about happiness in the past hundred years perhaps none is more so than that genes account for the lion's share of an individual's happiness. Behavioral geneticists, and others who study the role of the contribution of genes to our traits and characteristics, express their findings in terms of heritability measures. Heritability estimates for happiness range from 40 to 80 percent.[1] In this section we will look briefly at the concept of heritability, and in the following section we will look specifically at the heritability of happiness.

Heritability estimates apply to traits or characteristics that exhibit variability. An example of a trait that does not exhibit variability is 'a beating

Happy-People-Pills For All, First Edition. Mark Walker.
© 2013 John Wiley & Sons, Inc. Published 2013 by John Wiley & Sons, Inc.

heart.' All living humans have hearts, and so this trait shows no variability. So, with no variability there is no heritability estimate. A trait that exhibits variability is the previously discussed case of human height. Some people are tall, and some short, so human height is subject to heritability estimates. The variation in height is due to two factors: environmental and genetic factors. Important environmental factors that determine stature include nutrition and serious disease in childhood. For instance, the gains in average height in the last few centuries are often attributed to better nutrition and fewer childhood diseases in comparison with our ancestors. On the genetic side, human height is influenced by a number of genes, making it a polygenic trait. A few human traits are determined by a single gene and so are monogenetic; for example, Huntington's disease is caused by a single gene mutation; but most traits are polygenic, like height, meaning they have multiple gene influences.

To get some idea of how heritability estimates are made, consider a couple of examples. The average height for a population of white males in North America is about 178 centimeters (Figure 7.1) and geneticists estimate that height is 80% heritable. So, if Bill is a white male in this population and stands 183cm, then he is 5cm above the average. Given a heritability estimate of 80%, then on average, 4cm of Bill's above-average height is attributable to genetics, and 20% due to environmental differences, so 1cm of height would be accounted for in terms of environmental influences, such as a good diet and lifestyle. On the other hand, there is almost no heritability to the trait of having a favorite professional football team – environmental influences explain why people prefer one NFL team to another.

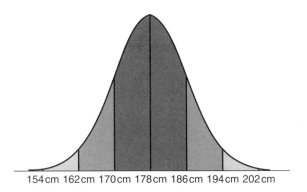

154cm 162cm 170cm 178cm 186cm 194cm 202cm

Figure 7.1   North American male height distribution graph.

To illustrate further, suppose Alvin and Simon are adopted siblings: both are in their early twenties and living in some relatively affluent city of North America. They have attended the same schools, had similar meals, and suffered the same childhood illnesses. In short, they have as many environmental influences in common as any biologically related siblings. You have a chance to bet on Simon's height with the following conditions: you may bet Simon is either 178cm tall or 194cm tall. If you are within 8cm, you will win one million dollars. Suppose you are told that Alvin is 194cm tall. If stature is mostly determined by environmental influences, it would make sense to bet that Simon is 194cm tall since, after all, they have experienced very similar environmental conditions. Yet even though Simon and Alvin share so many environmental influences smart money would say to bet that Simon is 178cm. Here's why: 68% of the population lies within 8cm of 178cm, whereas only about 16% of the population lies within 8cm of 194cm. So, if we had to bet whether some person randomly drawn from the target population was within these two groups, it would be wise to take the 178cm bet. Almost two thirds of the population lies within 8cm of this number, whereas only 16% lies within 8cm of 194cm. Knowing that Alvin and Simon are not genetically related, and how little influence environmental influences have on height, smart money will go with the 178cm bet. Most of Alvin's above-average height will be attributable to genetic factors. Since Alvin and Simon are not genetically related, the same reasoning applies where we simply choose a person at random. We do not know anything about the biggest determinate of Simon's stature, his genetics, so we ought to put our money on the bet with the largest pool of candidates.

Here is a second bet. For another million dollars you can bet on the height of Theodore who is the identical twin brother of Alvin, raised by a different family in a different relatively affluent city in North America since birth. Thus Theodore and Alvin have far fewer environmental influences in common than Alvin and Simon, but they are genetically identical. Should you bet that Theodore is within 8cm of 194cm or within 8cm of 178cm? Even though only 16% of the population falls in the taller category, smart money would bet on Theodore being within 8cm of 194cm precisely because of the large genetic influence on height. On the other hand, if you had to bet whether Simon likes the same football team as Theodore or Alvin, you should bet on Simon favoring the same team as his adoptive brother rather than that of his biological brother. As we said, a favorite NFL team is not a highly heritable trait: it is something that is more likely caused and explained by environmental factors.

An often overlooked factor is that heritability estimates are always relativized to some population, and therefore relativized to an environment. Thus, a study done by D. F. Roberts and colleagues found that heritability of stature in West Africa is only 65%, which differs significantly from the figure of 80% for white North Americans.[2] Part of the explanation for the difference may lie in differences in population genetics, but undoubtedly most of the difference is due to greater environmental differences experienced by the population of West Africa, as opposed to the comparatively homogeneous environment of the white North American populations. In the case of stature, where nutrition and disease in childhood are large determinants, the more homogeneous a population's environment the higher the heritability estimate. This may seem counterintuitive, since heritability is a measure of the effects of genes on traits and it may seem that genes should have less of an influence if the environment is more homogeneous. The anomaly disappears when we consider that heritability is used to explain differences in traits: any differences in stature that remain in a population where every child is adequately fed, and equally protected from disease (and so on for other environmental influences), will mean that most of the remaining differences in height will have to be explained in terms of genetics.

7.2   Genetics of Happiness

How do you explain your present level of happiness? Most people asked this question will cite things like a good (or bad) relationship, income, educational attainment, and so on. Suppose we know these relevant facts about you, and suppose too that unbeknownst to you, you have an identical twin. We have available your twin's happiness score on the same test taken ten years previously. Which of these measures: your education, income, status or your twin's score ten years previously, is the best predictor of your present level of happiness? No doubt you have guessed what Lykken and Tellegen found: "The reported wellbeing of one's identical twin, either now or 10 years earlier, is a far better predictor of one's self-rated happiness than is one's own educational achievement, income, or status."[3] What this means is that in the typical case, a large measure of one's happiness over the course of a lifetime, compared with the population average, depends on how one fares in the "genetic lottery."

It is important to note what heritability measures of happiness – even the highest estimate of 80 percent – do not say. In particular, some confusion arises with talk of a 'happiness set point,' which to some suggests that one's level of happiness is set in stone and cannot, at least for long, be affected by the circumstances or decisions of one's life. While there may be some misunderstanding of this in the popular press, no serious researcher has ever suggested anything remotely like this. Rather, suppose Happy Harry has a high set point for positive affect, and Sad Sam has a low set point for happiness. It is quite consistent with the set point theory that if Happy Harry loses his wife, his dog runs away, he is fired and severely disabled, then Happy Harry will no longer be happy. Likewise, if Sad Sam wins the lottery and a Nobel Prize in the same month that he gets married, then it is quite possible that he will be very happy. No serious proponent of the happiness set point theory denies this. Nor do set point theorists need to postulate that Happy Harry's level of happiness will necessarily return to the previous set point. If Happy Harry is tortured on the rack every day for the rest of his life in his solitary isolation cell, then he is not going to be very happy. What the set point theory does predict is that if Happy Harry and Sad Sam experience similar life events – both have a good job, a stable relationship, and the same educational attainment, Harry's higher set point (based ultimately on genes) will mean that he will be happier than Sam on average, even though there will be days when Sam is happier than Harry. Admittedly this understanding of the happiness set point is not nearly as dramatic as sometimes advertised. But the loss in dramatic effect is offset by the gain in plausibility. It would be nothing short of astounding if nothing environmental could have a profound effect on happiness. Even traits as rigidly set as adult height can be affected by environmental factors like serious accidents and height-increasing surgery.

The most common cited heritability estimate is that happiness is about 50% heritable. Sonya Lyubomirsky illustrates the point nicely with a picture on the dust cover of her book *The How of Happiness*, which features a pie, 40% cut away (Figure 7.2).[4] This 40%, we are told, is within our control. Lyubomirsky says that 10% influence is environmental factors that we do not have individual control over – broadly social aspects of our environment. And of course 50% is due to genetics, so again we have no control.

The 50% heritability is the most commonly cited measure, so what do we say about the 80% heritability estimates? In general, it is wise to go with the opinion of the majority of experts in a field where one is not an expert

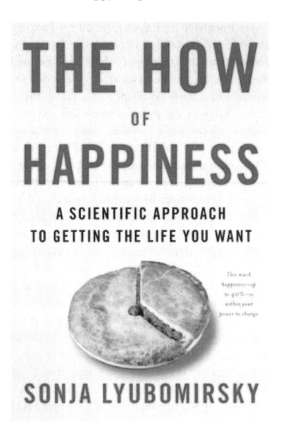

Figure 7.2   The cover of *The How of Happiness*.

oneself, suggesting we adopt the 50% figure. However, in this case, David Lykken has made a convincing argument in "A More Accurate Estimate of Heritability" that the higher number of 80% is much closer to the truth.[5] The paper begins with a comment which, as far as I can tell, is intended to be an amusing jab at many of his colleagues. "One of the attractions that psychological research still has for the young is that there remain so many easy and obvious improvements to be made in its theories and methods."[6] He adds:

> One example is the almost universal but erroneous assumption that a single measure of a trait constitutes the lasting sum or product of genetic and environmental influences and that, apart from an inevitable but (usually) small amount of measurement error, that single measure reflects the trait's stable value or intensity.[7]

I'll try to translate his claim and argument into a more familiar idiom. Consider first a typical adopted twin study, of the sort that Lykken himself built a considerable reputation on, on a trait like height. As indicated above, such studies are done by locating grown identical twins adopted by different families. With a relatively stable trait like height, it is necessary only to gather the information once. If someone is 180cm tall, we do not expect there to be much change in height if we measure his or her height again a year later – assuming that the person is an adult, of course. If Jim and Tim are identical twins reared apart, we would not be in the least surprised to find that Jim and Tim are both very close to 180cm tall.

Single measures do not work as well with traits that are known to fluctuate over the course of a typical adult life. Imagine a questionnaire is sent out to identical twins, Ted and Jed, raised apart. Ted reports weighing 160 lbs., while Jed is 180 lbs. These results may suggest that weight is not highly heritable, because of the large 20 lb. difference. But suppose it turns out that Ted was about to attend a high school reunion, and so lost 10 lbs. on a crash diet, while Jed gained 10 lbs. on a Caribbean cruise just before completing the survey. These short-term results may mislead about the facts that they each tend to weigh about 170 lbs., and that our survey is picking up short-term fluctuations. Suppose we took a second measurement five years later and this time they both weigh 172 lbs. The average measurement for Ted is 166 lbs. and 176 lbs. for Jed. The point then is that the averaging of several measures rather than taking any single measure is likely to better indicate an underlying set point. With two measures the calculated difference in their weight is reduced by half. In other words, weight will look much more heritable using multiple measures. The same point applies to measuring chronic positive affect: temporary ups and downs will lead us to underestimate any genetic component to a disposition to a certain level of positive affect if only one reading is taken.

We are now in a position to appreciate what Lykken means in the passage quoted above. A single measure of weight does not accurately reflect the stable value or intensity. The initial single measures of Ted and Jed's weight do not fully capture their disposition to a certain weight. Thus Lykken seems to be correct when he says, "twin and family data based on one-time measurements *must* underestimate true heritability."[8] As Lykken points out, it is understandable why researchers do single measures of traits: doing multiple measures is hard and expensive. The relevance of all this to happiness studies, of course, is that measurements of heritability of happiness are sometimes done with single measures and sometimes with multiple measures. Not surprisingly, the higher estimates of heritability, in the 80% range, are multiple measures whereas the lower estimates, in the 40–50% range, are single measures of trait.

It is important to clarify what this argument shows. Lykken and colleagues claim a higher heritability of happiness trait using multiple measures than single measures. However, as Lykken notes, there are so few multiple measure studies that replication of his findings is relatively sparse.[9] So, it may be that heritability is not as high as 80%, but it seems almost certain that single measures that estimate in the 40–50% range underestimate the heritability of happiness as a trait.

7.3   Environmental Influences on Happiness

It is worth thinking for a moment about the non-genetic component of happiness. As we have said, the notion of heritability is typically seen as a composite of two factors: genetics and the environment, where 'environment' simply means all non-genetic influences. So, unlike genetics, which is univocal in picking out a single causal influence, the notion of environment is an umbrella term for a variety of causal influences such as nutrition, family life, peers, work, love, socio-economic status, weather, and so on. Psychologists distinguish between environmental influences that one has intentional control over, and those that one does not.[10] For example, winning the lottery or becoming paralyzed are mostly matters of luck, something that one does not have a lot of intentional control over. One of the more surprising results of happiness research is how little some such events change one's happiness. It is true and hardly surprising that lottery winners and accident victims initially have a huge swing in their happiness levels. What is surprising is that often, within a year or two, they return reasonably close to their previous levels. So, if Jill is on the lower end of the normal range of happiness and she wins the lottery, happiness researchers will predict that her happiness level will see an immediate increase. They will also predict that within a year or so, her happiness level will return to its "natural level," which, as we said for Jill, is at the lower end of the normal curve. So, the television commercials that show people being extremely happy just after winning the lottery are correct. What such commercials do not show is that the winners' happiness levels return within a year or so to their baseline states. Other events, such as losing a spouse, seem to have a midterm effect on happiness, perhaps five years or more.[11]

In terms of making people happier, attempting to manipulate the non-intentional aspects of their environment is not particular promising, for several reasons. First, by definition, 'non-intentional' circumstances include things that we as individuals have little or no control over (at least in the short term), such as "a person's national or cultural region, demographics (e.g., gender and ethnicity), personal experiences (e.g., past traumas and triumphs), and life status variables (e.g., marital status, education level, health, and income)."[12] Second, while non-intentional influences do prevent third-party interventions, these typically would be macroscopic changes that would take considerable effort and time to implement. For instance, it has been suggested that the reason Northern Europeans tend to be happier than their US counterparts has to do with the more egalitarian economic systems of the former. Supposing that something like this is true (and this is far from uncontroversial), still there is a large issue of whether the US should reform its economic system, and how victory might be won against countervailing forces. Third, even if we could advise individuals to do something about that which they cannot control, it is likely to have the least effect. Recall that the influence of circumstances is the smallest piece of Lyubomirsky's pie. She estimates it at about 10%, but given our previous discussion of Lykken's argument that single measures of variable traits will underestimate heritability, the effect of circumstances on happiness trait may be much less than 10%. For if heritability is higher than the 50% estimate, then this necessitates a reduction of the estimate of environmental influences on variation in happiness. None of this is to suggest that we should not at least consider political changes to promote wellbeing, only that we should be realistic about the effective size of such efforts.[13]

Lyubomirsky and others have convincingly argued that there is hope for intentional interventions to increase happiness and that it comes from a burgeoning subfield of psychology: positive psychology. One aim of this subfield is to use the techniques and power of scientific psychology to investigate which (if any) intentional techniques can be used to make people happier. In some sense the proposal is not entirely novel: at many bookstores one can find shelf after shelf stocked with self-help books that promise to make readers happier. No doubt some of the advice contained therein is good; the trouble is that there is little beyond anecdotal evidence: "the author tried this technique and became happier and so should you." I take it that the reader will see the problems with this sort of methodology.

Positive psychology attempts to bring the rigors of the scientific method to bear on the question. Here is an example of an empirical investigation of the effectiveness of strategies conjectured to boost happiness.[14] The research used the classical design of randomized assignment on experimental and control groups. The control (placebo) group was asked to write about early memories each night for a week. Five experimental groups were composed around the following tasks: (1) write a letter of gratitude to someone who had been kind to them; (2) write down three good things that happened each day for a week; (3) write and reflect for a week on a story of "you at your best"; (4) identify signature strengths and use one strength each day in a new way for a week; (5) identify signature strengths and use them more often for a week. Exercises (2) and (4) caused increased happiness for six months, the entire length of the study. The gratitude exercise had a more pronounced and immediate boost in happiness but the effect faded more rapidly than with (2) and (4). The study, then, shows in a scientifically rigorous way that happiness can be improved with effort. Other avenues of attitudinal and behavioral reform shown by this science to be causally efficacious include trying to cultivate a sense of optimism, 'living in the present,' savoring life's joys, committing to goals, and practicing religion and spirituality.[15]

But this raises an important question: if positive psychology provides us with a means to enhance our happiness, why should we pursue happy-people-pills? There are two related answers to this. First, genetics (at least on a population level) is the largest single factor in happiness variation. Notice that this is true even using the more conservative figure of 50 percent heritability that Lyubomirsky and others cite. Again, if Lykken's argument is correct, that single-trait measures are likely to underestimate the heritability of any genetic predisposition to positive affect, then this only strengthens the case for attacking the genetic component to happiness.

Second, clearly it is not a matter of one over the other. If you will forgive the somewhat trite analogy, if happiness is a rowboat, the question is like asking which oar should we pull: the oar of positive psychology or the oar of genetics? The greatest advances will be made if we pull both. Indeed, I am a big fan of positive psychology: I believe it should get more funding and would encourage more researchers to pursue this line of inquiry. (The field also seems to attract more than its fair share of practitioners whose scientific credentials are marginal – to put it politely. I am talking about investing in the *science* of positive psychology.) So, the question is not whether positive psychology can help, which I think it can, but whether it is all we need in our pursuit of happiness. The heritability research above indicates that this is not likely to be so. Positive psychology may help us each maximize our potential given our genetic endowment, but it is not going to fundamentally change our genetic endowment. Thus, we are almost certain to get better results if the two oars of happiness, the biological and the non-biological, pull in the same direction.

7.4   PGD and Genetic Technologies

There are at least three promising technologies we could use to change the biological basis of happiness: pre-implantation genetic diagnosis, genetic engineering, and advanced pharmacology. Of course the topic of this book is advanced pharmacology, but it is worth pausing to consider, albeit very briefly, the other two.

At least from a technical rather than an ethical perspective, the most straightforward means to leverage the knowledge that there is a biological component to happiness involves using pre-implantation genetic diagnosis (PGD). PGD is presently used most commonly for screening for genetic diseases. Couples having difficulty conceiving will use IVF technology to create embryos in the lab and then one or more embryos will be implanted in the mother's womb. Often the embryos are tested for genetic diseases such as Down syndrome and cystic fibrosis. Couples may choose not to implant such embryos. Some IVF clinics offer future parents the chance to choose other embryos for non-therapeutic reasons; for example, some presently offer prospective parents the chance to choose embryos on the basis of gender. Prospective uses of PGD include selecting embryos with a greater chance of high IQ, athletic ability, perfect pitch, and so on. If researchers are able to discover genes associated with happiness, parents could potentially choose to implant embryos with a genetic disposition to greater positive affect.

Of course, it would be the crudest form of genetic determinism to think that parents have guaranteed the future happiness of their child. Choosing genes associated with high potential for positive affect is merely to open the first of a number of doors, for example absence of trauma in utero, good nutrition, a nurturing environment while growing up. So, selecting an embryo with a genetic predisposition for high chronic positive affect does not guarantee the remaining doors will be opened, but given the role of genes in our happiness, not choosing to open the first door will affect the prospects for future happiness.

A second possibility is to use genetic engineering to alter genes associated with happiness. Unlike PGD, germline engineering is a technology whose development lies in the future. Still, if we could identify genes associated with happiness, and we had a safe and reliable method for genetic engineering, then this would be one route to happy-people-pills. Using genetic engineering we could add or subtract gene sequences from each zygote to ensure the greatest chance of hyperthymia.

There are several obvious problems with using these technologies as a means to implement happy-people-pills. First, the relevant knowledge and technology are beyond us at present. Both PGD and genetic engineering require us to know which gene sequences are associated with happiness, which as yet we do not. This does not conflict with what we said above, that we know there is a strong heritable component to happiness, for knowing that a trait is heritable is not the same as knowing where the associated gene sequences lie on the human genome. And while knowledge of the associated gene sequences would be sufficient to perform PGD for selection of embryos disposed toward hyperthymia, it would not be enough for genetically engineering happiness. Genetic engineering requires in addition that we understand how to reliably manipulate the genome, something that is beyond our present abilities.

Second, even if we had the relevant expertise, there are large ethical questions involved in the use of PGD and genetic engineering. One thing that separates them from the use of advanced pharmacology is that they necessarily involve using technology on beings that cannot consent to treatment. Pharmacology can be and is used on patients who cannot consent, for example children, but of course, it is also often used to treat consenting adults. However, PGD and germline engineering will inevitably be used on the earliest human life, on beings who cannot consent.

Third, even supposing the technical and moral hurdles could be passed, these technologies offer no help to all those living today. By their very nature, PGD and germline engineering can help only future persons. This is not to say that these technologies ought not to be pursued, only that their widespread implementation is not likely to lie in the near future.

7.5   Research Proposal: Happy-People-Pills

The most promising strategy to create pharmacological agents to make the rest of us hyperthymic would be to develop a drug using the hyperthymic as a model. By seeing what makes them tick, what makes them different from the rest of us at the biological level, we will have a good bull's eye to aim for in creating happy-people-pills. The proposal, in other words, is to reverse-engineer the hyperthymic and put in pill form what they have by nature.

Let me describe in very broad strokes how the investigation might proceed. The first step in this research proposal is to identify the hyperthymic. Psychological inventories for happiness, selected for their congruence with the understanding of happiness in Chapter 3, should help differentiate the hyperthymic from the non-hyperthymic. We noted previously that happiness as a trait falls on a normal curve, so there is no reason to suppose that there is some clear-cut boundary between the hyperthymic and the rest. Scientists will have to operationally define 'hyperthymic' along the lines of: "For the purposes of this study, 'hyperthymia' is understood as the top 5% (or 7% or 10%, etc.) on the positive mood inventory."

The second step would be to deploy a variety of genetic and physiological tests. The genomes of the hyperthymic would be sequenced, as would the non-hyperthymic, to serve as a comparison class. Physiological measures including levels of various neurotransmitters would be tested in the hyperthymic and the non-hyperthymic.

The third step is to mine these data for commonalities using a combination of two strategies. The top-down approach looks for neurochemical and neurophysiological differences between the hyperthymic and the non-hyperthymic. Questions such as: "Do they differ in their levels of serotonin?," "dopamine?," "glutamate?," and so on. The bottom-up strategy involves comparing the genomes of the hyperthymic with the rest of the population to see if any gene sequences appear more frequently, or less frequently, in the hyperthymic population.

Looking for associated genes will likely not be a simple task. We noted previously that hyperthymia is almost certainly not a single-gene characteristic following Mendelian laws of inheritance. For example, some genetic diseases, such as Tay Sachs, are single-gene-recessive, and so for a child to suffer from Tay Sachs he must inherit the recessive gene from both parents. Since hyperthymia is likely not a single-gene characteristic, optimism cannot be based on success in finding single-gene diseases. Rather, optimism for success can be based on the confidence which underlies the search for genes associated with psychiatric disorders that are not single-gene-traits. These are known as 'multiple-gene disorders' or 'complex genetic disorders.' For example, research shows that persons who have half their genes in common with a person diagnosed with schizophrenia have about an 11 percent chance of developing schizophrenia, which is about eleven times the average rate for the general population. Children have half their genes in common with each parent, and siblings have half their genes in common, so someone with a sibling or a parent who is schizophrenic is at eleven times the risk of developing schizophrenia as the general population. This is well below the 25 percent one would expect if schizophrenia were associated with a single recessive gene. Even identical twins have a slightly less than 50 percent concordance rate. If your identical twin has schizophrenia, then your chances of having it are about 50/50.[16] Of course, shared environmental influences may explain some of this higher incidence, but there is much consensus for a large genetic influence.[17] Researchers have found two possible candidate genes, neuregulin-1 and dysbindin, that might explain some of the incidence of schizophrenia.[18] Interestingly, both genes are thought to contribute to structural connections between nerve cells.[19] This means that a study at the chemical level, investigating simply neurotransmitters for example, may have missed this result. We will return to this point shortly.

One of the main difficulties in attempting to work out the genetics of complex genetic disorders is that different genes may cause the same condition, and the mere presence of some genes does not inevitably lead to the condition. So, if, as seems likely, hyperthymia turns out to be a "complex genetic characteristic," influenced by a number of genes and environmental conditions, then progress in finding genetic correlates will not be straightforward. But the fact that some progress has been made with complex genetic disorders like schizophrenia provides some optimism that progress could be made.

The search for genetic correlates is likely to become easier with the falling price of genetic testing and computing power. The Human Genome Project catalogued many of the three billion or so nucleotides that make up the human genome. It is estimated that there are about three million common variations in the three billion nucleotides, and these variations account for much of the genetic diversity between humans. If the DNA of a group of hyperthymics is tested against the DNA of the rest of the population, genetic linkages may be found using statistical programs. Obviously this is a staggering amount of data, but something that is decreasingly expensive to crunch with more sophisticated statistical programs.

Imagine for the moment that genes associated with happiness were discovered. Developing pharmacological agents requires us to understand how genes contribute to hyperthymia. For example, if it is discovered that the hyperthymic have genes that result in increased levels of serotonin or dopamine, then pharmacological agents might be developed to mimic these effects. If the genetic differences point to structural differences in the nerves, as is the case with some genes associated with schizophrenia, then this will be the catalyst to seek pharmacological agents to mimic these variances.

Top-down and bottom-up approaches are not antagonistic; indeed, much good may come from pursuing both simultaneously. As noted above, the bottom-up process of looking for genetic differences led to the discovery of physiological differences in patients with schizophrenia. We can imagine genetic sequencing of the hyperthymic may lead to similar results. Conversely, differences in, say, levels of serotonin or dopamine may guide researchers in a top-down manner to look for genetic differences associated with their production.

There is, of course, no guarantee that we can discover the genes or their functions, or mimic their effects pharmacologically. Again, some optimism that this might be possible comes from current research into the genetics of mental disorders like Alzheimer's and schizophrenia. To treat these afflictions requires overcoming the same sorts of obstacles: namely, identifying the associated genes, understanding the causal role of the genes in manifestations of Alzheimer's and schizophrenia, and, finally, developing pharmacological agents to overcome these genetic influences. Since the same obstacles stand in the way of generating pharmacological agents to create hyperthymia, we ought to be similarly optimistic (or pessimistic) about the technical possibility of creating pharmacological agents for hyperthymia and the prospects of treating these devastating diseases. Since many leading researchers are optimistic about the prospects for developing pharmacological agents to treat schizophrenia and Alzheimer's based on genetic knowledge,[20] we should hold out similar optimism for this approach to happy-people-pills.

Indeed, the methodology described here is borrowed entirely from how researchers currently tackle these diseases. There may be large ethical differences between therapy and enhancement, but at the biological level there is no difference in how research should proceed. Considered simply as scientific programs, eliminating all social and ethical considerations, the prospects for success or failure are exactly the same for both. Assuming time and money are not being wasted now by the cadre of scientists investigating the genetics of schizophrenia and Alzheimer's disease, there is not a single scientific reason why we should not initiate a program today to reverse-engineer the hyperthymic and attempt to develop pharmacological agents based on this knowledge.

7.6   Antidepressants: the Healy Study

The proposal to develop pharmaceuticals based on reverse-engineering hyperthymia is for a medium-term project. Estimates of how long it will take to develop advanced pharmaceuticals for treatment of schizophrenia are in the order of 5–20 years (although, as we will note below, only a range can be endorsed because it depends on the quantity of resources devoted to the task). Is there anything more immediate we might do?

I take it that it is fairly obvious that alcohol and street drugs like marijuana and cocaine are not going to fill the gap in promoting happiness. In terms of recreational use, I take no position on these drugs (at least in this work). Still, as permanent mood boosters they have obvious problems that prohibit them being considered as plausible candidates for fulltime enhancement. It is pretty hard to keep a job, one's health, and one's family when one is permanently drunk or stoned. The most plausible stopgap possibility, I want to argue, is to experiment with antidepressants on the normally happy.

The number of people currently taking antidepressants to treat depression is subject to some debate, but a figure of one in eight adults in the US is one of the more conservative estimates.[21] If it is thought that antidepressants should be universally prescribed for the depressed, then they may be under-prescribed, because up to 20 percent of Americans suffer from depression.[22] This multibillion-dollar industry has created such household names as 'Prozac,' 'Paxil,' 'Zoloft,' 'Celaxa,' 'Lexapro,' and 'Effexor.' Certainly, for some patients, taking antidepressants has made all the difference: lives marred by oppressive and ubiquitous depression have been turned around with their use. One only needs to read any number of case studies where individuals find relief from their use that years of therapy never succeeded in providing.[23] Even critics of happy-people-pills concede that pharmaceuticals can be of enormous therapeutic value.[24]

Like many pharmacological agents, there was evidence that antidepressants were effective in treating depression long before we had any idea exactly how they work. Indeed, the original discoveries were made quite by accident: drugs that were originally designed to treat other illnesses such as tuberculosis were found to have mood-boosting properties.[25]

One of the many intriguing aspects of antidepressants is that it often takes weeks, sometimes months, before they have any clinical effect. This in itself should signal how unlike they are to alcohol and street drugs: imagine drinking several beers a day but not getting drunk for six weeks. Nor is it the case that antidepressants simply build up. The rate at which antidepressants are purged from the body is measured in hours, not days. Indeed, pharmaceutical companies typically search for a way to make them work for a longer period of time; for example, one can purchase Prozac in a once-a-week formulation. An emerging explanation is that antidepressants promote the growth of new neurons in the hippocampus, the emotional center of the brain.[26] This is quite an exciting discovery that offers a tidy explanation for why antidepressants often take weeks to work: it takes time for new neurons to grow.

Unfortunately, on enhancing the moods of healthy individuals, there is limited research. Perhaps the best-known is the study by Dr. David Healy mentioned in the first chapter. Recall that Healy had healthy volunteers – mostly from the medical profession – try two antidepressants in a "cross-over" study. Either Zoloft or Reboxetine was randomly (and blindly) given to participants for two weeks, followed by two weeks where subjects took nothing, then the study concluded with participants taking the other anti-depressant for two weeks. Recall, too, Healy's surprising findings:

> Our focus group met two weeks after the study ended. We already knew that almost everyone had preferred one of the two drugs. But two-thirds rated themselves as having done "better than well" on one or other of the drugs. Although this was a study of well-being, antidepressants weren't supposed to make people who were normal feel "better than well." Not even Peter Kramer had said this. The argument of his famous *Listening to Prozac* was that people who were mildly depressed on Prozac became better than well.[27]

The fact that two thirds of these "normal and healthy" volunteers felt "better than well" sounds like good news for happy-people-pills. Indeed it is, but the news is certainly not all good. For a start, the use of antidepressants is somewhat hit and miss. In the study mentioned by Healy, two thirds of the volunteers felt better than well, so the effects of the drugs were not uniformly positive. And indeed, some subjects felt better on one antidepressant and not on the other, indicating that the effects of the drugs are quite variable or that the desirability of the effects varies with users. Of course, in itself this is not a decisive criticism; it simply suggests that at worst some experimenting might have to be done by normally happy individuals before they find an appropriate pharmacological agent.

However, antidepressants have unwanted side effects for some individuals, including reduced interest in sexual activity, nausea, constipation, and weight gain. The most disturbing result of Healy's healthy-volunteers study is that Zoloft dramatically increased the risk of suicidal ideation; specifically, two of the healthy volunteers began to have thoughts of suicide while on Zoloft. The Healy study illustrates the need to answer two important questions: Are antidepressants causally efficacious in boosting the moods of healthy volunteers? What side effects do antidepressants have on healthy volunteers?

7.7   The Efficacy of Antidepressants on Healthy Volunteers

The paucity of studies of the effects of antidepressants on healthy individuals is underscored by a recent meta-study by Repantis, Schlattmann, Laisney, and Heuser.[28] It is important to clarify that this is not to say that there were few studies involving antidepressants and healthy volunteers. Indeed, one unexpected result was that the literature search conducted by the researchers revealed a large number of pertinent studies: 135. However, very few of the studies were done specifically to test for enhancement; most tests were conducted to examine possible side effects. So, information about enhancement effects was almost invariably incidental to the main goal of most of these studies. Of course this in itself is not necessarily a problem, for often studies designed with one goal may be mined for other purposes. Nevertheless, in most cases this led to two important shortcomings. One was the length of the studies. It is well documented that in tests of the therapeutic efficacy of antidepressants they often take weeks to show measurable results. The meta-review found that only 17 studies of the 135 went on more than two weeks, and only one study lasted six weeks, which is the usual length of study for efficacy in treating depression. In other words, if we were looking for the efficacy of antidepressants to treat depression, only one study is of an appropriate length. A further problem is the tools for measuring the efficacy of treatment. Since the studies were not designed specifically to track mood enhancement in healthy volunteers, many studies may have missed crucial data. For example, using the Hamilton Depression Scale to measure the efficacy of an experimental drug to treat depression may make sense, but the same scale is probably not going to be a very good instrument for detecting mood enhancement in healthy volunteers, since it is designed to detect differences at the low end of the mood scale.

Despite these shortcomings, the authors of the meta-study found that

> For most of the outcomes an effect emerging over time could be found. Most interesting was the positive effect on mood that continuously increased over time. If the trials had been longer and had had more assessment points, one could speculate that this effect would persist or even become stronger or that a ceiling effect would emerge. One should also take into account that the majority of the studies included in this systematic review were not on enhancement and, therefore, the participants did not have any particularly high expectations that would generate a placebo effect. Nevertheless, a placebo effect did exist. However, there was still a small placebo-verum difference that was statistically significant at the last assessment point. Consequently, it is important to note that antidepressants even in healthy, non-depressed individuals seem to be able to heighten mood.[29]

As the authors repeatedly note, this conclusion must be tempered with the fact that almost no direct research has been conducted on the question, and that few of the studies meet the gold standard for research in this area: placebo-controlled, double-blind, long-term research.

The fact that there is even suggestive evidence that antidepressants may boost mood in the healthy may strike some as unlikely, given some of the skepticism about antidepressants in therapeutic applications. The question of the efficacy of antidepressants to treat depression seems to erupt with almost cyclical regularity. A few years ago a firestorm was precipitated in part by a meta-study by Irving Kirsch and his colleagues.[30] They remark: "there seems little evidence to support the prescription of antidepressant medication to any but the most severely depressed patients." Obviously, even if antidepressants aren't effective in treating the mildly depressed, it does not follow that they might not be effective in boosting the moods of the healthy. Still, the finding suggests that we ought to be at least suspicious of any claim of boosting the moods of the healthy if we have been so radically deceived about the efficacy of antidepressants to treat the depressed.

The words "radically deceived" are not used lightly. As noted, antidepressants are a multibillion-dollar industry, and have gone, in a generation, from being infrequently prescribed to the first line of attack on depression; in many cases, they displace other types of therapy altogether. However, there are two problems worth mentioning with accepting Kirsch and colleagues' findings.

The first is a difficulty raised by Erick Turner and Robert Rosenthal about the relationship between the Kirsch team's findings and their conclusion. In a study that predates the Kirsch study, Turner and Rosenthal found an effect size of 0.31,[31] while Kirsch's team found an effect size of 0.32. So, their data are in very close accordance, but their conclusions are surprisingly different. The conclusion of the Turner team's study was basically that the effect size of antidepressants is oversold in many journal publications. This conclusion is much more modest than the conclusion offered by Kirsch et al.: "there seems little evidence to support the prescription of antidepressant medication to any but the most severely depressed patients." Obviously there is a huge difference between the claims that the efficacy of antidepressants is exaggerated and the claim that there is little evidence of their efficacy. Clearly, too, the later conclusion makes for much better press, but how did the two studies come to such different conclusions? In their review of the findings of Kirsch et al., Turner and Rosenthal offer a compelling explanation. The Kirsch study used the standard for clinical efficacy from the UK's National Institute for Health and Clinical Excellence (NICE): a medium effect size of 0.5 is required for clinical efficacy. Once this definition is accepted, the logic is inescapable: 0.32 is less than 0.5, so antidepressants are not clinically effective.

The trouble is that the NICE definition is not particularly convincing in this context. Imagine you are depressed and you see your health practitioner who says that the only treatment available is antidepressants, but they are not clinically effective according to the NICE definition, even though clinical studies have shown a small (0.31) effect. Surely the correct response would be: "to hell with the NICE definition. If antidepressants are the only game in town then even a small effect size is better than none." Of course any hope for relief would have to be tempered by the realization that the established effect size applies to populations. There is the real possibility that antidepressants may have no effect on your depression. On the other hand, they might turn your life around. Now contrast this with the case where your health care practitioner in the future tries to sell you some new expensive antidepressant which Kirsch and colleagues have shown to have an effect size of 0.51, and so meets NICE's definition of clinical significance. Even though it meets this definition of clinical efficacy, still you would be right to ignore this if a new cognitive talk-therapy was available for free, was fast-acting and had an effect size of 0.95. So, Kirsch and colleagues are able to reach their stunning conclusion by adopting a stunningly unmotivated definition of clinical effectiveness.[32] (Just to clarify: I am not saying that there is no point in NICE's definition, only that it is entirely irrelevant for the purposes under discussion.)

The second criticism is not indigenous to Kirsch's meta-study, but is a much more pervasive weakness of almost all pharmacological studies. As was suggestive even in the small Healy study, a pattern that emerges is that people react quite differently to antidepressants. This is confirmed in clinical practice: psychiatrists may prescribe some combination of two or three antidepressants to be taken simultaneously. Since psychiatrists do not know which will work best for their patients in advance, this is usually done by trial and error. Obviously this can be very trying for patients. If there were only ten antidepressants that patients might try, there are 630 combinations that a patient might try. As we noted, the full effect of these drugs may take weeks if not months. Finding the right combination can be quite arduous for patients.

The fact that one size does not fit all has profound implications for how any future research on pharmacological agents for enhancement ought to proceed. Consider how a typical study for therapeutic efficacy might be done. We start with 100 patients all diagnosed as depressed. We randomly assign 50 to a control group and 50 to the experimental group. The control group receives a placebo, while the experimental group takes the pharmacological agent under investigation. Suppose we are using the Hamilton scale, where 14 corresponds to mildly depressed, 25–54 to severely depressed, and 6 and less to healthy. Suppose the average for the two groups is 14 at the beginning of the study, and we find after six weeks that the control group's and the experimental group's average is 12. The conclusion of this study then would be that the new drug is not effective. Both groups showed mild improvement, but each result can be explained in terms of the placebo effect. Suppose, however, that we find upon further investigation that there is more variance in the experimental group; for example, 25 patients' scores actually get worse and rise to 20 (+6) and the other half reduce to 4 (−8) in the normal range. When we average these out, the experimental group would improve by 2 points, exactly the same as the control group. But using this gross measure would fail to reveal the fact that it appears that half were harmed by the antidepressant (their scores went up), while the other half benefited (their scores went down). In this artificial case, the results are so polarized that any researcher could see it without advanced statistical methods.

If we start out with the assumption that one size does not fit all, then a better experimental methodology would be as follows. Start by administrating to all 100 test subjects the experimental drug for phase 1 of the experiment. Given the assumption that it may be harmful to some, have little effect on others, and help others, the second phase of the experiment would take as subjects only those whose depression scores improved by some margin. Say 50 subjects' scores improved by 8 points; they would move to the second phase of the study. Here we would introduce a placebo control: 25 would be randomly assigned to a placebo group while the others would continue taking the experimental drug. After a few weeks the averages between the groups would be compared to see if the initial improvement was merely a placebo effect or whether the drug was causally efficacious. If the scores of the placebo group are no different, then we would have good evidence that the drug does not work; if there is a difference, then we have good evidence of the efficacy of the drug.

This sort of methodology is somewhat unorthodox and more expensive to test, but it would give us a much better idea of whether pharmacological agents are effective for some subpopulation. So, this would not necessarily undermine the conclusion that any chosen antidepressants have a small effect on the general population (for example, the conclusion of the Turner and Kirsch studies above). But for individual patients this is not particularly useful information. The study design proposed here would allow us to say something like this to patients: "If you try this antidepressant, there is a 50/50 chance that it will do nothing or make things worse for you. However, if the drug works, then it is likely to work quite well for you." For example, on a population level the small effect found by Kirsch et al. of 0.32 could be because of a very strong effect in one third of the population and no effect (or negative effect) in the other two thirds of the population, for any given antidepressants. Obviously it is not particularly helpful to be told that some pharmacological agent benefits half the population if you do not know which half the patient is in. As noted, presently this typically means trial and error at the individual level.[33]

There may be suspicions of circular reasoning here in the study design, but I think it is misplaced. A positive experimental outcome would not conclude that the drug works on those patients whom it works for, but rather that the drug works on patients whom it *appears* to work for. The first phase sorts out those whom it appears to work for, and the second phase assesses whether it does work on those whom it appears to work for. Drug companies are not likely to be enthusiastic about such an approach. Not only is it more expensive to run clinical experiments, but also it would be an admission that the drug is not for everyone in the target group of their marketing efforts.

Obviously the same methodology should be used for testing for efficacy with enhancement. The results from the Healy study confirm why this would be important. As he noted, two thirds felt better than well, but not everyone did. And for each drug, only one third felt better. The proposed two-stage testing would first select only those who appear to benefit from the test drug, and then in the second stage test those who appear to benefit from the drug by randomly assigning them to a control and an experimental group.

7.8 Side Effects of Antidepressants on Healthy Volunteers

In terms of side effects, the authors of the enhancement study reported that "no evidence of a significant adverse event profile could be found. Antidepressants seem to be relatively safe in healthy individuals and had a high acceptability in a population that had a rather uncertain and small anticipated benefit."[34] This may seem surprising given how often unwanted side effects of antidepressants are discussed. Two points are worth mentioning in this connection.

First, the qualification "significant" is important in their conclusion. The meta-study on enhancement also confirmed that antidepressants seem to have some negative side effects. Of the 135 studies, 84 reported side effects and 20 reported no adverse effects. Among the adverse effects were nausea, diarrhea, dry mouth, epigastric pain, sleep disturbance, restlessness, tremor, headache, dizziness, fatigue, and drowsiness. However, often symptoms disappeared quite quickly. Also of note is that not everyone experienced the adverse effects equally. Some subjects showed no ill effects, while others suffered terribly and dropped out of the study altogether.

The second reason we ought not to be too surprised that healthy volunteers seem to handle antidepressants with relatively few adverse effects can be explained in part by the nocebo effect.[35] The nocebo effect is the antipode of the placebo effect. Subjects taking a sugar pill (the classic placebo) may experience symptomatic relief simply because they expect to. Similarly, some subjects taking a sugar pill experience adverse effects because of the expectation of side effects. So, just as some of the clinical effectiveness of antidepressants is due to the placebo effect, some of the adverse effects are due to the nocebo effect. The relevance of this is that it has been established that the placebo and nocebo effects are stronger in some segments of the depressed population, so it is not surprising to find that healthy volunteers do not seem to experience as many adverse reactions to antidepressants as the clinically depressed.

Although not pleasant, these side effects are a lot less worrisome than the suicide ideations noted in the Healy study. Readers of Healy's book, *Let Them Eat Prozac*, will find a tale of nefarious activities by major pharmaceutical companies. To call the industry corrupt is an understatement. Part of the problem, and only a part, is that the drug companies run their own trials, and publish the most flattering data and work hard to suppress the damaging data. So we need to be on guard in assessing research.

Newer studies tend to be more reliable, given new standards for transparency and reporting in many medical and scientific journals. And some of the newer data suggests that there may be no increased risk for suicide, at least with the newer antidepressants.[36] More surprising, given all the recent uproar about the role of antidepressants in suicide, is research that indicates that certain classes of antidepressants may actually reduce suicide.[37] Bear in mind that these new studies do not change the fact that pharmaceutical companies withheld pertinent information, especially in the 1990s, and so are culpable of putting profits before people.

One of the things we should remember is that even if the suicide rate does not change, it may affect which individuals commit suicide: antidepressants might relieve symptoms in one patient and cause suicidal ideation in another. The good news here is that with increasing awareness that antidepressants might have this effect, there is hope that the suicide rate will go down. Healy's study makes a good illustration of this point. When he conducted the trial there was little expectation that antidepressants might cause suicidal ideation, and so the two participants in the study who experienced these adverse effects did not immediately reveal the trouble they were experiencing to those monitoring the study. If the experiment were repeated today, with more widely publicized knowledge of this possible effect, participants forewarned would be in much less danger. Thus, just knowing the possible effect should help reduce the number of suicides. We will deal more with the issue of side effects in Chapter 10.

7.9   Open-Source Mood Enhancement

We saw above that the conclusion by Repantis and colleagues sounded fairly positive for the idea that antidepressants boost the moods of the normally happy: "Consequently, it is important to note that antidepressants even in healthy, non-depressed individuals seem to be able to heighten mood." Again, this conclusion is qualified by the authors on the basis that there are almost no studies specifically designed to address this question. So, it is far too early to conclude definitively that antidepressants boost the moods of healthy volunteers. What little evidence we have, however, is suggestive and this area is certainly worthy of further study.

Consequently, we should welcome fully transparent studies by big pharmaceutical companies that show the efficacy or lack thereof of antidepressants on healthy volunteers. Transparency has been a real problem for big pharmaceuticals for a long time. Some of these problems have been mentioned, but it will help to have a more inclusive list: not reporting negative findings, underreporting negative symptoms, lack of reporting of conflict of interest, names being included on papers of persons who did not participate in research, and names not being included, and so on. Individual pharmaceutical companies have to take some of the blame, but there is a systemic problem that makes it hard for individual companies to do the right thing. Suppose company A becomes more transparent, while companies B and C continue business as usual. Company A may suffer a serious setback in sales, and face a backlash from investors for doing the right thing. This is not to say that company A does not have such a moral responsibility, only that we should predict trouble when it is so hard to do the right thing. In any event, this is not the place to rehearse all the problems with the pharmaceutical industry or canvass systemic changes to it.

Even if there weren't problems of transparency in the industry, pharmaceutical companies have little incentive to study the effects of antidepressants on healthy individuals unless there is some expectation of a return on their investment. (Love of humanity is not a huge motivational force in the drug industry – or other industries for that matter.) This means that the only antidepressants that might get tested for enhancement purposes are ones under patent, that is, the more expensive ones.

An alternative that may get around some of these problems is an open-source approach. Let me describe how it might work with a specific example and then list some possible advantages. Let us suppose that 32 people decide to cooperate to test the enhancement potential of drug X. The role of researcher is assigned to two, while 30 people volunteer as subjects. One researcher is tasked with packaging and numbering three months' worth of an antidepressant for 15 people, as well as placebos for 15 individuals for three months. The second researcher distributes the pills to the subjects, but is kept ignorant of which gel caps contain the placebos and which contain the antidepressant. At random intervals a text message is sent to the 30 individuals asking them to report back on their mood and any side effects. After three months the code is broken to find out who was taking the placebo and who had the antidepressant. The numbers are then crunched to see what the effect size, if any, is. (Of course the study could also incorporate the two-part methodology for testing efficacy noted above, but we will ignore the complication to keep the illustration simple.)

The beauty of the system is that it could be done on a shoestring budget: the major expense would be three months' worth of antidepressants for fifteen people. If the antidepressant is off patent, the cost for the entire experiment may be less than $5,000 (assuming people use their own cell phones, labor is voluntary, and a personal computer is used to crunch the data using freely available software). Obvious safeguards could and should be built in: a check-up from one's physician before participation, and perhaps a family member also reporting occasionally on the subject's condition.

We are not in a position to assert that this open-source project should be initiated, but at this point, we can conclude that there is no technical reason why the experiment could not be run. The results would be as scientifically valid as any research done by big pharmaceutical companies; indeed, since the researchers do not have a monetary stake in the outcome there would be less worry about researcher bias.

There are several advantages to this proposal. One is simply more reliable data. The more experiments done under transparent conditions, the more data, and more reliable data, there will be. There is little danger of an inflated effect size, as so often happens when big pharmaceutical companies get to manage what data are released, since we will suppose that the data (positive or negative) will be published online. Another benefit is that adverse effects are more likely to be reported, and researchers will be more motivated to seek information on adverse effects. A third positive is that off-patent drugs could be tested. As we said, there is almost no incentive for companies to run new clinical trials once a drug is off patent (and cannot be re-patented). A fourth advantage is the increased likelihood of testing combination therapies. Researchers recently tracked a 40 percent increase in the average number of medications prescribed, with the median doubling from 1 to 2 medications in a ten-year period.[38] Thus, clinical practice has far outstripped controlled studies, for obvious reasons, not the least being that there is little financial incentive to research the practice. Also, there is a combinatorial explosion once testing of multiple medications is tackled. Imagine there are only two drugs to be tested, A and B. To test them individually requires two tests, and in combination a third test. But now consider four antidepressants, A, B, C, and D. To test their efficacy where single prescription is the norm four tests must be run. The number of additional tests where clinicians commonly prescribe multiple combinations rises to 10: AB, AC, AD, ABC, ABD, ABCD, BC, BD, BCD, CD. We noted above that with 10 drugs there are 630 combinations, and because dozens of drugs are commonly prescribed, this means that there is a very large pool of combinations. An open-source project could help with large research holes.

Just in case there is any mistake, I am not saying that we should all go on antidepressants today. Rather, I am advocating responsible testing of antidepressants. I am not averse to all individual experimentation, but the most useful data would come from placebo-controlled, double-blind studies. It need hardly be mentioned that such experiments face formidable legal hurdles in some jurisdictions. Some problems lie in the fact that in many jurisdictions medical health care practitioners are the only legal means to obtain antidepressants. At least part of the problem here could be circumvented by co-opting family physicians to prescribe antidepressants or placebos in consultation with the researchers. Of course this would make the study "single blind," since the family physician would know whether her patient was receiving the placebo or the antidepressant. The other major problem is the legal gray area of enhancement itself. These are realities that need to be dealt with. However, if social and political obstacles can be met, then open-source testing of enhancement offers an inexpensive means to scientifically test the efficacy of the enhancement potential of antidepressants.

Notes

1. Lykken and Tellegen, "Happiness Is a Stochastic Phenomenon"; Lykken, *Happiness*; Tellegen et al., "Personality Similarity in Twins Reared Apart and Together"; Stubbe et al., "Heritability of Life Satisfaction in Adults."
2. Roberts, Billewicz, and McGregor, "Heritability of Stature in a West African Population."
3. Lykken and Tellegen, "Happiness Is a Stochastic Phenomenon."
4. Lyubomirsky, *The How of Happiness*.
5. Lykken, "A More Accurate Estimate of Heritability."

6. Lykken cites himself ("What's Wrong with Psychology, Anyway?") in support of this comment.

7. Lykken, "A More Accurate Estimate of Heritability," 168.

8. Ibid., 173.

9. Ibid.

10. Lyubomirsky, *The How of Happiness*.

11. Lucas and Donnellan, "How Stable is Happiness?"

12. Boehm and Lyubomirsky, "The Promise of Sustainable Happiness."

13. For concrete suggestions see Bok, *The Politics of Happiness*, and Diener, Lucas, and Schimmack, *Well-being for Public Policy*. Haybron, *The Pursuit of Unhappiness*, has a few cryptic suggestions.

14. Seligman et al., "Positive Psychology Progress."

15. Lyubomirsky, *The How of Happiness*.

16. Sullivan, "The Genetics of Schizophrenia."

17. National Institute of Mental Health, "Genetics and Mental Disorders"; Merikangas and Risch, "Will the Genomics Revolution Revolutionize Psychiatry?"

18. Stefansson et al., "Neuregulin 1 and Schizophrenia"; Straub et al., "Genetic Variation in the 6p22. 3 Gene DTNBP1, the Human Ortholog of the Mouse Dysbindin Gene, is Associated with Schizophrenia."

19. Barondes, *Better Than Prozac*, 109.

20. See Barondes, *Better Than Prozac*, for a popular review.

21. Shim et al., "Prevalence, Treatment, and Control of Depressive Symptoms in the United States."

22. President's Council on Bioethics, *Beyond Therapy*, Ch. 5, n. 16.

23. For examples of such case studies see Kramer, *Listening to Prozac*, and Barondes, *Better Than Prozac*. We will deal with skepticism about the efficacy of antidepressants below.

24. President's Council on Bioethics, *Beyond Therapy*; Fukuyama, *Our Posthuman Future*.

25. Healy, *Let Them Eat Prozac*; Barondes, *Molecules and Mental Illness*.

26. Santarelli et al., "Requirement of Hippocampal Neurogenesis for the Behavioral Effects of Antidepressants"; Malberg et al., "Chronic Antidepressant Treatment Increases Neurogenesis in Adult Rat Hippocampus"; Kodama, Fujioka, and Duman, "Chronic Olanzapine or Fluoxetine Administration Increases Cell Proliferation in Hippocampus and Prefrontal Cortex of Adult Rat"; Warner-Schmidt and Duman, "VEGF is an Essential Mediator of the Neurogenic and Behavioral Actions of Antidepressants."

27. Healy, *Let Them Eat Prozac*, 280.

28. Repantis et al., "Antidepressants for Neuroenhancement in Healthy Individuals."

29. Ibid., 158.

30. Kirsch et al., "Initial Severity and Antidepressant Benefits." Kirsch has followed this up with a book treatment of the subject: Kirsch, *The Emperor's New Drugs*. Kirsch's book is critically reviewed by Bloom ("Placebo Versus Antidepressant. Review").

31. Turner et al., "Selective Publication of Antidepressant Trials and Its Influence on Apparent Efficacy."

32. Ibid.

33. It has been argued by Joyce, Mulder, and Cloninger that a psychological inventory of temperament predicts which depressed patients respond to drugs which augment norepinephrine, and which respond better to drugs that augment neurotransmission by serotonin ("Temperament Predicts Clomipramine and Desipramine Response in Major Depression"). As we shall see in the next chapter, there is evidence that genetic testing might also help predict response to antidepressants.

34. Repantis et al., "Antidepressants for Neuroenhancement in Healthy Individuals," 159.

35. Barsky et al., "Nonspecific Medication Side Effects and the Nocebo Phenomenon."

36. Simon et al., "Suicide Risk During Antidepressant Treatment."

37. Ludwig, Marcotte, and Norberg, "Anti-depressants and Suicide."

38. Mojtabai and Olfson, "National Trends in Psychotropic Medication Polypharmacy in Office-based Psychiatry."

References

Barondes, S. H. *Better Than Prozac: The Future of Psychiatric Drugs*. Oxford: Oxford University Press, 2003.

Barsky, A. J., R. Saintfort, M. P. Rogers, and J. F. Borus. "Nonspecific Medication Side Effects and the Nocebo Phenomenon." *Journal of the American Medical Association* 287, no. 5 (2002): 622–7.

Bloom, F. E. "Placebo Versus Antidepressant. Review: *The Emperor's New Drugs: Exploding the Antidepressant Myth*." *Cerebrum* June (2010).

Boehm, J. K. and S. Lyubomirsky. "The Promise of Sustainable Happiness." *Handbook of Positive Psychology* (2009): 667–77.

Bok, D. *The Politics of Happiness: What Government Can Learn from the New Research on Well-Being*. Princeton, N.J.: Princeton University Press, 2010.

Diener, E., R. Lucas, and U. Schimmack. *Well-being for Public Policy*. New York: Oxford University Press, 2009.

Fukuyama, F. *Our Posthuman Future: Consequences of the Biotechnology Revolution*. London: Profile, 2003.

Haybron, D. *The Pursuit of Unhappiness*. New York: Oxford University Press, 2008.

Healy, D. *Let Them Eat Prozac: The Unhealthy Relationship Between the Pharmaceutical Companies and Depression*. New York: New York University Press, 2004.

Joyce, P. R., R. T. Mulder and C. R. Cloninger. "Temperament Predicts Clomipramine and Desipramine Response in Major Depression." *Journal of Affective Disorders* 30, no. 1 (1994): 35–46.

Kirsch, I. *The Emperor's New Drugs: Exploding the Antidepressant Myth*. Sydney: ReadHowYouWant, 2010.

Kirsch, I., B. J. Deacon, T. B. Huedo-Medina, A. Scoboria, T. J. Moore, and B. T. Johnson. "Initial Severity and Antidepressant Benefits: A Meta-analysis of Data Submitted to the Food and Drug Administration." *PLoS Medicine* 5, no. 2 (2008): e45.

Kodama, M., T. Fujioka, and R. S. Duman. "Chronic Olanzapine or Fluoxetine Administration Increases Cell Proliferation in Hippocampus and Prefrontal Cortex of Adult Rat." *Biological Psychiatry* 56, no. 8 (2004): 570–80.

Kramer, P. *Listening to Prozac*. New York: Penguin Books, 1993.

Lucas, R. E. and M. B. Donnellan. "How Stable is Happiness? Using the STARTS Model to Estimate the Stability of Life Satisfaction." *Journal of Research in Personality* 41, no. 5 (2007): 1091–8.

Ludwig, J., D. E. Marcotte, and K. Norberg. "Anti-depressants and Suicide." *National Bureau of Economic Research Working Paper* 12906, 2007.

Lykken, D. T. *Happiness: What Studies on Twins Show Us About Nature, Nurture, and the Happiness Set-point*. New York: Golden Books, 1999.

Lykken, D. T. "A More Accurate Estimate of Heritability." *Twin Research and Human Genetics: The Official Journal of the International Society for Twin Studies* 10, no. 1 (2007): 168–73.

Lykken, D. T. "What's Wrong with Psychology, Anyway?" In *Thinking Clearly About Psychology, Volume 1: Matters of Public Interest*, edited by D. Cicchetti and W. M. Grove, 3–39. Minneapolis: University of Minnesota Press, 1991.

Lykken, D. T. and A. Tellegen. "Happiness Is a Stochastic Phenomenon." *Psychological Science* 7, no. 3 (1996): 186–9.

Lyubomirsky, S. *The How of Happiness: A Scientific Approach to Getting the Life You Want*. New York: Penguin Books, 2008.

Malberg, J. E., A. J. Eisch, E. J. Nestler, and R. S. Duman. "Chronic Antidepressant Treatment Increases Neurogenesis in Adult Rat Hippocampus." *Journal of Neuroscience* 20, no. 24 (2000): 9104–10.

Merikangas, K. R. and N. Risch. "Will the Genomics Revolution Revolutionize Psychiatry?" *American Journal of Psychiatry* 160, no. 4 (2003): 625–35.

Mojtabai, R. and M. Olfson. "National Trends in Psychotropic Medication Polypharmacy in Office-based Psychiatry." *Archives of General Psychiatry* 67, no. 1 (2010): 26–36.

National Institute of Mental Health. "Genetics and Mental Disorders: Report of the National Institute of Mental Health's Genetics Workgroup." National Institutes of Health, 1998.

President's Council on Bioethics. *Beyond Therapy: Biotechnology and the Pursuit of Happiness*. New York: Dana Press, 2003.

Repantis, D., P. Schlattmann, O. Laisney, and I. Heuser. "Antidepressants for Neuroenhancement in Healthy Individuals: A Systematic Review." *Poiesis & Praxis: International Journal of Technology Assessment and Ethics of Science* 6, no. 3 (2009): 139–74.

Roberts, D. F., W. Z. Billewicz, and I. A. McGregor. "Heritability of Stature in a West African Population." *Annals of Human Genetics* 42, no. 1 (1978): 15–24.

Santarelli, L., M. Saxe, C. Gross, A. Surget, F. Battaglia, S. Dulawa, N. Weisstaub, J. Lee, R. Duman, O. Arancio, C. Belzung, and R. Hen. "Requirement of Hippocampal Neurogenesis for the Behavioral Effects of Antidepressants." *Science* 301, no. 5634 (2003): 805–9.

Seligman, M., T. A. Steen, N. Park, and C. Peterson. "Positive Psychology Progress: Empirical Validation of Interventions." *American Psychologist* 60, no. 5 (2005): 410–21.

Shim, R. S., P. Baltrus, J. Ye, and G. Rust. "Prevalence, Treatment, and Control of Depressive Symptoms in the United States: Results from the National Health and Nutrition Examination Survey (NHANES), 2005–2008." *Journal of the American Board of Family Medicine* 24, no. 1 (2011): 33–8.

Simon, G. E., J. Savarino, B. Operskalski, and P. S. Wang. "Suicide Risk During Antidepressant Treatment." *American Journal of Psychiatry* 163, no. 1 (2006): 41–7.

Stefansson, H., V. Steinthorsdottir, E. Thorgeirsson, R. Gulcher, and K. Stefansson. "Neuregulin 1 and Schizophrenia." *Annals of Medicine* 36, no. 1 (2004): 62–71.

Straub, R. E., Y. Jiang, C. J. MacLean, Y. Ma, B. T. Webb, M. V. Myakishev, C. Harris-Kerr, B. Wormley, H. Sadek, B. Kadambi, A. J. Cesare, A. Gibberman, X. Wang, F. A. O'Neill, D. Walsh, and K. S. Kendler. "Genetic Variation in the 6p22.3 Gene DTNBP1, the Human Ortholog of the Mouse Dysbindin Gene, is Associated with Schizophrenia." *American Journal of Human Genetics* 71, no. 2 (2002): 337–48.

Stubbe, J. H., D. Posthuma, D. I. Boomsma, and E. J. C. De Geus. "Heritability of Life Satisfaction in Adults: A Twin-family Study." *Psychological Medicine* 35, no. 11 (2005): 1581–8.

Sullivan, P. F. "The Genetics of Schizophrenia." *PLoS Medicine* 2, no. 7 (2005): e212.

Tellegen, A., D. T. Lykken, T. J. Bouchard, K. J. Wilcox, N. L. Segal, and S. Rich. "Personality Similarity in Twins Reared Apart and Together." *Journal of Personality and Social Psychology* 54 (1988): 1031–9.

Turner, E. H., A. M. Matthews, E. Linardatos, R. A. Tell, and R. Rosenthal. "Selective Publication of Antidepressant Trials and Its Influence on Apparent Efficacy." *New England Journal of Medicine* 358, no. 3 (2008): 252–60.

Warner-Schmidt, J. L. and R. S. Duman. "VEGF is an Essential Mediator of the Neurogenic and Behavioral Actions of Antidepressants." *Proceedings of the National Academy of Sciences of the United States of America* 104, no. 11 (2007): 4647–52.

8

Arguments for Happy-People-Pills

In this chapter we will canvass several arguments for happy-people-pills. Much of the groundwork has already been laid. The outline of a theory of wellbeing articulated in Chapters 3, 4, and 5 dovetails nicely with the social science research canvassed in Chapter 6. The argument turns on the idea that happy-people-pills will promote such fundamental prudential values as happiness, achievement, and virtue. Since happy-people-pills will promote wellbeing, this is a powerful reason to permit their use. I don't mean to suggest the argument is completely one-sided: in the following chapter we will consider arguments opposed to the use of happy-people-pills.

8.1 Autonomy

One of the most telling criticisms of *Brave New World* is that the citizenry lack autonomy. In this section the case will be made that, far from diminishing autonomy, happy-people-pills will enhance autonomy. Indeed, they will free us from "slavery" to the genetic endowment bestowed upon us by nature.

A brief examination of autonomy etymologically is quite suggestive: its roots mean something like "self-law-giver" or "self-governance." The history of the concept is often traced back to Kant, but its roots reach deeper in history.[1] Its importance for our self-understanding can hardly be overstated. It plays a vital part in contemporary (Western at least) political and ethical thought, and is often cited as a central value in bioethics.[2]

Happy-People-Pills For All, First Edition. Mark Walker.
© 2013 John Wiley & Sons, Inc. Published 2013 by John Wiley & Sons, Inc.

Not surprisingly, analyses of this important concept differ, but, as Marina Oshana argues, the idea that personal autonomy is often understood "as the condition of being self-directed, of having authority over one's choices and actions whenever these are significant to the direction of one's life,"[3] seems to capture what many see as essential to the idea that "autonomous agents are self-governing agents."[4] While there is little agreement about how to philosophically explicate the concept of autonomy, there is a reasonable consensus about when autonomy is absent.

Slavery is a paradigmatic case. Slaves have little ability to choose and execute a life plan, and so lack much in the way of autonomy. Another obvious example of loss of autonomy is incarceration: it is pretty hard for most to execute a life plan while in jail. Likewise, indoctrination leads to a loss of autonomy. We said that socialization in *Brave New World* has a large element of indoctrination. The point of indoctrination there is to ensure that the citizenry adopt the sort of life promoted by the state: Alpha-type lives for Alphas, Beta-type lives for Betas, and so on.

Controlling the emotions of others would be a comparable infringement upon autonomy. So, consider the machinations of Dr. Evil. Some time ago, he slipped a long-acting hyperthymic pill into Anna's coffee, and a dysthymic pill into Brianna's beverage. Slowly, over the course of several months, Anna moves from the "C" range on the happiness curve to the "A" range, while Brianna moves in the opposite direction, from the "A" range to the "C" range. Let us suppose that the pills act slowly enough that neither notices any dramatic change over the course of any particular week, and nor do their intimates. However, over the course of many months, Brianna finds her former zest for many activities is gone; she describes herself as "dragging a bit." Her change is both emotional and cognitive: she finds uninteresting and unenjoyable many things she formerly found interesting and enjoyable. For example, she used to like to go dancing on Saturday evenings but now she often spends them alone watching television. For Anna, the effect is quite opposite. Over several months she notices that she is more upbeat, she goes out more, meets new friends, and in general is more inclined to try new things.

Dr. Evil is guilty of violating the autonomy of Anna and Brianna. It is clear that he has greatly influenced their respective life plans in a manner that they did not authorize. This is not to say that they are worse off for the violation. While there is little reason to suppose that Brianna is better off, there is *perhaps some* argument that Anna is better off. But even if we could be convinced that she is better off, this does not show that Anna's autonomy was not violated: Anna did not authorize affecting her moods and emotions with the hyperthymic pill, and so Dr. Evil has clearly violated her autonomy.

If we turn the example around, we can see that if people are presented with the opportunity to take happy-people-pills, their autonomy will actually increase. If Anna decides that she wants to enjoy the fruits of having positive moods, and the downstream consequences of higher average positive moods, then the opportunity to take happy-people-pills provides her with more significant choices in selecting and executing a life plan. Formerly, no one had a choice about what to do about the genetic contribution to happiness. Now she has a choice: to live *au naturel* with the biological component of happiness bequeathed to her from the roulette wheel of nature, or to take happy-people-pills to boost her happiness and enhance her genetic endowment.

It is worth noting that the claim that happy-people-pills are autonomy-enhancing is not based simply on the fact that they provide a new choice. Some new choices are not autonomy-enhancing, as in that from the thief that jumps from behind the bushes and offers the brand new choice: "your money or your life?" Other new choices may be so insignificant that they do not affect autonomy to any appreciable degree; for example, your favorite restaurant adds a new wine to their list, but it is a type you dislike and would never order. It is true that you have more choice in this instance, but hardly one of much significance.

In contrast, the ability to alter moods is a much more significant choice because moods are both ubiquitous and deep. By 'ubiquitous' I mean that we are almost always in some mood or emotion. Almost invariably, our emotional state can be described as one or more of the following: aggravated, amused, annoyed, anxious, apathetic, bitchy, blah, blissful, bored, calm, cheerful, chipper, content, cranky, depressed, drained, ecstatic, energetic, excited, giddy, gloomy, happy, hopeful, hyper, irritated, lethargic, melancholic, mellow, optimistic, peaceful, refreshed, rejuvenated, satisfied, stressed, or tired. (As noted earlier, I take no position on which of these might be better described as a mood or as an emotion. Also, some items on this list are perhaps synonymous, and the list is not exhaustive.) To say that moods are deep is to invoke a metaphor, but it is hard to explain this metaphor without using others. Moods tend to "color" the way we experience the world, the way we reason, and the way we act. The earlier example of waking up on a spring morning in Canada may serve as illustration. Recall that in both cases you wake up to the exact same sound: birds chirping. In one case you find the noise objectionable, in the other you experience the same sound as pleasant. In both cases you reason to yourself about the challenge of starting a koi pond. In one case you judge the task objectionable, in the other a stimulating challenge. Likely it will mean quite different actions on your part: starting or ignoring the task. So the koi pond example is but a small illustration of the weighty effect moods can have on our experience and cognition.

To get some idea about the profoundness of having more control over our emotional states it may help to look at other examples that are both ubiquitous and deep. But our first obstacle is that they are not so easy to come by. It is easy to think of examples that are ubiquitous but not deep, or deep but not ubiquitous. Getting a tattoo is ubiquitous but not deep. The small tattoo on your shoulder is always there, but you never think about it much. The decision to see a movie about the genocide perpetrated by Pol Pot may affect you deeply, but over the course of a few weeks or months the experience no longer remains quite as vivid or troubling. While not entirely analogous, marriage and education are plausible candidates for things that are ubiquitous and deep. Of course not all marriages are ubiquitous and deep; some are for mere convenience and for short periods of time. But others do seem deep and ubiquitous: a marriage may change a person's thinking from mostly the first person singular to mostly the first person plural. No longer is it: "What should I do?" but "What should we do?" At least for some, getting a university education has an effect that is ubiquitous and profound. (Of course, for many others, universities are merely institutions for higher earnings.) So, happy-people-pills are autonomy-enhancing because they allow us to take control of something deep and ubiquitous, our emotional states, in a manner hitherto impossible. It is autonomy-enhancing in the same way that being able to choose a spouse enhances autonomy as compared with an arranged marriage, or the way that opening up universities to women and the less well-off enhanced the autonomy of many.

One obstacle to appreciating how autonomy-enhancing happy-people-pills could be is the assumption that we are largely responsible for our happiness or unhappiness. This assumption is so common it deserves a name: "the fallacy of deserved happiness." This fallacy is readily apparent once we realize the falseness of the idea that happiness floats free of all genetic influences and environmental influences over which we have no control. Take a concrete example: Alexis is not very happy. She is not clinically depressed by any stretch of the imagination, but unhappier than most; she is a "D" or a low "C" on our happiness scale. The fallacy of deserved happiness says that if she is unhappy she must be responsible for this. We can predict with almost apodictic certainty that those who know Alexis will make the following sorts of remarks:

> *Alexis never pursued opportunities for further education or training, and so it is not surprising that she is now stuck in a job that does not make her happy. And Alexis never seems to make many friends, and when she does it is never for very long. Every relationship she enters into inevitably blows up. We have talked to Alexis about this, yet she does not seem prepared to make the changes in her life that might bring her increased happiness. Her unhappiness is due to the life choices she has made, and the fact that she is not prepared to make positive changes, so she deserves whatever unhappiness she is experiencing.*

The first thing we might ask is whether it is true that people are always the authors of whatever happiness or unhappiness they experience. Consider that people are likely to revise an assessment of responsibility in light of information about strong environmental influences. In Alexis's case, suppose it is discovered that she was brought up in an appalling environment: her father was physically and sexually abusive and her mother was cold and unsupportive. Most, I think, would reverse the judgment that she is responsible for her unhappiness, for if at least some of the reason for her unhappiness is factors that she had little influence over she can hardly be said to be responsible for these influences. What we can conclude from this is that it is not always the case that a person can be said to be responsible for their own happiness, because some environmental events are beyond the control of the individual.

If we grant this in the case of environmental influences, then it seems we ought to, on pain of inconsistency, say the same about the strong genetic influences upon positive affect, which is to say that our folk psychology is wrong on this point: we do not have nearly as much control over our happiness as is often supposed. Happy-people-pills are a means by which we need no longer be merely passive with respect to our biological inheritance. It is something that we shall soon be able to control and so increase the sphere in which we may take authorship of our lives.

At the risk of sounding hyperbolic, the suggestion can be put in an even stronger form: happy-people-pills are a means of ending slavery to our emotional disposition. The analogy may be a bit much, but the point is that we have only so much control over something that affects us on such a profound level. This should not be taken to suggest that we have *no* intentional control over our happiness. As we have seen, some of the recommendations of positive psychology may help us to that end, as might societal changes. But there are severe limits to how much of our emotional lives we can control at present. The more we wrest control of our emotional lives from nature, the more autonomy we have. If the analogy is overdrawn, it is not because moods and emotions are merely trivial: as we have said, moods and emotions are deep and ubiquitous, affecting how we perceive and reason about our world and our lives. Where the analogy is stretched, perhaps, is in the thought that this is a form of slavery, for that seems to imply that nature (from whence our biology originates) is master.

The point may be accepted – it is too much to think of nature as enslaving, no better than complaining about the tyranny of the law of gravity. So it is at best a metaphor to say that we are enslaved at present to our biological natures. Be that as it may, the thought process issues a fair warning to the future: perhaps nature cannot be said to enslave us, but those who oppose the increase of autonomy through the use of happy-people-pills will be guilty of a form of slavery. It would force upon us something deep and ubiquitous: the biological natures we find ourselves with. We will return to this point in Chapter 10.

It will help to offer one clarification of the argument and respond to one objection. The clarification is that the argument should not be taken to imply that those presently low in positive affect lack autonomy. If we think in terms of having or lacking autonomy, this is what might be thought of as a threshold concept of autonomy. For example, sometimes the question of whether a patient is competent to make a medical decision turns on the question of whether the patient is autonomous or not. This is typically understood as a threshold concept: certain standards such as being sufficiently informed and sufficiently rational are prerequisites to meeting the threshold. There is no suggestion in our discussion that those low in positive affect are not autonomous. In our example we are assuming that Anna is autonomous prior to being offered the choice of happy-people-pills and so meets the threshold standard. However, this is consistent with the claim that the chance to take happy-people-pills will *increase* her autonomy.

The objection is this: if autonomy is enhanced by having the choice to have more positive moods, then autonomy could be further enhanced by having even more choices for significant life options: the choice to take an "unhappy-people-pill." Then, instead of only two choices, there would be three: to accept one's moods *au naturel*, to take happy-people-pills or to take unhappy-people-pills. But if this is the case, so the objection goes, then surely something has gone wrong with the argument.

The objection may be taken in one of two ways: either that control of our happiness is not autonomy-enhancing, or that it is not wellbeing-enhancing. Let us take these in turn in reference to an example. Let us imagine Suzie was born with the genes associated with hyperthymic persons, and was raised in an environment that allowed this genetic predisposition to be realized. Suzie, then, is hyperthymic, but finds herself wishing that she experienced more negative moods. It seems that she believes she would be a better artist if she could experience negative affect to a much greater extent. This is based on her belief that her artistic hero, Edvard Munch, experienced powerful negative emotions and this contributed to his great art.

It is hard to see how having access to unhappy-people-pills eliminates Suzie's brief that such pills contribute to her autonomy. This is not, obviously, to say that we think a decision to take such pills would make things better for her, but it is to say that it allows her more significant options to execute a life plan. Specifically, the hyperthymic like Suzie, even if their lives are in general more enviable than most, still have no more or less control over their emotional lives than the rest of us.* So, if hyperthymic pills are autonomy-enhancing for those in the lower normal range of happiness, then it seems by the same token that unhappy-people-pills are autonomy-enhancing for the hyperthymic. This is not an embarrassment for the argument, but a natural consequence of the general principle that greater control of our emotional lives means more autonomy.

The objection is probably better understood as the idea that more autonomy may not add to our wellbeing; in particular, having unhappy-people-pills may make us more autonomous, but not better off. This version of the objection is entirely consistent with the main argument of this work. The claim that we have made about the prudential goods on our long list is that, other things being equal, the more we have of each, the better off we are. If people destroyed other aspects of their lives with unhappy-people-pills, if the pills caused marriages to fail, people to lose

---

* At least as far as we know – this is an empirical conjecture. The assumption, in other words, is that the degree to which the hyperthymic can effectively will themselves to be unhappy is about the same as the degree to which the rest of us can effectively will ourselves to be happy.

their friends, and so on, then this would be some argument that the gain in autonomy is not worth the cost. But this is no objection to the main argument. For then we can simply say that while access to happy-people-pills and unhappy-people-pills enhances autonomy, only the former improves wellbeing overall.

We will canvass in the next chapter two objections involving authenticity and identity that are related to the notion of autonomy. For the moment, we can conclude that we have made at least a prima facie case for the idea that happy-people-pills will enhance autonomy.

8.2   Individual Wellbeing

The argument that the use of happy-people-pills will promote many aspects of wellbeing is perhaps fairly obvious at this point. Some of the earlier chapters have provided the necessary premises; it only remains to draw the conclusion. Briefly, the argument may be stated thus. In earlier chapters (3, 4, and 5) we gave an account of individual welfare that included a long list of intrinsic benefits: positive affect, friendship, health, knowledge, virtue, desire-satisfaction, etc. Since positive moods promote many of these items, and happy-people-pills will boost moods, happy-people-pills should increase individual welfare. Since the promotion of individual wellbeing is a positive moral good, this provides a powerful reason to suppose that use of happy-people-pills is a positive moral good.

It may help to illustrate the argument with an example. Suppose Juanita is a person you know who, by your estimation and that of professional psychologists, is not clinically depressed, but by no means the happiest person. Let us say she is slightly below average – she scores a low "C" – on our happiness normal curve. Suppose Juanita begins taking happy-people-pills. What should we predict will be the effects on her wellbeing?

Obviously, one thing we should predict is more positive moods and emotions. Perhaps not immediately, for it is not clear how long it would take happy-people-pills to elicit an observable effect. We noted above that the use of antidepressants on depressed patients often takes several weeks to show any effect, while in Healy's healthy volunteer study the antidepressants showed almost immediate effect. Conservatively we might suppose that within a few weeks we could expect to see Juanita more cheerful on average and for her to report feeling "brighter" moods with an extra spring in her step. If this prediction holds true, then it alone counts as a positive development in her wellbeing, since, as we have said, greater frequency of positive moods and emotions, other things being equal, is a positive in terms of wellbeing.

We noted previously that research indicates that happier people are likely to have more friends; so one of the downstream consequences of taking happy-people-pills that we should predict for Juanita is that she will have more friends. I term this a 'downstream consequence,' since obviously it is absurd to suppose that happy-people-pills will somehow magically cause friends to appear in Juanita's orbit. Rather, the build-and-broaden model mentioned earlier suggests that one way she may make more friends is that positive moods increase the likelihood that we will approach novel situations. In more positive moods Juanita is more likely to strike up a conversation with someone than if she avoids them while in a foul mood. Approaching people in this way is usually a necessary first step to making friends. Conversely, research shows that others are more likely to approach those whom they perceive as happy. Positive moods are friend-magnets.

The same research suggests that we ought to predict for Juanita more success in her love life, more educational attainment, more volunteering, and better mental and physical health. We should also predict improvement in other aspects of happiness. Recall, we said that happiness has three components: positive moods and emotions, positive attitudes, and sensory pleasure. Our best model of how pharmacology works says that it will most directly affect moods and emotions. However, it seems a likely conjecture that positive moods and emotions should have downstream consequences for both positive attitudes and sensory pleasure. Consider that as Juanita has more success in her love life and other aspects of her life, she will have more to be pleased about. Even prior to such increase in success, it seems a likely conjecture that positive moods and emotions will make it easier for people to focus on the positive and more likely that they will do so. If you are in a good mood, you are more likely to be pleased that the glass is half full than displeased that it is half empty. And so, positive moods and emotions should promote the positive attitudes identified by attitudinal hedonism: being pleased about something. Similarly, it is easy to imagine persons taking greater sensory pleasure – in the sip of a fine wine, or a gourmet meal – when they are in a good mood.

Admittedly, some of this is conjecture: scientists have not investigated the different aspects of happiness exactly as outlined in Chapter 3. There is some empirical support, however. We noted above that positive affect and life satisfaction ratings have been found to correlate at around 0.40 to 0.50 in undergraduates and 0.52 in business students.[5] We also noted that there is considerable overlap between some life satisfaction instruments and attitudinal hedonism. I'm not saying it is a sure thing that if scientists investigate the different aspects of happiness discussed they will find that positive moods and emotions cause an increase in attitudinal pleasure and sensory pleasure. I am saying it is a very good bet.

So, thinking about the effects of taking happy-people-pills, we ought to predict a broad range of improvements in Juanita's wellbeing. From here the argument is a cinch: other things being equal, if wellbeing increases we ought to see this as a significant moral positive.

There are several caveats that are worth mentioning. First, these predictions about Juanita are made on the basis of Juanita being representative of the population. Obviously if we have more specific information about Juanita, these predictions may fail. For example, if we know that Juanita has been diagnosed with terminal cancer we might revise a prediction of better health outcomes for Juanita. Presumably her health will decline over time, not improve. Equally obvious, happy-people-pills will not be the cause of her decline in health, and perhaps her health may be better than it would have been otherwise, since we know that positive moods help cancer patients. What most people might expect from happy-people-pills, then, will vary depending on their individual circumstances.

Relatedly, these predictions are based on statistical generalizations. Juanita may well gain in some of the predicted areas and lose in others. Suppose after taking happy-people-pills she gets out of an unsatisfactory relationship and finds and marries her soul mate. They decide to quit their jobs, sell everything, and sail around the world in a small sailboat with the goal of raising money for the needy. Juanita's income would go down in this case, not up. The number of friends she has may actually go down rather than up, since she may lose contact with people during her long voyage. In this case Juanita may well be better off overall, she may be happier, and in a more successful relationship, while meeting the challenge of sailing around the world, even if she is not more successful in every department of her life. So, there is no guarantee that people will excel at everything. The previous predictions are based on population averages.

We should not predict that everyone will benefit. A prisoner being tortured on the rack is probably not going to be helped by happy-people-pills. Indeed, it is entirely possible that taking happy-people-pills will occasionally make the lives of some worse. Suppose Juanita takes happy-people-pills and her community discovers this and ostracizes her – perhaps it runs against the community's religious beliefs. Being excluded in this way may make her worse off. It cannot be stressed enough that there is no ironclad guarantee that life will be better for each consumer of happy-people-pills. But life offers little in the way of such guarantees. The same point applies to any generalization about how to increase individual wellbeing. Getting married usually makes people better off, but it may not for everyone. More education usually makes people better off, but it may fail to do so for some. Still, it is true that usually getting married and usually getting more education makes people better off.

Third, we have just examined some possible external constraints on increased happiness, but there may be internal ones as well: if individuals do not like the effects of happy-people-pills, then this should count as strong evidence that happy-people-pills do not improve the wellbeing of the individual. If Juanita says that she does not like the positive moods, then this would certainly count against Juanita continuing to use them. If she says something to the effect that "when I am in 'the flow of the moment' I do not mind being on them. It is not like they are a constant source of awfulness such as, say, a broken rib, but I just don't feel comfortable on happy-people-pills." We might take such avowals as at least some evidence that they have not added to her overall wellbeing. I suspect that this sort of initial reaction might not be uncommon, especially if it is not possible to slowly ramp up the dose of happy-people-pills. For suppose it is possible to increase the dosage of happy-people-pills slowly over six months, taking 1/6 of a pill daily for the first month, 1/3 for the second month, and finally up to a whole pill daily in the sixth month. Juanita, her friends and colleagues might not notice any difference on a week-to-week basis, but after six months everyone may notice a difference compared to the Juanita of six months earlier. (The daily dosage is merely illustrative. The weekly formulation of Prozac suggests that it may be possible for the frequency to be much less.)

Even if it is not possible to slowly ramp up their use, I suspect people will eventually become quite used to them, and indeed prefer their newfound positive moods. So, an initial feeling of "strangeness" perhaps should be expected, and perhaps counted as a short-term negative. Consider that the same thing happens when we change our external environment. It only took me a few days to get to the point in my new house where I could walk around in the dark and not bump into things. But this is not the same as feeling comfortable in a new place. It took months before I felt fully comfortable. As of this writing, I've been at my new university for almost a full year, yet it really doesn't feel like home yet. I'm not saying that my situation in my new university is not better in some objective sense – here I have the prestige of occupying an endowed chair, whereas back at my old university I was dangling on a yearly contract. I'm talking about the "feel" of the place, and it doesn't quite feel like home. I'm not sure I can describe this feeling other than with strained metaphors like "in my bones it does not feel like home." My point here is simply that it can take some time to adjust to our external environment, and so I wouldn't be surprised if there was an adjustment period with happy-people-pills as well. If people never acclimate but always feel uneasy about the increased positive affect, then this would certainly count against the use of happy-people-pills. I see no reason why this should be so, and it seems exceedingly unlikely, but it is not something we can dismiss out of hand. Most likely some people will like the feel and others won't. But this shouldn't surprise us: there are very few invariant human responses.

Fourth, it is important to emphasize a point made earlier: that happy-people-pills are not some elixir that people need only take for wellbeing to descend on them like manna from heaven. If people in the lower range of happiness are going to have the same level of wellbeing as those in the upper range, they are going to need to do so the old-fashioned way: they will need to work at it. The causal claim is this: happy-people-pills will increase the likelihood of broaden-and-build behavior; those lower on the happiness curve will be more likely to dig in and do what it takes to enjoy higher levels of wellbeing. Making friends, getting more education, getting a better job will all require effort on the part of individuals. True, some of the causal paths between increased positive affect and higher levels of wellbeing may be more immediate, such as the connection with better health. Here the broaden-and-build model is less applicable. Positive affect is thought to boost immune response, and the mechanism here is not likely to require much intentional activity on the part of agents. On the other hand, there is every reason to expect that intentional activity will be required to gain further education, make friends, get involved in charity, enjoy a good marriage, and so on. Still, increased positive affect will increase the likelihood of persons making such efforts.

If the reader will forgive the analogy, happy-people-pills are like the water for the garden that is our life. No one can garden where there is no water. But water is only one ingredient to successful gardening. People taking happy-people-pills ought not think they can simply sit back and passively watch their lives bloom, but neither should we expect people to do well in a severe drought, as is the case with the clinically depressed, or in a mild drought of happiness like those in the lower range of happiness.

8.3   Additive Wellbeing

We have argued that happy-people-pills will increase the prudential good of individuals. It seems an obvious inference that happy-people-pills ought to improve society's good. After all, it is hard to imagine the good of society and individual good as completely independent variables. It seems perverse to say country X is a model for the rest of the world to emulate and esteem, yet everyone in X is unhappy and achieving little. So, it seems a natural inference that society as a whole should benefit from the use of happy-people-pills if, as we have said, individuals will benefit from the use of happy-people-pills. We will think of this as the 'additive argument.'

There are cases where the simple additive argument of the previous paragraph does not hold. A famous example by Fred Hirsch nicely illustrates the point: "If everyone stands on tiptoe, no one sees better."[6] The trap here is perhaps obvious: if no one else is on their tiptoes then it is to your advantage to stand on tiptoes in order to see better than your flatfooted peers. So, on an individual basis, standing on one's tiptoes adds to one's wellbeing. Yet, the point does not generalize, for if everyone else is on tiptoes, then you will not see any more than if you were flatfoot. Why would people stand on their tiptoes if it were just going to make everyone worse off? Clearly, the answer is that early adopters (those first on their toes) will be at an advantage. This advantage is quickly eroded as others attempt to adopt the same advantage. How do we avoid backing into a situation like this where everyone is worse off? The obvious answer in a case like this is to institute some public norm: "thou shalt not go on tiptoes," for not only does no one see better when everyone is on tiptoes, but everyone is in fact worse off: it is hard to be on tiptoes for long. Where a tiptoes arms race (as it were) threatens, everyone is better off if there is a societal norm to prohibit such a race. The example, then, shows that the inference from "each to all" does not hold. It may be the case that something might benefit each person, if done by him or her alone or by some few, but if everyone does the same thing no one benefits. Indeed, as this example illustrates, individually and collectively, people suffer.

One thing to notice about Hirsch's example is that it involves exclusionary goods or what Hirsch calls a "positional" good. Not everyone can be in a position to have a clear view over everyone else. For some to see over others, others must fail (at least in Hirsch's example). Some goods for individuals are defined even more explicitly in terms of their relation to the good of others, for example 'the most popular in the graduating class,' or 'the greatest scientific achievement' and other such superlative goods. If our only reason to take happy-people-pills was to win the race to achieve such exclusionary goods, then at the individual level it may help some, but at the societal level there would be no benefit. Assuming that we do not allow ties, there will always be one most popular person in the graduating class, and only one greatest scientific achievement. Of course the problem here is that it is simply impossible to boost the number of such superlative honors. Even an omnipotent being cannot make it the case that everyone in the graduating class is the most popular.

Fortunately, not all goods are exclusionary, and we may see societal benefit in the use of happy-people-pills for promoting such non-exclusionary ends. For example, it is conceivable that if everyone in the graduating class took happy-people-pills, then the average number of friends might rise. Notice that the trait 'average number of friends' is not defined in exclusionary terms. My having more friends does not preclude you from having more friends since the comparison here is not to each other, but to a baseline number of friends. Nor are friends a scarce good like beachfront property: not everyone can own beachfront property, but everyone could have more friends. Similarly, the idea that happy-people-pills might make us healthier does not introduce any exclusionary aspect. If we say that happy-people-pills make a population healthier, we are comparing this to some baseline.

Interestingly, most of the social science research we canvassed previously was ultimately measured in non-exclusionary terms. Thus, there is no reason to suppose that if my wellbeing is increased by happy-people-pills, this should preclude others from also increasing their wellbeing. In addition to health and friendship, there is no logical contradiction in everyone having better marriages, being more altruistic, being better corporate citizens, being more energetic, etc., so long as 'more' and 'better' here are measured in terms of some baseline. Nothing can change the fact that only 10 percent of all people will be in the top 10 percent of physical health, but we could all become healthier in non-comparative measures like blood pressure, days sick with the flu, etc. Exceptions to the additive nature of wellbeing are the exclusionary categories of 'better job' and income discussed in Chapter 6. Recall the study by Staw, Sutton, and Pelled which showed a correlation between desirable jobs – those higher in terms of autonomy, meaning, and variety as rated by trained observers – and happiness, and the correlation between happiness and income in Oshi, Diener, and Lucas.[7] There are only so many high-paying jobs that provide high levels of autonomy, meaning, and variety. The scarcity of such jobs means that not everyone can have a good job any more than everyone can have beachfront property. The fact that happy-people-pills cannot solve this problem is at best a limitation, not a criticism, of happy-people-pills. That said, it certainly would not be out of the realm of possibility that, over the medium and long term, a happier workforce that is better educated and more productive might generate more good jobs.

So, while the inference from each to all is not always justified, it is so in the vast majority of instances we have looked at. So, in general, the more individuals are able to make their lives go better by improving their happiness and achievement with happy-people-pills, the more society as a whole should benefit.

8.4 Multiplicative Wellbeing: Virtue and Pro-social Behavior

In the previous section we looked at an argument that says that at a societal level wellbeing is, for the most part, additive. In this section we will examine an argument that happy-people-pills can be multiplicative: their use should encourage the acquisition and exercise of pro-social virtues. So, not only will happy-people-pills benefit those who take them, but they should also promote the good of others.[8]

The first step in our argument, that our world could use more pro-social behavior, is one that I take to be generally accepted. There can be no doubt that our world is, morally speaking, a fixer-upper. To cite but a few examples: today millions of children in the two-thirds world will go to bed hungry, today women on every populated continent will be raped, today more of the environment will be destroyed by human activity, and today – even in the most materially wealthy nations – many elderly persons will find themselves alone and unable to care for themselves. Of course, unfortunately, such examples could be enumerated seemingly without end. Yet, it seems our world could be much worse but for the concern and industriousness of some: people volunteer their time to collect money for organizations like Oxfam for the express purpose of helping underprivileged children. Volunteers at universities walk women home from campus late at night. Community groups spend weekends cleaning up polluted rivers.

The volunteer association, Meals on Wheels, provides hot meals to shut-ins, etc. True, as with just about any human activity, not all efforts to help others are successful. Sending a truckload of electric can-openers to impoverished areas that have no electricity or canned food may be well-meaning, but not particularly helpful. Despite such blunders, overall our world is better for (most of) these efforts. Admittedly, some have disputed this claim. Thomas Malthus, for example, thought that feeding the poor would do more harm than good in the long run. Garret Hardin famously updated the case in the 1970s with his (in)famous article: "Lifeboat Ethics: the Case Against Helping the Poor."[9] It is not my intention to argue the point here; rather, let me simply record my agreement with the widely held view that most pro-social efforts most of the time have a net positive benefit for recipients.

We noted above the large body of empirical literature that indicates a correlation between happiness and pro-social behavior. For instance, recall the conclusion in this connection of the meta-study by Lyubomirsky, Diener, and King: "happy people are inclined to be kind and charitable people."[10] While these studies indicate a correlation between happiness and pro-social behavior, it is a truism that correlation is not causation, and so it is worth revisiting for a moment the question of causation. We noted that correlation is necessary for causation (in the absence of confounding variables), and so to this extent these studies provide *some* indication of a causal connection. Further evidence of a causal connection stems from longitudinal studies. A panel study (which involves following the same subjects over time) by Thoits and Hewitt showed that an increase in happiness follows an increase in pro-social behavior.[11] Additional evidence of a causal connection comes from a large-scale natural experiment reported by Meier and Stutzer.[12] The reunification of Germany caused the collapse of much of former East Germany's volunteer structure. Controlling for other variables, Meier and Stutzer found that reduced opportunities for volunteer work led to a decrease in happiness.[13] More traditional experiments also support this conclusion: for example, even small 'random acts of kindness' significantly boost subjects' happiness.[14]

The evidence we have just examined suggests that the arrow of causality runs from pro-social behavior to happiness. However, longitudinal and experimental evidence also suggests that happiness causes pro-social behavior. Thus, the panel study mentioned earlier found that those who are happier at an earlier time are more likely to exhibit pro-social behavior in the future.[15] A number of laboratory experiments also confirm the idea that happiness causes pro-social behavior. The results are sometimes summarized as the 'feel good, do good' phenomenon. For example, experimenters might arrange it so that an experimental subject 'just happens' to find a coin. This typically provides a boost to positive affect in subjects, and the subjects are subsequently more likely to engage in pro-social behavior.

We said that our world is often made better by pro-social efforts. So, it seems reasonable to suppose that our world would be better still if there was even more pro-social effort. That is, other things being equal, if more children were fed, if more people volunteered to help escort women home late at night, if more people worked to save the environment, if more people helped deliver hot meals to shut-ins, etc., our world would be morally better.

Scientific research on happiness and pro-social behavior indicates that we are in the enviable position where moral obligations and enlightened self-interest are not antagonistically related. For example, we might suggest that if people want to be happier they should engage in pro-social activities; for example, volunteering a few hours a week might improve their positive affect.

The multiplicative conclusion follows: those taking happy-people-pills should benefit by exhibiting more pro-social behavior. To exhibit pro-social behavior is to exercise virtue: traditionally pro-social behavior might be linked to the virtue of benevolence. The argument of Chapter 5 suggests that (other things being equal), to the extent that consumers of happy-people-pills are more benevolent, they are better off. Acting benevolently in turn benefits others. So, the multiplicative effect is a strong moral reason to suppose that we ought to use happy-people-pills.

Notes

1. Brender and Krasnoff, *New Essays on the History of Autonomy*.
2. Dworkin, *The Theory and Practice of Autonomy*; Taylor, *Sources of the Self*; Beauchamp and Walters, *Contemporary Issues in Bioethics*.
3. Oshana, "How Much Should We Value Autonomy?," 100.
4. Buss, "Personal Autonomy."
5. Lucas, Diener, and Suh, "Discriminant Validity of Well-being Measures"; Staw and Barsade, "Affect and Managerial Performance."
6. Hirsch, *Social Limits to Growth*, 5.
7. Staw, Sutton, and Pelled, "Employee Positive Emotion and Favorable Outcomes at the Workplace"; Oishi, Diener, and Lucas, "The Optimum Level of Well-being."

8.   Economists sometimes refer to these as 'network' effects. See Buchanan (*Beyond Humanity?*) for further exploration of the idea that biological enhancements may have network effects. Network effects are often illustrated with examples of unintended positive externalities. The classic example is a network of telephones. Every additional telephone in a network provides more potential places to call for everyone else in the network. In this section I am speaking about intentional positive externalities, so it is not exactly the economists' paradigm for network effects.

9.   Hardin, "Lifeboat Ethics."

10. Lyubomirsky, King, and Diener, "The Benefits of Frequent Positive Affect," 828.

11. Thoits and Hewitt, "Volunteer Work and Well-being."

12. Meier and Stutzer, "Is Volunteering Rewarding in Itself?"

13. Ibid.

14. Boehm and Lyubomirsky, "The Promise of Sustainable Happiness"; Switzer et al., "The Effect of a School-Based Helper Program on Adolescent Self-Image, Attitudes, and Behavior"; Fordyce, "A Program to Increase Happiness."

15. Thoits and Hewitt, "Volunteer Work and Well-being."

References

Beauchamp, T. L. and L. Walters. *Contemporary Issues in Bioethics*. New York: Wadsworth, 2003.

Boehm, J. K. and S. Lyubomirsky. "The Promise of Sustainable Happiness." *Handbook of Positive Psychology* (2009): 667–77.

Brender, N. and L. Krasnoff. *New Essays on the History of Autonomy: A Collection Honoring J. B. Schneewind*. Cambridge: Cambridge University Press, 2004.

Buchanan, A. E. *Beyond Humanity? The Ethics of Biomedical Enhancement*. Oxford: Oxford University Press, 2011.

Buss, S. "Personal Autonomy." In *The Stanford Encyclopedia of Philosophy* (Fall 2008 edn.), edited by Edward N. Zalta. http://plato.stanford.edu/archives/fall2008/entries/personal-autonomy/.

Dworkin, G. *The Theory and Practice of Autonomy*. Cambridge: Cambridge University Press, 1988.

Hardin, G. "Lifeboat Ethics." *Psychology Today* 8, no. 4 (1974): 38–43.

Hirsch, F. *Social Limits to Growth*. Cambridge, Mass.: Harvard University Press (1976).

Lucas, R. E., E. Diener, and E. Suh. "Discriminant Validity of Well-being Measures." *Journal of Personality and Social Psychology* 71, no. 3 (1996): 616–28.

Lyubomirsky, S., L. King, and E. Diener. "The Benefits of Frequent Positive Affect: Does Happiness Lead to Success?" *Psychological Bulletin* 131 (2005): 803–55.

Meier, S. and A. Stutzer. "Is Volunteering Rewarding in Itself?" *Economica* 75, no. 297 (2008): 39–59.

Oishi, S., E. Diener, and R. E. Lucas. "The Optimum Level of Well-being: Can People Be Too Happy?" *Perspectives on Psychological Science* 2, no. 4 (2007): 346–60.

Oshana, M. "How Much Should We Value Autonomy?" *Social Philosophy and Policy* 20, no. 2 (2003): 99–126.

Staw, B. M. and S. G. Barsade. "Affect and Managerial Performance: A Test of the Sadder-but-Wiser vs. Happier-and-Smarter Hypotheses." *Administrative Science Quarterly* 38, no. 2 (1993): 304–31.

Staw, B. M., R. I. Sutton, and L. H. Pelled. "Employee Positive Emotion and Favorable Outcomes at the Workplace." *Organization Science* 5, no. 1 (1994): 51–71.

Switzer, G. E., R. G. Simmons, M. A. Dew, J. M. Regalski, and C. H. Wang. "The Effect of a School-Based Helper Program on Adolescent Self-Image, Attitudes, and Behavior." *Journal of Early Adolescence* 15, no. 4 (1995): 429–55.

Taylor, C. *Sources of the Self: The Making of the Modern Identity*. Cambridge, Mass.: Harvard University Press, 1989.

Thoits, P. A. and L. N. Hewitt. "Volunteer Work and Well-being." *Journal of Health and Social Behavior* 42, no. 2 (2001): 115–31.

9

Ethical Objections

The focus of this chapter is on ethical objections to happy-people-pills. The objections form something of a mixed bag; they include the claims that happy-people-pills will lead to emotional inappropriateness, to instrumentalizing our emotions, false happiness, inauthenticity, loss of identity, and unfair distribution. Certainly there is no pretense that absolutely every objection to happy-people-pills is answered here; rather, I consider what I take to be the strongest objections on the basis of my reading of the literature and from having spoken on this topic a number of times. Showing how these criticisms may be dispatched should strengthen the case for happy-people-pills.

9.1   Emotional Inappropriateness

When our loved ones are coping with injury or imminent death, it seems entirely appropriate to grieve and be worried. When we hear about children and innocent civilians dying from an errant bomb, we do, and should, feel sad. A world of happy-people-pills, so the objection goes, precludes such emotionally appropriate responses. A world where we are happy when faced with tragedy seems to be a world where we have lost something of great importance. As Leon Kass notes, there is something wrong with attempting to achieve total psychic tranquility. Feelings of shame, remorse, horror, and disgust are entirely appropriate in certain circumstances:

Happy-People-Pills For All, First Edition. Mark Walker.
© 2013 John Wiley & Sons, Inc. Published 2013 by John Wiley & Sons, Inc.

And yet, there seems to be something misguided about the pursuit of utter psychic tranquility, or the attempt to eliminate all shame, guilt, and painful memories. Traumatic memories, shame, and guilt, are, it is true, psychic pains. In extreme doses, they can be crippling. Yet they are also helpful and fitting. They are appropriate responses to horror, disgraceful conduct, and sin, and, as such, help teach us to avoid them in the future. Witnessing a murder should be remembered as horrible; doing a beastly deed should trouble one's soul. Righteous indignation at injustice depends on being able to feel injustice's sting. An untroubled soul in a troubling world is a shrunken human being. More fundamentally, to deprive oneself of one's memory – including and especially its truthfulness of feeling – is to deprive oneself of one's own life and identity.[1]

Kass's argument is a paradigmatic case of offering a false dilemma: either we keep our current emotional states or we "seek utter psychic tranquility." Surely there is some middle ground here. With this same logic we could discourage efforts to feed the starving in the two-thirds world because no one wants to see them die from obesity. Clearly it is not vain to hope that we might have more positive emotional states without supposing this requires utter psychic tranquility. After all, aiming for enhanced emotional states is not necessarily the same thing as aiming for psychic tranquility. For there is nothing to say enhanced emotional states do not require a range of emotional states. We may want, for example, to be able to experience sadness in order to appreciate Mozart's Requiem Mass or Joy Division's "The Eternal," while still holding out for a bit more in the way of positive moods in our daily life.

The irrelevance of the criticism of "utter psychic tranquility" should also be apparent from the fact that our goal for our model is hyperthymic people, and there is no indication that the hyperthymic are emotionally one-dimensional. It is sheer fantasy to suppose that the hyperthymic laugh when they see a traffic fatality or that they do the limbo at their spouse's funeral.

Also, there is good statistical evidence that the hyperthymic experience negative emotions. For example, as Lyubomirsky, King, and Diener note, the top 14 percent of those completing the World Value Survey (1994) reported experiencing negative emotions or moods within the last few weeks.[2] Diener and Seligman found similar results among college students: the happiest students, that is, those who experienced positive moods the most, also had the full range of positive and negative moods:

Members of the happiest group experienced positive, but not ecstatic, feelings most of the time, and they reported occasional negative moods. This suggests that very happy people do have a functioning emotion system that can react appropriately to life events.[3]

Kass's criticism seems to trade on the stereotype that pharmacological agents will necessarily produce a blunted emotional response. Perhaps what critics have in mind here is the *soma* taken by denizens of *Brave New World*. However, there is no reason to suppose that all pharmacological agents would have this effect. Indeed, there is some evidence that some of the current generation of antidepressants belie this claim. In the aforementioned study on healthy volunteers, Healy found:

> Chasing the question of whether Zoloft caused emotional blunting, half the group said it had given them a "nothing bothers me" feeling. Reactions were split about this: Some liked the effect; others found it made them emotionally dead. Reboxetine, in contrast, didn't seem to make anyone feel indifferent – calm, perhaps, but not indifferent. Its effects were better described as energizing – again, good for some but not for others.[4]

So even with the current stable of drugs, the loss of emotional appropriateness or "emotional blunting" is not a universal side effect, since it seems not to apply to half of the study group when taking Zoloft, and to none when taking Reboxetine. Advanced pharmacological agents like happy-people-pills should provide even better control over the emotional blunting problem, for those for whom it is a problem.

Emotional blunting is not inherently bad. The Stoics, for example, put some premium on just this. For some a little emotional blunting may be an improvement: it is entirely appropriate to be annoyed by a scratch on your new car, but if this so upsets you that your weekend is ruined, a little blunting may be just what you need. Being emotionally insensitive – being emotionally blunted – is not desirable, nor is being too emotionally sensitive. Ideally, we would like to be in the mean between the extremes. As we have noted, many of the hyperthymic fall into this range. The goal in creating happy-people-pills should be to make sure we are still emotionally sensitive (but not too sensitive).

9.2   Instrumentalization

It may be wondered whether the previous response fully captures what critics are worried about in thinking about emotional appropriateness.

Consider an analogy. Suppose a baseball coach convinces a player that he will hit a home run on the next at-bat. Suppose further that if the player believes he will hit a home run, his chances of hitting a home run increase from 15 to 16 percent. Has the coach encouraged the appropriate belief? In one sense, yes. The batter convinced of success is more likely to achieve his goal. However, the belief is not appropriate in the sense that we think that beliefs should be truth-directed: beliefs should aim to be true and this explains in part why we value beliefs. It is inappropriate for the player to believe he will hit a home run when the belief's truth-directedness is at issue: after all, there are good reasons for thinking the batter will not hit a home run. The reason, of course, is that the odds are much higher that he won't hit a home run. The coach may justify this coaching strategy by saying that false beliefs may be effective. But even if we grant this, it still shows that there is some loss to the player: he has lost some of the value we often associate with beliefs: namely, their truth-directedness. His belief has been instrumentalized: truth has been sacrificed for increased batting efficiency. This is not to say that this sacrifice is not in the player's interest, but it is to say that his increased batting efficiency comes at some cost.

Similarly, positive moods and emotions may be effective in achieving certain ends, some of which were described in Chapter 6, but this does not show that positive moods or emotions are appropriate to the circumstances. Nor does the point made in the previous section, that the hyperthymic experience both positive and negative emotions, answer the objection. For if happy-people-pills boost our moods in general, then it may well be that some lives are such that a preponderance of positive moods is inappropriate. Think of the Deltas in Huxley's *Brave New World*, who have been intellectually stunted by alcohol during gestation. It seems wrong for the Deltas to be happy about their situation, although of course the Deltas have little control over how they feel about the matter. The appropriate response seems to be one of sadness: their intellects and opportunities have been purposely limited by society. No doubt it might help the Deltas cope with their situation if they try to remain happy, but this is to point out the instrumental value of happiness in coping. It does not show that they should be happy about their situation. So, even if it is granted that happiness has instrumental value in achieving certain types of perfectionist goods, it does not change the fact that one cost of happy-people-pills may be that people are happy in situations where happiness is not the appropriate emotional response.

In order to reply to this criticism, it will help to recall an earlier example. In the first chapter we heard Dr. Friedman relate the story about a woman who had come to see him who had suffered great personal tragedy. She had lost her husband and her job within the last year. Despite the terrible circumstances, the woman had not sought out Friedman as a patient herself but for advice about her son, who was having a difficult time coping with the loss of his father. Friedman had found that the woman was much more resilient:

> Despite crushing loss and stress, she was not at all depressed – sad, yes, but still upbeat. I found myself stunned by her resilience. What accounted for her ability to weather such sorrow with buoyant optimism? So I asked her directly.
>
> "All my life I've been happy for no good reason. It's just my nature, I guess." But it was more than that. She was a happy extrovert, full of energy and enthusiasm who was indefatigably sociable. And she could get by with five or six hours of sleep each night.[5]

Interestingly, the first sentence sounds almost like a contradiction: "Despite crushing loss and stress, she was not at all depressed – sad, yes, but still upbeat." After all, it seems a legitimate question to ask how someone could be both sad and upbeat. It is hard to know for sure, but it seems likely that the distinction between attitudinal hedonism and emotional state theory might explain this apparent tension. It is plausible to assume that she was very displeased by the loss of her husband and her job. This attitudinal displeasure explains her sadness. On the other hand, the "hardwiring" or biological predisposition to positive moods and emotions attributed to her by Dr. Friedman explains why she is still "upbeat".

With this in mind, we can see an important difference between the Deltas and the woman who came to see Dr. Friedman. The Deltas are biologically manipulated in vitro and indoctrinated to take great attitudinal pleasure in their situation. Recall that through hypnopaedia they are encouraged to think that they are fortunate to be in the ideal class. They are pleased with their lot. It is safe to assume that the woman in Dr. Friedman's office was not pleased in losing her husband and her job. So, this woman and the Deltas are happy in the affective component of happiness but only the Deltas have cognitive happiness about their situation: they are attitudinally pleased about their lot. Since we are thinking about boosting moods, not indoctrinating people, the Deltas introduce extraneous concerns. The upshot of this is that we must be sure that we are focusing on instrumentalizing moods and emotions, not propositional attitudes. This shows why the optimistic batter and the Deltas are not good analogies: they have incorrect propositional attitudes.

Is there something inappropriate about the woman being emotionally upbeat? I think it will help to parse this into the short term and the long term. In the short term it might not be entirely appropriate to be upbeat about the loss of her husband. Nothing in what Dr. Friedman relates says that she was upbeat at her husband's funeral. And as we have seen above, the hyperthymic have both positive and negative moods, and so there is every reason to suppose that this woman was emotionally down in the short term when her husband died. So, our question resolves down to whether it is inappropriate for the woman to be emotionally upbeat in the longer term, specifically, in the same year that her husband died.

I see no reason to suppose that this is inappropriate. We do not need to actually believe in an afterlife to speculate what the reactions of the dead might be. In this case we can imagine that her husband might be shocked or disappointed if he observed her from the afterlife experiencing joy at his dying. On the other hand, we can imagine the late husband would be glad that she is able to maintain an upbeat emotional outlook despite her attitudinal displeasure at his death. To be emotionally down later that same year would be harmful and serve nothing. Furthermore, it seems we have an expectation that people will "renormalize" after a certain amount of time, that is, they will eventually emotionally bounce back. The length of the interval seems to be dependent upon a number of factors including the nature of the calamity – a small fender bender should not dampen moods and emotions in the same way as the loss of a loved one – and perhaps cultural expectations as well. Not only do we have this expectation, it seems it is a rightful expectation: we are and should be concerned about those who do not bounce back. With the woman who went to see Dr. Friedman, it sounds like she is on her way to bouncing back.

Finally, it seems part of the reason for thinking that there is nothing to this criticism is that it is not clear what emotional reaction is appropriate to "life in general". In other words, we have expectations about the appropriate emotional responses to specific events: joy at the birth of a child, grief at the loss of a loved one, but little expectation about an emotional reaction to routine and daily events. Suppose you are a sanitation engineer: your job involves dumping garbage cans into the back of a truck 40 hours a week. Suppose there are no other big events going on in your life. Is it more appropriate for you to feel emotionally down most of the time, or is it more appropriate for you to feel emotionally up most of the time? The question hardly makes sense. We seem to have little expectation about what the correct emotional reaction is to "life in general". We can think of reasons you might be down: the job involves backbreaking, smelly work that is not held in high social esteem. We can also think of reasons you might be up most of the time: at least you have a job, you don't bring home a briefcase full of work, your job allows you to stay fit, etc.

So, when we think about the emotionally inappropriate objection, it seems to have little traction. In the short term, we expect the hyperthymic to experience grief in response to tragic events just like the rest of us. In the long term, we expect people to renormalize their emotional states, and there is no apparent standard for an emotional response in the typical case to "life in general."

9.3   False Happiness

A frequently expressed concern is that by taking a pill one would achieve only a "false happiness", not the "genuine happiness" that most seek. Imagine, for example, someone who is not clinically depressed but feels that she would like to experience greater levels of subjective wellbeing. After taking the pill she says, "I feel happy, extremely happy in fact. But I feel this way because of the pills I take. If I did not take the pills I would not be so happy, and so the happiness I experience is not genuine. I would like to experience authentic happiness: happiness that is not due to a pill but a happiness that originates with me." Kass and the President's Council on Bioethics make the same point in connection with therapeutic uses of antidepressants. They say that patients receiving pharmacological therapy

> worry about using artificial means to change their psyches, a concern that springs ultimately from their desire that feelings and personalities not be artificial and false but genuine and true. Their worry, also widely shared, about having one's experiences of the world mediated by a drug is, at least in part, a worry about having one's real experience distorted. Even the expressed concern over "taking the easy way out" may involve not so much an opposition to ease, but a concern about distortion and self-deception.[6]

Why do patients feel that their experiences are "distorted", not "genuine or true"? As noted above, it is not known exactly how all antidepressants work, but the naive answer seems to be that they affect the neurochemistry and the neurological structures of our brains. This seems to support the worry about distortion and self-deception: but for these pills, the neurochemistry and structure of my brain would be different.

But surely the rallying cry can't be that we should have experiences, moods, and emotions free of neurochemicals and neurological structures: we know that even without pills our experiences are mediated by neurochemicals in our brains. Without neurochemicals we would have no experiences at all; for example, if all the serotonin, norepinephrine, dopamine, etc. were to be vacuumed from our brains, we would have no experience, no moods, no emotions at all. We would be brain-dead. So, why think that pills make all the difference? The President's Council on Bioethics suggests an answer:

> While such drugs often make things better – they often help individuals achieve some measure of the happiness they desire – taking such drugs may also leave many of the same individuals wondering whether their newfound happiness is fully *their own* – and in this sense, fully real.[7]

So, the answer seems to be that the neurochemistry of my brain not affected by pills is my own, whereas a brain affected by pills is not fully real. But why should we accept their answer? After all, universalized, such a judgment seems fairly harsh. It would say that persons who take SSRIs or other antidepressants are not genuinely happy: their happiness is distorted and not fully their own. In other words, this would mean that people who take SSRIs for debilitating depression never experience genuine happiness. Here the President's Council on Bioethics seems ambivalent. They want to say that those who do suffer from debilitating depression can experience genuine happiness with SSRIs, but they do not explain why someone of a normal level of subjective wellbeing who uses pills to enhance his or her happiness is not similarly genuinely happy.

The therapy/enhancement distinction may be of some use in explaining the difference. The proposal then would be that false happiness is not at issue when mood boosters are used for treating depression but is at issue when they are used for enhancement. While the distinction may tell us *when* mood boosters lead to false happiness – in the case of enhancement – and when they don't – when used for therapy – it does not tell us *why*. Why does therapy not lead to false happiness but enhancement leads to false happiness? One suggestion might be that in the case of therapy we are restoring someone's happiness: people fall into depression and so antidepressants help them return to their true level of happiness. The idea of restoring, however, won't do the trick, for it is both too wide and too narrow. It is too narrow because it does not explain why someone with lifelong depression can use antidepressants for therapeutic purposes. If the idea of restoring means returning to one's former level of happiness, then life-long depressed patients could not be "restored", because they have always been depressed. Also, restoring is too wide because it does not prohibit enhancement. Imagine someone who has, until recently, been hyperthymic – an A+ on our happiness curve. However, her dog left her and her husband ran away. Now she is less happy. She has fallen into the A− range. It seems she should be a candidate for mood boosters to restore her to her former level. But of course this would be a case of enhancement. So, the therapy/enhancement distinction is of no help in this case.

Not only does the President's Council on Bioethics not have an answer; but also I think this line of criticism hides a crucial ambiguity. To see this, consider a parallel with sex-change procedures. Imagine Chris undergoes plastic surgery and hormone replacement therapy in order to change from being phenotypically male to female. After these procedures (let us concede) there is a clear and undeniable sense in which her looks are "not genuine and true": her morphology is to some extent artificial in the sense of not being entirely the product of the usual genetic and environmental influences that contribute to human sexual dimorphism.[8] But I believe that many of us would accept that there is a sense in which Chris's post-sex-change appearance is truer or more genuine. The reason that we might say this is that her new appearance is an expression of the sorts of looks she believes are more appropriate. In other words, plastic surgery can be seen as an expression of the person you want to be, and therefore more authentic, than the looks provided by the environment and genetics.

What this indicates is that there are two distinctions at work here: artificial versus natural, and authentic versus inauthentic. The first might be understood along the lines of bodily integrity: "the natural" happens in and to the human body (including the brain) on its own, whereas "the artificial" occurs when intervention breaks the bodily boundary, as in surgery or pills. 'Authentic' in this context means reflecting the individual's priorities, values, and decisions, while 'inauthentic' means not doing so. Applying this to Chris, we should say that her looks are artificial (and so not 'genuine' or 'true' in this sense) but authentic (and so genuine and true in the other sense), since they reflect her values and her self-understanding. So, there is no contradiction in saying that Chris's looks are artificial (created by plastic surgery) and authentic (chosen by her to represent her understanding of herself).

Applying this distinction to taking happy-people-pills we might say that someone who chooses to do so will experience artificial happiness, but the happiness might also be authentic. Although the pill is modeled on those that are naturally hyperthymic, the pill would artificially create hyperthymia in those with a genetic predisposition to lower normal levels of happiness. The parallel with plastic surgery is that someone may have their appearance artificially changed by surgery; others might have the good fortune of obtaining their attractive features through winning the genetic lottery. We could also say that those taking the happy-people-pills are authentically happy, because their happiness would be more in line with their own self-understanding of the person they want to be. Someone whose genetics are relevantly different from the naturally hyperthymic might say that they would like to be the sort of person who is generally in a positive mood, and so the hyperthymic pill allows them to be the sort of person they would like to be.

The point is not that greater happiness *necessarily* leads to a more authentic realization of one's self, any more than plastic surgery *necessarily* leads to a more authentic realization of one's self. Many people are satisfied with their looks, including those who do not fit societal norms of beauty. For such individuals, there is not a great divide between what they are naturally and their authentic looks. To force those who are pleased with the looks they have received through genetic inheritance into plastic surgery, designed to make them "more beautiful" with respect to some social norm, would be to create looks that were both artificial and inauthentic. Again, we say 'artificial' because plastic surgery is (by assumption) artificial, and 'inauthentic' because such a change does not reflect the priorities and self-understanding of the individual. Similarly, surreptitiously adding happy-people-pills to a normally happy person's diet would be to create artificial happiness that is inauthentic.

A final example that vividly demonstrates how authentic and artificial can be distinguished is by considering, again, the case of Suzie, who is genetically predisposed to positive moods. Recall that she believes she would be a better artist if she could experience negative affect to a much greater extent. This is based on her belief that her hero, Edvard Munch, experienced powerful negative emotions and this contributed to his great art. In this case, we might say that Suzie's very high chronic positive affect is natural but not authentic: she does not identify with the positive emotions that she experiences. Indeed, if we could make a pill for chronic negative affect then she might take the unhappy-people-pill to artificially introduce into herself the negative emotions she ascribes to her hero. If she did so, then her chronic negative affect would be authentic and artificial.

The upshot here is that proponents of happy-people-pills would do well to concede to critics that artificially creating happiness would not lead to authentic happiness for all. For if we understand 'authentic' as meaning 'in accordance with the values, goals, and beliefs of the person', then it is clear that for some, authentic happiness means living within whatever constraints one's genome dictates. But if the "not real happiness" objection is to apply to every single individual that might seek to improve positive affect through technological means, it must be the case that every use of technology to compensate for how one fares in the genetic lottery results in an inauthentic happiness. It is this judgment that we have said cannot be supported. Even if we allow that technology introduces an artificial happiness, there are good reasons to suppose that the resulting happiness is authentic (at least in many cases), and so, in this sense, the happiness is real.

9.4   Inauthenticity

There is an argument that turns our previous thinking on its head. It says that the choice to use happy-people-pills is likely to lead to inauthenticity. Thus, Carl Elliott writes:

> We can see something of these ideas in the conflicted attitudes that many Americans have toward Prozac. On the one hand, if the way to lead a meaningful life is to search for self-fulfillment, and self-fulfillment is achieved through a life of honest work and householding, then it makes sense to embrace a drug like Prozac, which offers the promise of doing better, more meaningful work in a happier, more enthusiastic way. Yet if living a meaningful life is also tied to living an authentic life – the life that is uniquely yours, which you discover and develop by looking inward – then a drug like Prozac can seem deeply problematic. What could seem less authentic, at least on the surface, than changing your personality with an antidepressant? What could be further from the "simple life" than a life dependent on cosmetic psychopharmacology?[9]

Elliott's worry is that the use of Prozac to enhance happiness will be to medically treat the philosophical insights of some. If we prescribe Prozac for the feelings of malaise associated with inauthenticity, then this is to pharmacologically treat inauthenticity. But it would be wrong to so treat inauthenticity; hence, we ought to be wary of using Prozac for the enhancement of happiness. Elliott's paradigms of persons suffering from malaise are like many of the characters that populate Walker Percy's novels (such as Will Barrett in *The Last Gentleman*). The contemporary predicament is worse in some ways, says Elliott. The "anchors of meaning" have fallen away: we can no longer appeal to the eternal verities to justify our lives, to answer the question of life's meaning. God, Being, History, Science, etc., provide no overarching theory and justification for the meaning and purpose of life. Faced with this "existential angst", people fall into a malaise. So Elliott wonders:

> Suppose you are a psychiatrist and you have a patient who has precisely this sense of alienation; say, an accountant living in Downers Grove, Illinois, who comes to himself one day and says, Jesus Christ, is this it? A Snapper lawn mower and a house in the suburbs? Should you, his psychiatrist, try to rid him of his alienation by prescribing Prozac? Or do you secretly think that maybe, as bad off as he is, he is better off than his neighbors? Because, as Percy puts it, even though he's in a predicament, at least he's aware of it, which is a lot better than being in a predicament and thinking you're not.[10]

Elliott's discussion has been influential; but it seems to rely on a very questionable premise. Let me begin with a purposively obtuse question: what is wrong with being an accountant, having a Snapper lawn mower and living in the suburbs? I sincerely doubt Elliott has anything against accountants or Snapper lawn mowers. I suspect Elliott would say that it is not *which* life is chosen, but *how* it is adopted. For example, ultimately, the accountant's life is not going to be any more meaningful if he gives everything to charity and goes to work for Sea Shepherd, throwing himself between baby whales and Japanese harpoons, or works as a volunteer in the impoverished two-thirds world. According to the theory of existential angst that Elliott outlines, each life is equally meaningful, or meaningless: from the grand perspective of Being, Time, or History, each is a tale told by an idiot: full of sound and fury, signifying nothing. So the criticism of the Snapper lawn mower life is not that it is intrinsically less meaningful than, say, a life in service to others. Such a view would depend on the idea that different lives have different levels of intrinsic meaning. This is precisely the sort of understanding – this objective ranking of the meaning of lives – that Elliott thinks is unavailable to us moderns. To make it an authentically lived life, one has to realize that there are no such objective rankings; we are, in the words of Nietzsche, "value legislators".[11] An authentic life is one that endorses the view that the meaning of life is chosen, and one must take responsibility for this. So, anyone who does not understand this through reflection is living an inauthentic life. But once we realize this we can see that there is no principled reason why one cannot live a life in suburbia with a Snapper lawn mower. If upon reflection you decided through "looking inward" that this is the life that you truly want – and you are not living it on the basis of false consciousness or pressures from the "Others" (to give this all a nice existentialist ring) – then a life in suburbia can be just as authentic as being a starving writer or saving children in the two-thirds world. Therefore, the problem with prescribing cosmetic mood enhancers is not that there is something necessarily wrong with that type of life, per se. Rather, the problem with prescribing mood boosters is that it interferes with living an authentic, and hence meaningful, life.

This is a serious charge but why should we believe it? Elliott seems to make epistemological and metaphysical arguments for this position, but both of them are open to question. The epistemological argument is contained in the thought process in which Elliott invites us to wonder whether as psychiatrists we should proscribe Prozac for the accountant to rid him of alienation. Recall Elliott says:

> Or do you secretly think that maybe, as bad off as he is, he is better off than his neighbors? Because, as Percy puts it, even though he's in a predicament, at least he's aware of it, which is a lot better than being in a predicament and thinking you're not.[12]

But this is a bit strange. For a start, it seems to invite us to decide for the accountant that his life goes better with the truth – that he is aware of his predicament – rather than positive moods. But this seems to be choosing for him, which makes one wonder whether this would be an authentic life. It would seem that even on this problematic understanding we ought to turn the question back to the patient: do you want the truth or do you want positive moods? After all, it would seem an open question whether the patient endorses truth or positive moods as being more in line with his values.

Second, why would Prozac stop him from understanding his alienation? Prozac is not supposed to distort cognitive functioning. Surely Elliott cannot be saying that only the morose can understand the philosophical point of alienation and the necessity in the postmodern world to be value legislators. This would be to simply confuse mood with depth: you need not be morose to think about meaning and meaninglessness. Presumably this is not what Elliott has in mind, but his discussion certainly calls to mind the amusing caricature of the brooding existentialist, chain-smoking in a coffee shop. I don't see why one needs to be brooding to appreciate the death of the eternal verities, History, Being, God, Nature, and Spirit. Certainly Nietzsche, the godfather of this way of thinking, thought that a joyful wisdom is possible. As the attending psychiatrist it would seem that an understanding of the state of alienation for us moderns might be achieved by means of some reading material and some Prozac. That way the patient need not decide between the truth and positive moods. So, the epistemic argument seems unfounded.

The metaphysical argument is that taking Prozac leads to a change in personality that leads to inauthenticity. The relevant passage, to quote again, is: "What could be less authentic, at least on the surface, than changing your personality with an antidepressant?" But how exactly does changing one's personality lead to inauthenticity? One might think the claim that changing one's personality leads to inauthenticity follows simply from the concept of authenticity itself. This seems to be L. L. E. Bolt's understanding of what Elliott is saying: "the idea of a meaningful life involves authenticity and uniqueness, discovering your own values by looking inward instead of being dependent on an antidepressant."[13] Bolt does not explain this comment further, but seems to suggest that authenticity precludes taking an antidepressant. I suspect Elliott endorses a weaker claim: people may feel forced to take mood boosters to accommodate themselves to conventional life – the Snapper mower again – rather than choosing their own lives. The idea seems to be that taking Prozac is a symptom of inauthenticity rather than the cause.

But if this is Elliott's understanding, it points to a diametrically opposed conclusion. If authenticity means not simply taking anything as "given", then choosing to alter one's personality through the use of mood boosters would be at least one means to achieve authenticity. The ethic of authenticity that Elliott cites seems more in line with saying "I have chosen this personality" than with saying "Nature handed me this personality (at least in part) and so choice does not come into it." The latter seems inauthentic because, if Elliott is right, personality is something that can be changed with mood boosters. Elliott seems to at least partially acknowledge this point because he does acknowledge that psychedelic drugs were often seen as a way of gaining greater authenticity:

> Intellectuals and artists may well have seen psychedelics as a path to a more authentic life, but they also saw them as a means of revolt – as a way of transcending conventional ways of living. Perhaps Prozac can also be a tool

of revolt (as Kramer says, by giving a person the energy to get up and do what needs to be done) but at least as often it seem to be a way of accommodating to conventional ways of life and making the best of them.[14]

Elliott's discussion seems to go a little off the rails here. Revolt is not necessarily a sign of authenticity: much of the so-called counter-culture of the sixties, for example, went along with the movement simply because it was what their friends were doing. The idea of revolt sounds more like a Romantic notion: saying that conventional life is inferior to other types of lives. But as we said, the life of the Snapper lawn mower in the suburbs is not inherently meaningless or inferior to other lives. It violates authenticity only if the life is not autonomously endorsed by the person whose life it is.

The argument also has a singular lack of support for its critical premise: that taking mood boosters is often a way to accommodate oneself to life in the suburbs. I'm not sure why Elliott thinks this is true. It is easy to imagine antidepressants having the opposite effect, which he attributes to Kramer: suppose happier people tend to have the energy and resources necessary to break with conventional life. Mood boosters may make it easier to accommodate to life in suburbia, but it is a reasonable conjecture that they are just as likely to increase the chances of a break with such a life.

Notice too that even if we accept his claim about who is likely to take mood boosters and for what reasons, it still leaves some, perhaps many, cases where taking mood boosters is done authentically. Elliott, recall, qualifies his discussion by saying "more often than not". Of course, not taking mood boosters is no sign that one is leading an authentic life: rejecting mood boosters may simply be a way to accommodate oneself to the societal expectation that mood boosters are a "crutch". In other words, the worry seems to be one of autonomous decision-making: people ought not to take mood boosters simply because society expects you to be happy. This would lead to what Elliott calls the "tyranny of happiness". But of course the point cuts both ways: one ought not to renounce mood boosters simply because society thinks the level of positive affect dispensed by the genetic lottery is natural, and so good. And this is a critical flaw in the argument: absolutely no reason is offered why mood boosters will interfere with gaining an understanding of an authentic life, and why, even if mood boosters alter personality, that personality cannot be authentically altered.

Ultimately, it seems to me that Elliott's argument boils down to the true but somewhat banal prescription that we ought not to take mood-enhancing drugs simply because we feel pressured by others or society to be happy, for this leads to inauthenticity.[15] Fair enough. But by parallel reasoning, we should not *refuse* mood-enhancing drugs simply because we feel pressure from society or others to not rely on such a "crutch". So, even if we follow Elliott in adopting an ethic of authenticity, it hardly decides the issue one way or the other.

Indeed, I have no formal studies on the matter, but my sense from speaking to a number of North American audiences about happy-people-pills is that there is far, far, far more social pressure not to rely on a "crutch" like pharmacology than there is to take pharmaceutical substances to be happy. Many audience members describe pharmacology in terms of a "crutch" or they say that the consumption of pharmaceuticals is indicative that "there is something wrong with you". So, I would say that the greater danger at this moment (at least in North America) is that people will inauthentically refuse to take pharmaceuticals to boost their moods, rather than that people will take pharmaceuticals because they feel pressure to be happy.

9.5 Loss of Identity

An even more radical criticism of happy-people-pills is that they ultimately alter the self or change one's identity. Several commentators have taken some of Elliott's work to express this criticism.[16] For example, Elliott suggests that "it would be worrying if Prozac altered my personality, even if it gave me a better personality, simply because it isn't my personality." The objection raises intriguing philosophical issues, but ultimately it is unsustainable. To see why, we will need to think about its two key premises: first, that mood enhancement causes a change in identity, and second, that a change in identity is morally problematic. Both premises are not plausible, at least in the form required by Elliott's argument.

The plausibility of the first premise turns on our understanding of 'identity'. One sense is what philosophers sometimes term 'personal identity', or persistence of numerical identity. Personal identity in this sense will tell us what conditions are required for the same person to exist from one moment to the next. The problem is familiar to philosophers, but for those not so acquainted, some insight can be had by considering the familiar fictional example of people switching bodies. One of my personal favorites is a schlocky episode in the original *Star Trek* series. Captain Kirk finds himself in the body of his jilted ex-lover, Dr. Janice Lester, after an alien "personality-swapping machine" is used on him. She, jealous of his power, takes control of his body, and his spaceship. The plot device has been used numerous times since, including in the movie "Freaky Friday" where a mother finds herself in her teenage daughter's body and vice versa. These works of fiction are premised on the idea that whatever makes individuals the individuals they are is only contingently related to the bodies that they find themselves in. Captain Kirk grew up in a male body, but for at least a short while he inhabited a female body. The question then naturally arises, what makes Kirk Kirk, if not his body? An answer going back at least to Locke, who used a body-switching example himself, is that it is psychological properties that are the basis of personal identity; for example, Kirk's memories, beliefs, desires, character traits, moods, and emotions are what make him Kirk, and these can, at least in principle, be transferred from body to body.

It is worth pausing to consider an alternate view on personal identity to the one presupposed in the aforementioned works of fiction. For they seem to presuppose the mind, soul or personality is the foundation of identity. However, some suggest that in fact what makes you you is the fact that a physical body persists through time. Applied to the *Star Trek* example, this theory says that there is no switching of numerical identity in the Kirk case. Kirk may act differently, and appear to have the personality and memories of his jilted lover, but Kirk never switched bodies, because Kirk simply is the body.

With this in mind, it is interesting that a literal reading of what Elliott says reveals that he is not talking about numerical personal identity. Consider again the relevant passage: "it would be worrying if Prozac altered my personality, even if it gave me a better personality, simply because it isn't my personality". The quote suggests that personality is separable from identity. Read in this way, it means Elliott would be the same person before and after taking Prozac. Elliott survives taking Prozac, but his personality has changed. This has an odd ring to it, but there is a way to explain it if one invokes the bodily continuity view of personal identity. Since there is one and the same body before and after taking Prozac, and that body is Elliott, clearly Elliott survives taking Prozac. Perhaps one need not invoke bodily identity, but some psychological continuity. For example, if we locate identity in continuity of memories, then since we do not think that Prozac wipes or otherwise seriously affects memories, Elliott survives taking Prozac: he has the same memories of his childhood after taking Prozac as he did before, even though he has a different personality. For our purposes it does not matter which view of personal identity Elliott endorses, what matters is that we understand that he is not suggesting that numerical personal identity is affected by taking Prozac.

Still, this leaves the question of what to make of the idea that taking Prozac results in a personality that "isn't my own". Once the connection with personal identity is severed, the reason for thinking that the resulting personality is not my own is puzzling. The problem can't be that there is a personality change. For, changing one's personality seems to be a goal of at least some interactions between patient and therapist. Seeing a therapist to alleviate one's depression, to stop obsessing about some imagined bodily deformity, to stop acting aggressively towards one's loved ones, is a conscious attempt by both patient and therapist to change the patient's personality. We might think that successful therapy results in a better personality for the patient, but this in itself does not suggest an answer. For in this case we typically think that the improved personality of the patient is different, but still his or hers. The same thought would apply to radical changes in personality brought upon by religious conversion or philosophical enlightenment. Elliott's argument seems to be that the personality is not mine because it is inauthentic. But this means that the change in personality objection looks to collapse into the inauthentic objection. In other words, there is no distinct identity objection on this understanding of Elliott.

Perhaps it may be thought that there is a problem of identity and that Elliott did not push far enough. There may be limits on how far one's identity can change even if the change is authentically endorsed. Aristotle, for example, says that in wishing for what is best for our friend, we should not wish that he become a god, for then he would no longer exist. Aristotle's point may be put in the first person so that we may connect it with the issue of authenticity: I cannot wish to become a god, for this is to wish the impossible. A god trying to honor this wish would run into the problem that I would have to be changed so radically that I would cease to exist. Similarly, I could not wish – in a good Kafka spirit – to become a bug, for then at some point in the metamorphosis I would cease to exist. This understanding leads to the following formulation of the identity objection: in taking Prozac there is such a radical transformation that one person ceases to exist and a new person is born. Thus we should not say that John is happier after taking Prozac, we should say that the old John is dead, and a new person now inhabits the body of John. This is an extreme view, and not one many of us would be willing to take seriously.

One reason not to take it seriously is to imagine that John kills someone and then begins taking Prozac immediately afterwards. Several weeks later the police use fingerprint evidence to identify the hand that pulled the trigger. When they come to arrest him, John says: "Oh, that was John I who did the killing. I'm John II. I have a new personality." Most of us would be reluctant to put an innocent person in jail, even to discourage others, so if we accept this view of personal identity, we would have to let John II go. But of course this is absurd. There is only the one John and he should go to jail. If he is on Prozac, this simply means that he may be a bit happier in jail than he might have otherwise been.

Even if we accept the radical position that taking Prozac results in a change of identity, this still would not establish the identity objection. For recall that the objection requires two steps: that identity is affected, and that this is morally problematic. And we have at least some reason to suppose that it is not morally problematic; indeed, it may be morally praiseworthy.

Consider first the general idea of altruistic suicide. A classic example is a soldier who dives on a grenade to save his comrades. A related example is this: suppose we believe that personhood begins in the second trimester of pregnancy. Barbara is in her first trimester and medical opinion has established that she will die if she takes the child to term (or to any point of viability). We encourage her to have an abortion to save her life. She says that she is willing to sacrifice her life for the sake of the future person who will be her child. She says that she would not criticize anyone else who had an abortion under these circumstances. She is not doing this out of a sense of duty. Rather, she says she is freely willing to make the sacrifice so that another may live. She agrees she is committing suicide, but she is doing so altruistically.

Certainly, not all sacrifices for others are morally unproblematic. But at least some sacrifices for others seem to be paradigms of morally praiseworthy actions. So, the defender of the identity objection must show that taking Prozac is not such a noble self-sacrifice. I might say: "Tonight I will take Prozac. Once it starts to make me less depressed, my life will end. So, soon we will see the end of Mark I. A new person, Mark II, will inhabit this body. He will appear very similar to me (Mark I), but he won't be me. He will have the same knowledge, skills, and memories, but he will be a different person. I have bequeathed all my belongings to Mark II so he will not be penniless. Indeed, in some ways, he will inherit a lot of my life. But Mark II will not be me. I am willing to make this sacrifice for him." Of course this sounds wildly over the top, but it is because we find it hard to believe that

Marks I and II are not one and the same person. But if we can somehow swallow this assumption, we can well imagine that Mark II would be very grateful for Mark I's sacrifice. Critics have done nothing to show that such sacrifices are morally problematic, and so the second step of the argument is unsupported.

9.6 Too Easy

One objection to this line of thought is that it makes achievement "too easy". John the Savage seems to express this point in debate with the Controller:

> " . . . in civilized countries," said the Controller, "you can have girls without hoeing for them; and there aren't any flies or mosquitoes to sting you. We got rid of them all centuries ago."
>
> The Savage nodded, frowning. "You got rid of them. Yes, that's just like you. Getting rid of everything unpleasant instead of learning to put up with it. Whether 'tis nobler in the mind to suffer the slings and arrows of outrageous fortune, or to take arms against a sea of troubles and by opposing end them . . . But you don't do either. Neither suffer nor oppose. You just abolish the slings and arrows. It's too easy."[17]

The objection may strike us as a bit perplexing: usually we consider it to be a plus when something is made easier, not an objection. However, the objection is really that happy-people-pills destroy the connection between effort and success.[18] If we simply pop a pill to be happy in an attempt to improve our wellbeing, then we will not have added the requisite effort. It is only through effort that our happiness is truly our own.

There are several responses to this objection. For a start, the idea that we shouldn't take the 'easy way out' seems to apply most forcefully to our most important goals. For example, suppose you wait three hours in a government office to pay a bill and then your friend tells you that was a great achievement on your part: it was a real testimony to your patience that you survived three hours in a crowded office with unpleasant bureaucrats. Indeed, kudos to you for not taking the easy way out and paying the bill online in a matter of seconds. When you ask why she did not tell you that the bill could be paid online, she says that she did not want to destroy the connection between effort and achievement. Before you kill her, you point out that there are many other more important goals you could have pursued in those same three hours, so you would have been willing to sacrifice the link between effort and the achievement of your goal in this case. Similarly, the goal of taking happy-people-pills is to boost our mood. Perhaps some mood boosting is possible through more laborious means, such as positive psychology. However, spending time doing positive psychology exercises has an opportunity cost: time spent on it could have been time spent on other goals. So, at best, this objection shows that we might have to sacrifice the connection between effort and achievement for one goal (more positive moods), but not for achievement of other goals like pro-social activity.

A second, complementary response reminds us not to forget that there is a limit to what positive psychology can do for us in terms of boosting our positive affect, just as there is a limit to what good nutrition and health can do for increasing the height of our offspring. The fact that happy-people-pills might help us increase our positive affect in no way challenges the fact that genetics plays a role in our happiness, any more than the fact that nutrition plays a role in how tall our offspring will grow undermines the idea that genes play a dominant role in how tall individuals grow. Or, to switch the analogy, the reduction of childhood death in developed countries since the nineteenth century has a lot to do with changes in cultural practices, for example hygiene practices. But these changes did not obviate the need for biological interventions such as antibiotics and immunization shots.

In terms of causality, the "too easy" objection seems to be doubly mistaken. As we have argued, the arrow of causality sometimes goes from happiness to achievement: positive affect causes achievement. (Of course the arrow of causality goes in the opposite direction as well.) Also, the "too easy" objection seems to have in mind some sort of magical mechanism for achieving. We have noted before that there is no reason to suppose taking happy-people-pills will automatically lead to achievement. It is worth revisiting this line of thought here. Suppose Juanita was never very happy. Not depressed, just not very happy. She found brief respite from this unhappiness when she met Anthony. After knowing him for only two weeks she moved to a new town to be with Anthony. Within a month she realized that Anthony is a real jerk. Now she is in a place where she is in a dead-end job, and has no life partner and no friends. Suppose she takes a happy-people-pill; how does this help her obtain the friends, marriage, and workplace success that she believes is important for having a good life? I'm sure the "too easy" objectors don't suppose that Juanita need merely take a happy-people-pill and friends and a spouse will simply pop into existence. This is magical thinking. The trouble is that it is hard to see what "too easy" in this context amounts to. It seems to me that if Juanita is going to make friends, find a spouse, and succeed in the workplace, she is going to have to do it the old-fashioned way. She will have to make friends by finding mutual interests with people she meets, and she will need to go through the rituals of dating and romance, and perhaps upgrade her workplace skills by taking night classes. None of this is magical, revolutionary or easy. While happy-people-pills will do none of these things for Juanita – she won't be able to send the happy-people-pills to night class to take notes for her, or go out and meet people for her at a singles event – they will provide Juanita an important tool for pursuing the good life. Happy-people-pills are not a substitute for the usual means of this pursuit; rather, happy-people-pills may provide Juanita the tools she needs to succeed. Recall the "build and broaden" model of how positive moods contribute to achievement: positive moods make us more inclined to build our repertoire of the skills necessary to succeed.

If the reader will forgive again the analogy, our lives are gardens and we are the gardeners. Positive moods are the water for our gardens. Some people are naturally (i.e., genetically) blessed with plenty of water, others find themselves naturally on more arid land. Happy-people-pills are the aqueducts that bring water to otherwise arid lands. Water makes it easier to be a good gardener, but still there is a lot more to a successful garden than simply water. People like Kass and Sandel seem terribly confused on this point. In terms of our analogy, they would be rebuking the subsistence farmer for having a well drilled on his property because easy access to water destroys the connection between effort and achievement. It may destroy the connection between effort and achievement in terms of getting water, but what is most significant about being a good gardener remains.

9.7   Just Distribution

The just distribution objection is that if happy-people-pills were developed, they would be too pricey for the average consumer, or at least too pricey for the poor. So, this would lead to an unjust situation where only the upper classes can purchase happiness and all its downstream benefits.

It is worth noting how antipodal this criticism is from those just mentioned. The earlier criticisms are united in the assumption that taking happy-people-pills would be harmful to, or at least not benefit, consumers. This criticism seems to assume that taking happy-people-pills would benefit those who partake, and that those who cannot afford it would lose out. This is worth noting because so often this criticism is mentioned alongside the others. However, if one thinks that happy-people-pills are harmful, then one should welcome the consequence that they might be expensive. Consider how we might react to someone who criticizes a new brand of cigarettes because they are more harmful to the health of the consumers than regular brands, and also complains that they are so expensive that only the rich will be able to afford them. The critic should welcome the consequence that they are more expensive if it means that fewer will be harmed.

The objection is one about how to distribute the benefit of happy-people-pills given that it might be costly. There is something to the reply that this objection is to an unfair economic system rather than to happy-people-pills, per se.[19] Certainly it is true that if we had a more egalitarian distribution of wealth, the objection would lose traction. For example, if we lived in a radically egalitarian society, then everyone would have the same amount of money, so either everyone could afford happy-people-pills or no one could. And so, it seems that this objection is based ultimately on our economic system rather than on an argument against happy-people-pills.

While this reply is plausible as it stands, notice that it does not tell us how to operate in our present political climate. That is, given that the great egalitarian revolution is not imminent, what should we do in our present circumstances? One might think that it is sufficient to say that happy-people-pills, like any consumer good, may be differentially distributed in a market economy where there are huge disparities in wealth. The inadequacy of this response is that happy-people-pills are not a typical consumer good. To see this, consider the difference between providing a luxury car and a four-year college education to Poor Joe. Given that the car is luxurious enough, and the college tuition fees modest enough, the price tag of the latter may actually be substantially lower. But to compare these two simply in terms of cost is to miss a crucial difference. A fancy car is not likely to do much in the long term for Poor Joe's financial situation, almost certainly not as much as a four-year college education will. And so, the fact that the market charges a lot for certain cars is less of a problem for overcoming economic inequalities than the price of higher education. To put the point negatively: the harm to the poor is greater if the market prices education, as opposed to luxury cars, out of the reach of the poor. Similarly, the harm to the poor is much greater if they cannot afford happy-people-pills than if they cannot afford a luxury car. The reason of course is that happy-people-pills will likely provide the consumer with numerous benefits, much more than any luxury car is likely to. So, the reply that happy-people-pills are just another typical consumer good that will be unevenly distributed is not adequate.

A more promising reply questions the premise that happy-people-pills will be expensive. At least in the long term, this premise is almost certainly false. No doubt many of us have heard how prohibitively expensive some antidepressants are. The question is whether this will be the case with happy-people-pills. The economics of the pharmaceutical industry is complex and contested. The litany of complaints includes the allegations that the big pharmaceutical companies make windfall products, innovate little, and exert undue influence on medical practitioners. Apologists point out that there are large development costs for any drug that must be recouped if there is to be innovation, and this cost must be recovered during the patent life of the drug. Everyone agrees pharmaceutical companies are able to charge such high prices because of the patent system. It is generally recognized that the production cost of most SSRIs is literally "pennies a pill", yet at one time, Prozac cost more than three dollars a pill.[20] There are a bunch of arcane laws pertaining to how long a patent can be enforced, and they vary from jurisdiction to jurisdiction, but, roughly, a patent provides a monopoly for twenty years. Naturally, it is a very sad day for manufacturers when their patent expires. Generic versions of Prozac can be had for as little as 20 cents a pill now, for example. One point that emerges is that if distributive justice is a problem, it is not likely to be much of a problem after a patent expires. True, this may be unfair while the patent is being enforced, if the critics are correct, but this is not a long-term problem.

A second point has to do with potential market. If we accept the argument that pharmaceutical companies must charge a lot to recover their investment, then we can see that the price they must charge to recoup their investment is related to the number of pills they sell. But this bodes well for happy-people-pills. The number of people who could potentially benefit from happy-people-pills is much larger than the number of people diagnosed with depression. As we noted, estimates for depression rates are in the 5–10 percent range, while the potential market for happy-people-pills is the entire population. So, if price is a function of the need to recover investment, there is less need to charge as much per pill if there is a larger market. This is not to say that big pharmaceutical companies would not charge exorbitant prices – this is the beauty of having a monopoly after all – but the high prices could not be justified solely in terms of incurred expenses.

Even if the patent system is in place, there is every reason to suppose that public options would be available for just distribution. The government could put an "enhancement tax" on pharmaceutical companies and consumers for happy-people-pills and use this revenue to make them more affordable for the rest of the population. There are even more radical options, such as nationalizing some of the pharmaceutical industry or publicly whipping pharmaceutical executives who authorize windfall profits.

It is worth noting that the just distribution objection ultimately has more traction on the economic left than on the economic right. If one is economically right, then one may think that the poor deserve their plight (because they are lazy or less naturally endowed with talents to compete in the market) or that the economically disadvantaged classes are an unfortunate consequence of the free market. So, in general, we should expect those on the economic right not to be particularly moved by this objection. The objection is more at home with the economic left. But, those on the economic left have a number of public options consistent with their view to eliminate or at least reduce any distributive injustice, some of which we noted above. Ultimately, the distributive justice objection is not a theoretical showstopper, but more a practical problem of influencing public policy in the short term. We will discuss this a bit more in the next chapter.

Notes

1. Kass, "Ageless Bodies, Happy Souls."
2. Lyubomirsky, King, and Diener, "The Benefits of Frequent Positive Affect."
3. Diener and Seligman, "Very Happy People," 84.
4. Healy, *Let Them Eat Prozac*, 182.
5. Friedman, "Born to Be Happy, Through a Twist of Human Hard Wire."
6. President's Council on Bioethics, *Beyond Therapy*.
7. Ibid.
8. There are obvious problems (Glover, "How Should We Decide What Sort of World is Best?") with drawing the distinction in this way; e.g., laser eye surgery then counts as an unnatural change. However, the point developed below is that even if we grant such a distinction to opponents of happy-people-pills, it is not sufficient to support their position.
9. Elliott, "The Tyranny of Happiness," 185–6.
10. Ibid., 180.
11. Nietzsche, *Beyond Good and Evil*, Section 211.

12. Elliott, "The Tyranny of Happiness," 180.
13. Bolt, "True to Oneself?," 288.
14. Elliott, "The Tyranny of Happiness," 180.
15. Elliott (*Better Than Well*) suggests Americans have attitudes toward mood enhancers that are in tension: seeing them both as necessary for the good life and also as a mere crutch.
16. Bolt, "True to Oneself?"; DeGrazia, "Prozac, Enhancement, and Self-Creation."
17. Huxley, *Brave New World and Brave New World Revisited*, 224.
18. Sandel, *The Case Against Perfection*; President's Council on Bioethics, *Beyond Therapy*.
19. DeGrazia, "Prozac, Enhancement, and Self-Creation."
20. Huskamp et al., "Generic Entry, Reformulations, and Promotion of SSRIs."

References

Bolt, L. L. E. "True to Oneself? Broad and Narrow Ideas on Authenticity in the Enhancement Debate." *Theoretical Medicine and Bioethics* 28, no. 4 (2007): 285–300.

DeGrazia, D. "Prozac, Enhancement, and Self-Creation." *Hastings Center Report* 30, no. 2 (2000): 34–40.

Diener, E. and M. E. P. Seligman. "Very Happy People." *Psychological Science* 13, no. 1 (2002): 81–4.

Elliott, C. *Better Than Well: American Medicine Meets the American Dream.* New York: W.W. Norton, 2004.

Elliott, C. "The Tyranny of Happiness: Ethics and Cosmetic Psychopharmacology." In *Enhancing Human Traits: Ethical and Social Implications*, edited by E. Parens, 177–88. Washington, D.C.: Georgetown University Press, 1998.

Friedman, R. "Born to Be Happy, Through a Twist of Human Hard Wire." *New York Times*, December 31, 2002, section F.

Glover, J. "How Should We Decide What Sort of World is Best?" In *Ethics and Problems of the 21st Century*, edited by K. Goodpaster and K. M. Sayre: 79–92. Notre Dame, Ind.: University of Notre Dame Press, 1979.

Healy, D. *Let Them Eat Prozac: The Unhealthy Relationship Between the Pharmaceutical Companies and Depression.* New York: New York University Press, 2004.

Huskamp, H. A., J. M. Donohue, C. Koss, E. R Berndt and R. G. Frank. "Generic Entry, Reformulations, and Promotion of SSRIs." *PharmacoEconomics* 26, no. 7 (2008): 603–16.

Huxley, A. *Brave New World and Brave New World Revisited.* Toronto: Vintage Books, 2007.

Kass, L. R. "Ageless Bodies, Happy Souls." *New Atlantis* 1 (2003): 9–28.

Lyubomirsky, S., L. King, and E. Diener. "The Benefits of Frequent Positive Affect: Does Happiness Lead to Success?" *Psychological Bulletin* 131 (2005): 803–55.

Nietzsche, F. *Beyond Good and Evil*, trans. Walter Kaufmann. New York: Vintage, 1966.

President's Council on Bioethics. *Beyond Therapy: Biotechnology and the Pursuit of Happiness*. New York: Dana Press, 2003.

Sandel, M. J. *The Case Against Perfection: Ethics in the Age of Genetic Engineering*. Cambridge, Mass.: Harvard University Press, 2007.

10

Happy-People-Pills and Public Policy

This chapter explores policy questions that arise from accepting our moral arguments for happy-people-pills. We will look at arguments from the liberty and justice point of view which support the policy prescription that society should permit the development of happy-people-pills. We will then turn to objections to such a policy based on adverse effects on health and society at large. Finally, we will address the question of how happy-people-pills ought to be justly distributed.

10.1 Liberty

An obvious reason to craft policy permitting the use of happy-people-pills is for the sake of liberty. Since, other things being equal, liberty is a good thing, we have at least some reason to permit individuals to use happy-people-pills. In some ways the conclusion is almost trivial if 'liberty' is to be understood in the sense that Locke attributes to Filmer: "every one to do what he lists, to live as he pleases, and not to be tied by any laws."[1] Not legislating against happy-people-pills provides more liberty to those who wish to use happy-people-pills, and so promotes the greater good. Thus, the conclusion is almost trivial, because the premise defines liberty in part in terms of absence of legal restraint. Still, the argument is not completely trivial, since it depends on the idea that liberty is good.

The 'liberty defense' of happy-people-pills is obviously reminiscent of arguments to legalize marijuana, cocaine, and other "street" drugs.

Happy-People-Pills For All, First Edition. Mark Walker.
© 2013 John Wiley & Sons, Inc. Published 2013 by John Wiley & Sons, Inc.

The liberty argument is probably worth considering for this reason alone. However, as we shall see, the liberty defense is only as good as a very specific political philosophical doctrine, one that is not shared widely, at least in practice. Thus, given the contested nature of the underlying political philosophical doctrine, for many the liberty defense does not provide much reason to permit the use of happy-people-pills.

Few will have issue with the claim that, other things being equal, the more liberty we have, the better off we are. However, the premise is not going to advance the debate to legalize street drugs, or even happy-people-pills for that matter. In the case of street drugs, critics charge that at least some people harm themselves and others by taking drugs. Tales of successful individuals falling from grace upon becoming addicted to drugs are the very stuff of anti-drug propaganda. So, it is clear then that the premise as formulated is too weak to carry the argument very far. A stronger premise is this: more liberty is always better. This premise will get us to the conclusion that there ought not to be laws against happy-people-pills and street drugs, but the premise itself is almost certainly false.

Complete liberty means there are no laws restraining our actions. But this liberty is likely to be purchased at great cost: we may have to fear for our own lives and the lives of our loved ones where laws do not restrain the liberty of others. We do not have to follow Hobbes down the road of complete servility, which says just about any loss of liberty is worth the price of peace, to see that liberty is not the only political value worthy of pursuit. Indeed, finding some middle ground between complete domination of the individual by the state in the name of peace, and complete liberty as promised by some forms of anarchy, is a central concern of modern political philosophy.

Assuming we do not want to go down the road of anarchism, we need to find a more plausible version of the liberty argument; fortunately we do not have to look far. A famous proposal made by J. S. Mill starts with the liberal premise that intervention in the lives of individuals is justified only to prevent direct harm to others. Thus Mill:

> The object of this Essay is to assert one very simple principle, as entitled to govern absolutely the dealings of society with the individual in the way of compulsion and control, whether the means used be physical force in the form of legal penalties, or the moral coercion of public opinion. That principle is, that the sole end for which mankind are warranted, individually or collectively, in interfering with the liberty of action of any of their number, is self-protection. That the only purpose for which power can be rightfully

exercised over any member of a civilized community, against his will, is to prevent harm to others. His own good, either physical or moral, is not sufficient warrant. He cannot rightfully be compelled to do or forbear because it will be better for him to do so, because it will make him happier, because, in the opinions of others, to do so would be wise, or even right…. The only part of the conduct of any one, for which he is amenable to society, is that which concerns others. In the part which merely concerns himself, his independence is, of right, absolute. Over himself, over his own body and mind, the individual is sovereign.[2]

The liberal premise, or the harm principle as it is often called, strikes a balance between permitting more liberty only when other things are equal, which is to say not very often, and the anarchist principle that says that more liberty is always better. The application to the debate over legalizing street drugs is pretty obvious. Marijuana and cocaine may physically or morally harm consumers but users do not directly harm others. Hence, the state is not justified in regulating the use of marijuana and cocaine. Present anti-drug laws are perniciously paternalistic according to this line of reasoning. The state in effect is saying that it knows better how citizens should live their lives than the citizens themselves. It is better to allow individuals liberty to find their own way in the world, says the Millian, even if this opens up the possibility that they may harm themselves.

Mill does allow that law can justly intervene in some cases of drug use:

in the frequent case of a man who causes grief to his family by addiction to bad habits, he deserves reproach for his unkindness or ingratitude; but so he may for cultivating habits not in themselves vicious, if they are painful to those with whom he passes his life, or who from personal ties are dependent on him for their comfort. Whoever fails in the consideration generally due to the interests and feelings of others, not being compelled by some more imperative duty, or justified by allowable self-preference, is a subject of moral disapprobation for that failure, but not for the cause of it, nor for the errors, merely personal to himself, which may have remotely led to it. In like manner, when a person disables himself, by conduct purely self-regarding, from the performance of some definite duty incumbent on him to the public, he is guilty of a social offence. No person ought to be punished simply for being drunk; but a soldier or a policeman should be punished for being drunk on duty. Whenever, in short, there is a definite damage, or a definite risk of damage, either to an individual or to the public, the case is taken out of the province of liberty, and placed in that of morality or law.[3]

One of the attractions of Mill's harm principle is that it offers a very general formula for balancing individual liberty against public goods like peace.

However, the harm principle has a contentious history. Critics wonder exactly what is meant by 'harm.' If it is only intended to cover physical harm, then the principle seems implausible: if I steal your car I do not physically harm you, so the state would not be justified in creating laws preventing the stealing of cars. Or if it can be arranged for you to be gently kidnapped, perhaps while you are asleep, the state ought not to intervene since you are not physically harmed. So, the principle must mean more than physical harm. But if harm means physical and mental harm, then the principle looks far too restrictive. If you insult my new shoes, then you may mentally harm me, in which case the state ought to intervene.

An obvious move here would be to ground the harm principle on something even more fundamental. Mill's utilitarianism is an obvious candidate. The idea would be to define 'harm' in terms of a certain level of pain. Thus, although kidnapping me and insulting my shoes may both cause mental rather than physical pains, the insult to my shoes is nowhere near as painful, and so won't count as harm. Unfortunately, this move will not do either. Many people might find it much more painful to hear their god insulted or their life's work ridiculed in the press than to suffer physical injury, such as a broken arm. The pain of hearing such remarks can be felt more deeply, and for much, much longer than the pain of some bone fractures that will mend in a few weeks. So, if we prohibit the harm of breaking bones because of the pain involved, then we ought to prohibit the pain of insults on the same grounds. Conversely, if insults do not count as harm, even though they can cause so much pain, then the reason for prohibiting the breaking of arms cannot be simply that a certain threshold of pain has been exceeded.

It might be thought that the Millian can simply respond that in a liberal society people *should not* be so pained by insults: this is one of the consequences of living in a society where liberty is a central political value. No one says that liberty is not without some costs, so freedom of expression opens us to the possibility of others criticizing or ridiculing all that we hold sacred or dear. This may be true, but notice how the Millian in this case has switched grounds: this is no longer a matter of arguing *to* a liberal society but *from* a liberal society. Ostensibly, Mill argues in *On Liberty* that we ought to adopt a liberal society because it is the only one consistent with the harm principle. The response under consideration argues exactly the opposite: we cannot consider insults as harms because this is inconsistent with the liberal state.

I have rehearsed some familiar problems with the harm principle simply to show that it is not nearly as straightforward as its sounds. So, a theoretical problem for the liberty defense of happy-people-pills is to formulate the harm principle, or some analogue thereof, in a way that is consistent and plausible.

A second and probably more serious problem is that even the spirit of the harm principle – that the state ought not to act paternalistically – is never endorsed in practice. Exhibit one is how little headway proponents of legalizing marijuana have made with legislators when invoking the harm principle. Rightly or wrongly, a considerable amount of legislative activity seems to be directed at saving people from themselves. Most people see little wrong with formulating paternalistic laws for others: pot laws are there, at least in part, to save potheads from themselves. So, a practical problem to accepting the liberty defense of happy-people-pills is that it requires adopting a political outlook that goes against the zeitgeist. If this were the best argument for permitting the use of happy-people-pills, then the prospects for happy-people-pills would be pretty dim in the foreseeable future.

10.2 Justice

Fortunately, we have available a much stronger argument. The justice argument contends that happy-people-pills will contribute to the wellbeing of many, so to prohibit the use of happy-people-pills would be an injustice.

The following analogy may serve as illustration of the justice argument. Imagine a small farming village built around a river. Families were originally settled by a lottery. Those who found themselves close to the river were the lucky ones, for they were able to grow wonderful crops with comparative ease. The rest were not so lucky: the further one lived from the river the harder it was to grow crops. No one died of starvation, but those furthest away from the river had to struggle hard and got much poorer results than their riverfront peers. So, they tended to achieve less, and be less happy, than the lucky living on the riverbanks, for they had to spend more time drudging water and performing other mind-numbing tasks. Imagine it was discovered that the entire village sat atop a massive aquifer, and that recently discovered well-digging technology could be used to easily increase irrigation. This opened up the possibility that many would be able to boost their crop production, and so too their wellbeing. Not only would they have more food, but they would also have more time and energy to engage in many activities in addition to farming. Clearly, any ordinance prohibiting the digging of wells to ensure the continued advantage of those living on the riverfront would be unjust: justice demands that others not be prohibited greater access to water. Of course the riverfront folk are analogous to the hyperthymic, while the rest of the town folk are equivalent to the non-hyperthymic. Any no-well-digging ordinance parallels laws to prohibit access to happy-people-pills. So, justice demands that we permit people to use happy-people-pills for a chance to increase their wellbeing.

We should consider an objection that will serve to illuminate the scope of the argument. Suppose Alexis suffers from depression as an adult and experts agree that her depression is the result of an abusive father and a cold, indifferent mother. Here there is good reason to suppose that Alexis's unhappiness is undeserved and unjust. Notice, however, it is wrong to argue that the same reasoning will apply to genetic influences upon happiness. In other words, imagine it was argued as follows: if we suppose that Alexis in fact grew up in a stable and nurturing environment, but that she inherited genes that influenced her low positive affect, then here too we would have to say that her unhappiness is unjust. The reasoning here is faulty because of a crucial difference between the two: in the case where Alexis's environment causes her low positive affect, there are agents to whom we can attribute responsibility, namely, her abusive father and indifferent mother. In the case where Alexis inherits genes that contribute to her low chronic positive affect, there are no agents to whom we can attribute moral responsibility. True, she inherited her genes from her parents, but her parents had no control over what genes they passed on.

Happy-people-pills progressives may accept this line of reasoning because it does not touch the main point: the injustice is *not* that some win the genetic lottery and some lose the genetic lottery, *but* that happy-people-pills conservatives would want to maintain the results of the genetic lottery even if compensatory mechanisms, such as a hyperthymic pill, could be developed. In the case of our river village, the claim of injustice is not that some ended up closer to the river – for this was settled by a fair lottery, let us suppose. Rather, the injustice would come in prohibiting the technology that would remedy this inequality. A more apt analogy is as follows: imagine Hira is a young child involved in a multi-car accident caused by a mudslide in a remote area. Twenty people died but Hira was miraculously thrown clear. Since it was assumed for good reason that Hira died along with everyone else, Hira was forced to fend for herself for a number of years, living off the land as a "feral child." Years later, Hira is found by hikers and undergoes a battery of tests by psychologists. Psychologists conjecture that her happiness, while in the low normal range, probably would have been in the hyperthymic range if she had had a nurturing environment in her formative years. In this case, her condition is not attributable to the culpable actions of anyone: no one was responsible for the mudslide, and there was every reason to suppose that she died in the car accident. In effect, Hira lost the "environmental lottery." Let us agree that no injustice has been committed. However, an injustice would occur if we insisted that Hira be prohibited from taking up an offer of special counseling to help her compensate for the impoverished environment she experienced. Surely blocking her from such counseling would raise howls of protest. The injustice here is not that she lost the "environmental lottery," but that she is prohibited from using a compensatory mechanism. Similarly, with happy-people-pills, the injustice is not that some win and some lose the genetic lottery, for there is little we can do about that (at this stage), but that the effects of the genetic lottery are enforced. The strong genetic component to positive affect means that people will experience a level of positive affect that they do not deserve. Given the value of happiness and achievement in an individual's life, we have a compelling prima facie reason to think that it would be unjust to prohibit individuals from using happy-people-pills to pursue these important goals.

Not permitting the people of the village to dig wells would be something akin to slavery. It would prohibit them from improving their wellbeing for no overriding moral reason. (I'm assuming here that there is no moral overriding reason like an increased chance of harming the rest of the community. Indeed, with greater productivity from well drilling, one would think the average level of wellbeing would rise for the whole community.) The comparison is perhaps a bit strained since of course many slaves have it much worse than the community on the outskirts of the village. Perhaps it might be thought more akin to indentured servitude; yet if the law prohibiting drilling has no statutory limit, then their fate seems worse than that of indentured servants: the villagers' reduced wellbeing is legislated in perpetuity. Other comparisons that might be drawn are to the oppression women suffered (and still do to some extent today, even in the so-called developed world) in terms of political and economic inequality. At least one reason why it is unjust to deny women the vote and to pay them less in the workplace is that these actions reduce their wellbeing in relation to what it would be in a more just society. Again, there are dangers here of simply drawing invidious comparisons. Slavery, indentured servitude, and gender oppression are all forms of oppression that have occurred in a variety of social configurations, and there is probably little value in trying to answer the question "Who had it worse?" Rather, we can be content with the conclusion that, whatever else they are, they are all forms of unjust oppression. To prohibit the development of happy-people-pills would be to instigate a new form of oppression: bio-oppression.

10.3   The Liberty Versus the Justice Argument

The liberty and justice arguments, at least on the surface, may appear to be very similar. Both arguments claim that there are limits to when the state can justly interfere in the lives of its members. They do, however, differ significantly. The liberty defense, based on the harm principle, is rooted in anti-paternalism: the state cannot legitimately intervene to stop harm to oneself; the state can intervene only to stop harm to others. The justice argument says that the state cannot justly intervene to stop the attainment of the wellbeing of its individuals unless there are overriding harms to others. The liberty argument, then, concedes that the activities it seeks to protect may be harmful to the individual, at least from the point of view of the state, whereas the justice argument makes no such concession to the activities it seeks to protect. So, the liberty argument applied to smoking marijuana says that potheads may be wasting their lives, but that is their business. The justice argument applied to happy-people-pills says that many will have better lives with happy-people-pills; so, the crucial difference is that the justice argument is compatible with paternalism in a way that the liberty argument is not.

Another way to see the difference in these two arguments is to note that street drugs are sometimes defended with the justice argument. Consider marijuana when used by patients undergoing cancer treatment. In this case, it is defended on the basis that it is integral to patient recovery. With this argument, proponents make no concession that marijuana is harmful (all considered) or merely "recreational." Rather, the argument is that to prohibit its use is a matter of depriving people of something that is fundamental to their wellbeing, namely, their health. Similarly, occasionally the argument is made that drugs are necessary for certain religious ceremonies. Ingesting mescaline made from peyote cactus is allowed in the US as part of a bona fide religious ceremony for aboriginals.

Here the brief in support of this practice does not concede that the peyote is harmful (overall) or merely for recreational use. Rather, the argument is that such uses are connected with religious practices that are understood to be central to wellbeing. It is not part of the present work to take a stand on the issue of whether street drugs should be legalized. But a little friendly advice to friends of marijuana and other drugs: given how little credence society attaches to the harm principle, the justice argument is where proponents of legalizing street drugs should make their case. That is, they should not concede that drugs are "merely" recreational; they should make the case that they are necessary for wellbeing. For instance, the role of drugs in the creation of art is well known. Everyone who likes music almost certainly appreciates at least one song created with the assistance of street drugs. Do you enjoy classical music, jazz, rock, blues, etc.? Then you are almost certainly helping some musician profit from their crime. You are an accessory after the fact.

10.4 Health Side Effects and Policy

One reason to deny the justice argument is that all drugs carry some risk, and so should only be used when absolutely necessary. So, by prohibiting happy-people-pills, governments are helping people avoid unnecessary risks. This objection is unashamedly paternalistic, but, as we have just seen, it cannot be rejected simply for this reason; otherwise we are back to the liberty argument rather than the justice argument. We will need to look at some general considerations of risk and policy before turning to the question of whether happy-people-pills can meet this objection.

Some people express outrage that the US government allows high school and college students to play football. The dangers of high school and college football are readily apparent to anyone who has seen even a little of the game, and it seems that every year the media reports cases of children and young adults dying in some horrific accident on the field. What may seem even more outrageous is that governments allow persons of all ages to engage in an activity that is nearly 200 times as dangerous. What is the activity that is 200 times as risky as playing football? Answer: riding in a car. Statistics show that 1 in 1.7 million high school and college players will die every year participating in football (about 5 deaths for over 8 million students involved annually), while there are nearly 200 deaths for 1.7 million yearly vehicle occupancies. Another activity that is 200 times as risky as football is the risk 50-year-old men take when using aspirin as a prophylactic against heart disease. They face a similar yearly risk of 200 deaths for every 1.7 million users.[4]

I don't mean to suggest that deaths in football accidents are not tragic, or that we should not do more to reduce them. Rather, in part it serves as a reminder that there is risk in everything we do. It doesn't take too long looking at tables of death stats to lead one to think that one should never get out of bed – until one realizes that a huge number of people die in bed. Of course it is somewhat banal to say that there is risk attached to all our activities, and that it is easy to get blinded by statistics; but these points do raise a more significant issue: why do we accept our current level of risk for various activities? Certainly it does not follow that because everything has risk attached to it, we ought not to worry about risks, or that there is nothing we can do to reduce them. Taking a bus, for instance, is about 50 times safer than driving a personal vehicle.[5] We could reduce our exposure to risk by renouncing all personal vehicles and taking buses. So, why don't we do this? The obvious answer is there are enormous benefits to having the convenience of a personal vehicle. That is, we accept the higher risks of personal vehicles for the sake of the benefits they provide. Consistency demands that happy-people-pills should be evaluated in the same manner: we should realize that taking them has some risk attached to it, but this needs to be weighed against the benefits they offer to recipients.

Unfortunately, in the case of happiness enhancement, this requires data that, for the most part, we lack. We saw in Chapter 7 that there is, at best, suggestive evidence that some of our current stable of antidepressants will enhance the moods of those in the normal range, and that, for the most part, the side effects when used for enhancement are generally mild or entirely absent.[6] Until we collect reliable data, it is nearly impossible to estimate the benefit (or lack thereof) of the current dispensary of antidepressants.

Still, it may be objected:

We know that antidepressants have side effects, and these risks are unacceptable when the antidepressants are used as enhancement. In the case of therapy, the risks are worth it, because the patient's wellbeing is in serious jeopardy. This is not the case with enhancement.

I will make two general comments about this, and address two specific ailments.

The first point is one made earlier: just as antidepressants seem to have variable efficacy in relieving depression, so too are the side effects variable.

One person may take an antidepressant and experience no side effects; another may experience terrible symptoms. On a population level, the side effects of antidepressants are comparatively mild. Recall, a partial list of possible symptoms includes nausea, drowsiness, sleep difficulties, weight gain, nervousness, fatigue, dry mouth, and blurred vision. Many patients find the symptoms disappear within a few days or weeks. This is not to downplay the side effects, but to say that cautious experimentation may avoid many of these problems. In fact, in the case of enhancement, where there is likely to be less urgency, people can start with very small doses to see if they react negatively or not. This is similar to the practice of physicians who typically start depressed patients on smaller doses and increase them as tolerance is demonstrated. In the case of enhancement, in order to minimize adverse reactions, we might start with even smaller dosages than in therapeutic applications, since the need is not as urgent. With time on their side, those experimenting with antidepressants for enhancement should have a reduced side-effects profile when compared with therapeutic cases. For instance, presently medical practitioners might prescribe 200 mg of bupropion (Wellbutrin) for patients seeking relief from depression. Depending on the patient and the prescriber, the dosage may be ramped up over a few days or weeks. For someone experimenting with bupropion as an enhancement, there is no reason to start with such a large dosage. One might start with 50 mg a day and work up from there.

Second, in general, advancing technology and knowledge has helped eliminate or ameliorate side effects. In part, this is because there is some tendency for a patent or license not to be pursued or granted if an experimental antidepressant does not have increased efficacy or a better side-effects profile.[7] Of course, the process can be (and has been) corrupted by politics and greed, but as a general tendency the trend over the last few decades is encouraging. Also, future patients may benefit from a less onerous testing procedure: a DNA sample might show indicators for compatibility. A little DNA obtained from some saliva may indicate that antidepressants A, B, and C are likely to cause side effects, whereas D, E, and F won't.[8]

One instance of the trend to a reduction of side effects can be seen in the oft-heard complaint that antidepressants can depress interest in sexual activity. For patients, this is usually of great concern because it tends to be a longer-term side effect than, say, nausea, which usually disappears in a few days. Again, this side effect is not universal, but for certain classes of antidepressants like SSRIs – the most commonly prescribed family of antidepressants – the reputation for reducing sexual interest is richly deserved. However, not all antidepressants are like this. Consider two examples.

The antidepressant amineptine was sold under the trade name 'Survector.' Far from suppressing sexual interest, Survector earned the name the "orgasm drug." Under pressure from the FDA, the drug was withdrawn from the European market in 1999, and was never commercially available in the US.[9] Ostensibly, the drug was taken off the market because of sporadic reports of abuse, but some suspect that it was mere prudery that motivated the decision. (Recall that this was an era before we were inundated with commercials for sexual enhancement products.) Interestingly, the studies that reported this connection also noted that most abusers of Survector had a history of drug abuse.[10] By this same reasoning, many other antidepressants ought to be withdrawn from the market. For instance, Venlafaxine, one of the more commonly prescribed SSRI antidepressants, ought to be withdrawn from the market because patients abusing Survector have gone on to abuse Venlafaxine.[11] The moral to be drawn here is not that Survector was particularly addictive, but that just about anything can be addictive for some. It seems that in practice this must be the current reasoning of health officials; otherwise it is difficult to explain why Venlafaxine (and other antidepressants) aren't withdrawn from the market for the same reason.

Wellbutrin is another drug that promotes sexual interest in many patients. The first publication about increased sexual response as a result of taking Wellbutrin came in 1987 in a placebo-controlled study.[12] As we have noted more than once before, on an individual basis there is a huge difference in response to antidepressants, so there is no reason to think that Wellbutrin is for everyone, but on a population level Wellbutrin has been shown to be as effective at treating depression with comparable non-sexual side effects as its blockbuster SSRI cousins such as Prozac, Zoloft, and Celexa. So, here is a billion-dollar question: Why did so many patients, for at least twenty years, suffer with the negative sexual side-effects of SSRIs when they could have been prescribed Wellbutrin by medical professionals? I'm not sure I know the full answer, but I would be surprised if the explanation did not involve money, prudery, politics, and more money.[13] I am not suggesting that we all run out and start taking Survector – which would be particularly difficult since it is no longer manufactured – or Wellbutrin, I am suggesting that it puts to rest the criticism that all antidepressants suppress sexual desire or performance.

The second side effect that deserves special consideration is suicide. The evidence that antidepressants might contribute to suicide *when used for enhancement* is very slim. The only evidence I am aware of is the study by Healy on healthy volunteers – the same study that did much to break the conspiracy of silence on the subject of the link between suicide and antidepressants in therapeutic cases. This is not to say that antidepressants do not cause thoughts of suicide when used for enhancement, only that the empirical evidence we have to work with is pretty scant.

It might be thought that we should simply extrapolate from what we know about the use of antidepressants in therapeutic situations with the depressed. However, this evidence does not help critics of enhancement, since, as noted above, some of the newer studies suggest that antidepressants may reduce the *overall* risk of suicide.[14] So, based on this evidence, a straightforward extrapolation to enhancement would say that they should reduce the incidence of suicide when used for enhancement. Also, as noted in Chapter 7, the fact that we now know there is at least this potential means that the incidence of antidepressants causing suicide should decrease. For instance, if this potential side effect had been known in the Healy study, the participants could have dropped out of the study earlier and significantly reduced their risk.

Also relevant here is the question of the overall risk of death, not just death by suicide. There is ample evidence, for example, that positive moods are correlated with beneficial health outcomes.[15] Any increased risk of suicide will have to be balanced against potential life-saving health benefits. For example, suppose it is discovered that while suicides increase with the use of antidepressants for enhancement, the risk of dying of coronary disease decreases with their use. We would have a situation similar to that of patients taking aspirin as a prophylactic against heart disease: it increases the chances of death by cerebral hemorrhage and the risk of gastrointestinal bleeding but lowers the risk from coronary disease. Imagine that it is discovered that there is an increase in suicide of two deaths per million users of happy-people-pills, but a reduction of death by coronary disease of ten in a million users. Overall, this would indicate a lower death rate with the use of happy-people-pills. Of course, I just made up these numbers. Going forward, what is required is careful and transparent collection of data about the incidence of side effects with the use of antidepressants and any new happy-people-pills. It is worth noting, however, that the link between happiness and health is already established; what is merely speculative at this point is whether and what side effects happy-people-pills may have.

We may summarize the discussion with three points: First, there is little evidence that current antidepressants present serious health risks when used for enhancement. Second, future developments promise a further reduction in side effects. Third, rational policy must balance any possible negative side effects with health benefits, and the promotion of wellbeing in general. In terms of policy, a high standard to use for comparison is the risk from driving a car. If the risk of dying or suffering serious injury from the use of pharmacological agents for happiness enhancement is equal to or less than that from driving a car, then rational policy should allow it. The reason to term this a high standard is that the comparison with driving risks significantly downplays the potential benefit of happiness enhancement. For, in general, the benefit of being able to drive is much less than the benefit of being happier and achieving more. Since the benefit of taking happy-people-pills is likely to be greater for most people than the benefit of driving, we should actually accept a higher risk of death or serious injury. However, the risks associated with driving provide at least one benchmark for rational policy.

10.5   A Social Experiment

A second reason to reject the justice argument is that doing so may have unforeseen and negative consequences. We simply do not know what will happen, according to this line of reasoning, if we alter human biology, on a large scale, with happy-people-pills.

At least this much of the objection seems sound: we do not know for certain the outcome of any social experiment, this one included. We don't know what it would be like to live in a world where those who live on the low side of the normal distribution of happiness are happier. We don't know what it would be like to live in a world where there is a concerted and successful effort to make ourselves happier and more successful through pharmacology. However, uncertainty is the traditional complaint against any change. Let's face it; most people are fearful of change. If for two hundred years a law required people to stick their head in a bucket of excrement every day, you can bet your life that there would be a hue and cry from many quarters against the radical proposal to repeal the law. Admittedly, this is to overstate the status quo bias somewhat, but it is a real human tendency. As illustration, it is always sad to read about nineteenth-century conservatives who fought to keep women politically subservient on the basis that such a radical change had unknown social consequences. The most histrionic of the nineteenth-century conservatives suggested that giving women the vote might lead to the collapse of civil society.

The point of this example is not that we know the happy-people-pills experiment will turn out positive in the same way that granting suffrage to women worked to such a spectacular degree. The point I want to make is much more limited: we have a long tradition of social experimentation – democracy, banning alcohol, legalization of abortion, the Internet, and so on – and the proposal to experiment with happy-people-pills is no different in this regard. The fact that it is an experiment is not sufficient for the objection; otherwise we would have to condemn our ancestors who tried the radical experiments in democracy and women's suffrage.

It may be protested that the bioconservatives need not be against all change – introducing reforms to reduce political tensions between the have and have-not nations, for instance, is not incompatible with bioconservatism – bioconservatives are united in opposing change to our biological natures. So, while the bioconservatives may say that the ends of prescribing happy-people-pills – greater happiness and achievement – are laudable, the means its proponents seek to achieve these ends, using science to alter our 'common biological nature,' are not morally laudable.

The qualification that bioconservatives are opposed to change to *our biology* is important if only to avoid the following embarrassing consequence for bioconservatives: if they are against happy-people-pills, then they ought to be against positive psychology as well, for both have the ambition to make people happier. The response by bioconservatives must be along the lines that positive psychology does not seek to alter our common biological nature whereas happy-people-pills do.

To assess this line of thought, consider first what it means to alter our 'common biological nature.' Obviously this objection would be mistaken if it were based on the idea that pharmacological agents would change our genomes.[16] So the objection about changing our common biological nature must be a comment about changing our phenotype. But if this is the case, then the objection seems to apply equally well to using positive psychology: while we do not understand exactly how such changes work, if positive psychology actually succeeds in raising the average level of happiness, then it will succeed in altering the biochemistry of our brains.[17] For example, suppose that studies show that subjects who regularly employ positive psychology experience more positive moods and have increased serotonin levels in their brains, along with other neurochemical and neurophysiological differences. If so, this would mean that positive psychology succeeds in changing our phenotype, for, if positive psychology works, it will change something about our brain physiology. So, explaining the difference between happy-people-pills and positive psychology because the former but not the latter alters our phenotype is mistaken. This is not to deny there is some difference between taking pharmacological agents and the psychological interventions suggested by positive psychology. The point here is that the moral difference cannot be explained in terms of altering our genotype or phenotype. Neither happy-people-pills nor positive psychology alters our genotype, and both alter our phenotype.

It will help to consider Fukuyama's response to this line of thought. His retort is basically that, unlike biological interventions such as pharmacology and genetic technologies, there is a limited amount that socialization or nurture interventions can do to change us. He is not committed to a crude genetic determinism; a better metaphor is that our common biology provides a common tether. Different societies are like a number of animals tethered to a post. They spread out seeking good grazing, but can only go so far from the common post they are tied to.[18] Fukuyama's fear then is that advanced pharmacology will, for the first time, allow us to uproot the common post. So, if we accept this line of thought, the real difference between cultural and biological interventions is that the latter are likely to effect much more profound changes. Of course, on pain of inconsistency, Fukuyama would have to resist any cultural changes that promised similar radical results. If positive psychology, for example, radically altered people's phenotype in a manner unprecedented by any other environmental interventions, then he would have to resist this form of intervention as well.

This tells us why attempts at cultural, rather than biological, improvement may be sanctioned – because the former are likely to change us much less: that is, they are not likely to be very effective in changing us; so they may be permitted. But none of this tells us why we ought not try to make wholesale changes. The justification Fukuyama offers for the view that wholesale changes are wrong lies in the idea of human dignity, which he grounds in his famous "Factor X":

> Factor X cannot be reduced to the possession of moral choice, or reason, or language, or sociability, or sentience, or emotions, or consciousness, or any other quality that has been put forth as a ground for human dignity. It is all of these qualities coming together in a *human whole* that make up Factor X.[19]

Unlike reductionist accounts of human dignity that would like to restrict it to a single factor, Fukuyama's analysis suggests a long list of attributes – moral choice, reason, language, sociability, sentience, emotion, consciousness – that comprise human dignity. Let us grant this account of human dignity, at least for the sake of the argument. How, then, does it follow that we ought not to use pharmacological agents and other technologies to enhance humans? Fukuyama offers two different responses, which I shall quote in full:

> If Factor X is related to our very complexity and the complex interactions of uniquely human characteristics like moral choice, reason, and a broad emotional gamut, it is reasonable to ask how and why biotechnology would seek to make us less complex. The answer lies in the constant pressure that exists to reduce the ends of biomedicine to utilitarian ones – that is, the attempt to reduce a complex diversity of natural ends and purposes to just a few simple categories like pain and pleasure, or autonomy. There is in particular a constant predisposition to allow the relief of pain and suffering to automatically trump all other human purposes and objectives. For this will be the constant trade-off that biotechnology will pose: we can cure this disease, or prolong this person's life, or make this child more tractable, at the expense of some ineffable human quality like genius, or ambition, or sheer diversity.[20]

The second response is:

> The utilitarian goal of minimizing suffering is itself very problematic. No one can make a brief in favor of pain and suffering, but the fact of the matter is that what we consider to be the highest and most admirable human qualities, both in ourselves and in others, are often related to the way that we react to, confront, overcome, and frequently succumb to pain, suffering, and death. In the absence of these human evils there would be no sympathy, compassion, courage, heroism, solidarity, or strength of character. A person who has not confronted suffering or death has no depth. Our ability to experience these emotions is what connects us potentially to all other human beings, both living and dead.[21]

Fukuyama's two answers boil down to these points: firstly, people applying biotechnology will inevitably concentrate on narrow ends and so harm our dignity by reducing the large array of factors that make up Factor X. Secondly, certain aspects of our dignity require "necessary evils": pain and death are not good in themselves but they are required for our moral virtue and emotional connection with others. Let us take these points in turn.

The first point is offered with absolutely no evidence. The crucial claim, remember, is that biotechnology seeks to make us less complex because of the "constant pressure that exists to reduce the ends of biomedicine to utilitarian ones – that is, the attempt to reduce a complex diversity of natural ends and purposes to just a few simple categories like pain and pleasure, or autonomy." Quite frankly, I have no idea what led Fukuyama to think that this is even remotely plausible. Researchers have suggested any number of possible enhancements for humans, including expanding intellectual, moral, physical, and emotional responses, so this part of his argument is quite baffling.[22] If there were any problem here, one would think that it is that too many enhancements are on offer, not too few.

The second reason is again completely unsubstantiated, but at least it is easier to see where Fukuyama is coming from. The idea that people must endure necessary evils is familiar from the history of the philosophy of religion. For instance, there is a long history of argumentation that God permits moral evil because he must do so in order that we may have free will, or, that suffering is necessary for building character. I think it is possible to challenge the general claim that we must endure such evils for the sake of some greater good, but I will grant it here for the sake of the argument. Does Fukuyama's conclusion follow? Certainly not. What he has not argued is the amount or *degree* of suffering that is required to achieve these greater goods. In other words, his entire argument rests on a false dilemma: either we leave humans completely unaltered by pharmacological and genetic technologies, or we will lose these greater goods that arise out of suffering. Our argument shows there are more alternatives here. Consider the hyperthymic: they enjoy more of the higher goods that Fukuyama celebrates than those in the lower range of the normal happy curve, yet they enjoy the benefit of a greater preponderance of positive moods. As we have noted more than once before, it is not that the hyperthymics' lives are characterized by a complete absence of negative moods. Thus, even if suffering is necessary for the attainment of higher goods, it seems that most of us have a suboptimal amount of suffering. At least the question should be asked, and Fukuyama does not even do this. Our argument is that we would do better to have *more* positive moods and attain *more* of the higher goods that Fukuyama celebrates. The way to do so, of course, is to use biotechnology to alter Fukuyama's Factor X.

Fukuyama seems to be more worried about changes in our social dynamics. In a well-known passage he writes:

> There is a disconcerting symmetry between Prozac and Ritalin. The former is prescribed heavily for depressed women lacking in self-esteem; it gives them

more of the alpha-male feeling that comes with high serotonin levels. Ritalin, on the other hand, is prescribed largely for young boys who do not want to sit still in class because nature never designed them to behave that way. Together, the two sexes are gently nudged toward that androgynous median personality, self-satisfied and socially compliant, that is the current politically correct outcome in American society.[23]

The social upshot is that Factor X is unhinged because it includes a broad range of personality types: some are more aggressive, others more passive, some happier, some sadder. Thus, according to Fukuyama, taking such substances alters the normal curves that characterize so many human traits that comprise Factor X.

It is very difficult to nail down exactly what dangers Fukuyama thinks are involved in narrowing the range of the normal curve. Reading the passage, one might think the problem is that taking these drugs serves the interests of others – how else should we understand the idea of "socially compliant"? But Fukuyama quickly retreats from this reading since he says that millions have actually benefited from these drugs. If the charge is simply that changing biology in this way will change our social dynamics, then this must be gleefully admitted. In the case of happy-people-pills, the hope is that it will be a change for the better. If the point is about loss of diversity, then this too should be gleefully admitted. Eliminating polio also narrows our diversity, and thankfully so. Nor is there any reason to suppose that a happier population will be any less diverse in other areas: the hyperthymic can be found dispersed amongst any number of occupations and social roles.

It is difficult to detect what threat to our social dynamics Fukuyama thinks the use of happy-people-pills might pose, other than the conservative's general worry that things might change, or change too fast. Since Fukuyama does not provide any concrete reasons for fear, his argument amounts to the usual conservative position that change is scary and bad. Can we do any better? Can we help the bioconservative out there by thinking of something more concrete to worry about? I'm not sure. The best I can think of, and even this, I believe, is so improbable that it really is almost not worth mentioning, is that if we get too many hyperthymic people we get a negative social dynamic like that of *Brave New World*. Suppose, despite all the evidence in Chapter 6 to the contrary, that once a critical mass of hyperthymic people is reached, they start to achieve less à la *Brave New World*. What would we do in this case? I suspect that some people would voluntarily stop taking happy-people-pills, just as many people stop smoking pot every day when they realize that they aren't accomplishing much with their lives. Governments may be forced to ban happy-people-pills, which no doubt would bring some protest, but governments have passed legislation to ban any number of drugs, so it is hard to imagine why this one might be any different. (And like the old joke that the marijuana movement would be much further ahead if so many of its activists did not smoke pot, so too if happy-people-pills breed apathy, governments will not have to worry about high-achieving activists.) Even this wildly implausible scenario – one that goes against all the empirical evidence we have at this point – is hardly civilization-ending.

Could the hyperthymic themselves be enhanced? In principle there seems to be no reason why not. As we noted, the hyperthymic are not characterized by having the highest emotional states all the time, so even within the normal parameters of human emotions there appears to be room at the top. Whether this is desirable or not cannot be decided simply by a priori speculation. We saw in Chapter 6 that there was some indication that there was a small tail-off in academic performance and income for the hyperthymic, so it may be that the hyperthymic are pretty close to the ideal in terms of wellbeing (at least without much more radical redesigns to human nature). Still, the question requires empirical investigation: there is no a priori reason to suppose that even some humans have been optimized for wellbeing. There are no evolutionary reasons for this either. Natural selection does not optimize for anything, and if it did optimize for anything it would be for having a large number of descendants who have a large number of descendants. It is not clear that the environmental pressures that hammered out the current human genome are relevant any longer. Those who were even happier than our current hyperthymic may have been eaten by saber-tooth tigers, and so weeded from the gene pool, but such environmental factors are no longer relevant.

What is required is experimentation: creating a positive mood-enhancing pill for the hyperthymic and observing the results. If the enhanced positive emotional states in the hyperthymic cause decreased acquisition of the long list of prudential goods, then this will give us some reason to consider the experiment a failure in terms of promoting wellbeing. If the enhanced positive emotional states in the hyperthymic cause increased acquisition of the long list of prudential goods, then this will provide us with some reason to think the experiment a success in terms of promoting wellbeing. Naturally, if the positive result transpires, the next task would be to see if pills could be developed to help the rest of us reach this state.

10.6   An Apollo Push

In this section and the next, we will examine the question of what role, if any, governments ought to have in the creation and distribution of happy-people-pills. We have argued that happy-people-pills are important for the wellbeing of many, but this in itself does not answer the question of just distribution of this good. This question is part of the larger and more familiar issue of what role, if any, governments should have in distributing goods such as health, education, and wealth; some favor a very restrictive role for governments, others argue for a more expansive role. Rather than trying to adjudicate this debate, or simply take sides, we will see what follows from each view of distributive justice. We will assume in this section that the more expansive role for government distribution is justified, and work with a more limited conception in the following section.

With some reluctance, which will be explained in a moment, we will think of 'welfare state liberalism' as the view that the state has a moral responsibility to reduce large inequalities of wealth by means of redistribution. One way to understand welfare state liberalism is in contrast with libertarianism, since libertarianism denies that the state should be so involved. Libertarianism is typically conjoined with (or partially defined in terms of) some form of relatively unfettered capitalism; for example, Nozick famously argued for such a view of distributive justice in his *Anarchy, State, and Utopia*. Rawls and other welfare state liberals would like to see at least some of the economic disparity generated by capitalism reduced: the most impoverished segments of society should have access to more resources, and these resources should come by and large from the richest segment of the population.[24]

Welfare state liberalism is not to be identified with 'left wing' as it is typically understood, since 'left wing' has a number of connotations that are not relevant for our purposes. For example, left versus right wing typically is used to divide people on economic *and* social issues. A typical left-winger might be for universal health care, pro-choice on the abortion issue, and for the legalization of marijuana, whereas the typical right-winger, at least in American politics, would take the opposing views on each of these issues. Our main focus here is on economic issues.

Another contrast that only partially overlaps is that between egalitarianism and non-egalitarianism. One problem is that 'egalitarianism' is probably too broad because, strictly speaking, it is about the desirability of people's condition being equal in some respect. However, the doctrine, as employed in contemporary political philosophy, is better understood as being about rectifying the inequalities of the least advantaged in society.[25] Think, for example, of the material disparity between a starving homeless person and a billionaire. With a magic wand one could institute equality by making everyone in the world a starving homeless person or everyone a billionaire. Equality would be served in either case, but the spirit of egalitarianism is better served by trying to make the worse off better than simply making the best off worse. Thus, in terms of actual policies, egalitarians tend to favor policies that seek to rectify social and natural inequalities by making the worse off better.

The egalitarian versus non-egalitarian contrast is, at least on some formulations, too specific in its recommendations for our purposes. If priority in policy is to always be given to making the worst off better, this will pit egalitarianism against, for example, utilitarians, who would tailor policy to maximize aggregate happiness. Imagine, for example, the decision to use educational funds in an impoverished school district either to hire 30 teachers with expertise in teaching special needs children, or 30 teachers who specialize in preparing students for college. It is calculated that, if the former are hired, only four special needs children will boost their reading scores from an average lifetime maximum of a grade 2 reading level to a lifetime maximum of a grade 3 level. Conversely, it is calculated that if the college prep teachers are hired, 300 more students per year will attend college. An egalitarian preferring to always concentrate on the worst off ought to prefer the former policy, while a utilitarian ought to prefer the latter, since so many more people can be helped in significant ways. Although they disagree on the specific policy here, both are welfare state liberals in our sense.

Why should welfare statists be interested in supporting the development of happy-people-pills? A prima facie case can be made by noting first that welfare state liberals advocate using the machinery of the state to distribute wealth in a manner that promotes the wellbeing of its citizenry.[26] Thus, most welfare state liberals believe that it is good to use state-mandated taxes to support access to higher education, particularly for the less well-off segments of society. As we have argued, happy-people-pills would increase the wellbeing of society as a whole. So there is at least a prima facie case for welfare state liberals to be interested in supporting the development of happy-people-pills, just as there is for welfare state liberals to support subsidized higher education.

The case for welfare state liberals supporting happy-people-pills, and higher education, is only prima facie because, after all, there are lots of ways of spending money to promote the wellbeing of citizens. Why should happy-people-pills or education rank high on a list of priorities for welfare state liberals? There is no argument that in all circumstances governments ought to support happy-people-pills. A country desperately short on food might be better served by its government investing public funds in the production of butter, whereas a country facing imminent invasion might be better served by investment in guns. Of course, in these circumstances, subsidized higher education is also probably not a priority. However, for developed nations not facing such immediate perils, investment in the development of happy-people-pills, I want to argue, should be seen by welfare state liberals as a sound use of public money.

In terms of investing in the development of a new generation of happy-people-pills, what is demanded by welfare state liberalism for the affluent industrialized nations is something like an Apollo push to this goal. By this I mean the massive mobilization of resources that were devoted to a single goal: landing people on the moon. Even to this day it is remarkable to think that in the 12 years from 1957 to 1969, humanity went from being almost earthbound to landing people on the moon. At its height, the Apollo project consumed about 5.5% of the US budget. In today's terms that would be equivalent to spending over 150 billion dollars annually on the development of happy-people-pills. I am not actually suggesting spending money on such a colossal scale. To put that number in some perspective, it is five times the estimated amount that the pharmaceutical industry in the US spends a year on research and development on all drugs (a little over 30 billion dollars).[27] This includes antidepressants, but also a wide gamut of other drugs such as antipsychotics, pain relievers and blood pressure-lowering agents.

To make the case, it will help to have some estimate as to the cost of development. It is difficult to say with any great precision, but we can put a lower and an upper bound on the estimate. Estimates as to how much it costs to bring a new drug to market vary quite substantially depending on how the costs are assessed, but are somewhere in the order of one hundred million to two billion dollars, while 800 million is a number that is commonly cited.[28] Since this is an average, it is at least conceivable that happy-people-pills – with a considerable bit of serendipity – might be developed for a few hundred million.

Despite the questionable accounting practices that underwrite some of these estimates, such estimates probably would underestimate the cost of developing happy-people-pills.[29] Most of the drugs that come to market are slight variants on existing drugs, and even those that are substantially new build on basic research that was not done by the pharmaceutical company itself, and so are not part of the estimates cited. The basic research needed to create a new drug from scratch may be far more expensive than that required for a typical drug launch. A more apt comparison can be seen in a call issued by Zaven Khachaturian, former director of the National Institute of Health's Office of Alzheimer's Disease Research, for an "Apollo Push" to cure Alzheimer's disease. He estimates a billion a year for ten years could conquer the disease.[30] This estimate is relevant because, as was argued in Chapter 7, the research program to develop happy-people-pills is similar in complexity to projects like curing schizophrenia and Alzheimer's disease. We will take this as our upper bound.

Now, a billion a year for ten years is a large number, but not impossibly big. With a national budget the size of that of the US, that sort of money can probably be found between the sofa cushions of congressional leaders. To put this number in some perspective, a billion a year represents 6% of NASA's budget, about 0.3% of the US government's allotment for higher education and 0.16% of military expenditures.[31]

None of this is designed to suggest that a billion a year for ten years is not a large sum of money, but simply to put this sum in scale. If we are trying to improve the wellbeing of millions, a billion a year does not go far. In the US, for instance, it would be equivalent to spending about three dollars per person for ten years. Giving everyone three additional dollars' worth of free education or medical care for ten years would unfortunately not make a perceptible difference. Alternatively, fewer people could be helped in a more substantial fashion; for example, give one in every seven thousand persons a chance at a $20,000 scholarship, and surely this would make a difference for those lucky enough to win; but the aggregate impact on the wellbeing of society as a whole would be tiny, for only one in seven thousand is helped by this policy. Consider that "in 2008 the Department of Education will administer over $90 billion in new grants, loans, and work-study assistance to help over 11 million students and their families pay for college."[32] A billion a year would only be a drop in the proverbial bucket compared to what the US government already spends, and so nationally would make, at best, little appreciable difference. The contrast with happy-people-pills could not be starker: it could be used by most of the population to enhance many aspects of wellbeing including academic achievement.

Notice too that investing in happy-people-pills research is a one-time cost. Once we have paid for the development of happy-people-pills we will have the benefits for all of eternity. The contrast here is with recurring costs. Adding a billion a year to existing grants, loans, and work-study assistance would help students only in the years the funds are provided. To permanently help the poor have better access to higher education would require expenditure in perpetuity.

Two other factors are important for assessing a public investment in happy-people-pills. One is the idea that the cost of development may be shared. There is no reason any one nation ought to bear the full cost of developing pills. An international consortium would reduce the burden of individual nations. Second, the benefit may be widely shared. Any nation or nations that develop happy-people-pills will be benefactors to all of humanity. All developed nations devote part of their resources to the wellbeing of people beyond their borders. To the extent that this is already considered morally salient, developing happy-people-pills will further this end.

Finally, it is worth noting that this research program would not necessarily require coming up with a billion dollars a year in new research money, since present research priorities could be reassigned. Psychologists, behavioral geneticists, and pharmacological researchers have a certain amount of discretionary money for basic research. These discretionary funds could be used to fund at least some of the research necessary to create happy-people-pills.

Thinking about how governments might promote wellbeing involves a number of empirical issues. A couple hundred years ago, Jeremy Bentham explicitly called for government policy to be directed at promoting the wellbeing of the citizenry, yet only recently have social scientists turned their attention to what factors might actually support such a goal.[33] One of the most surprising results from recent scientific attention is the "Easterlin Paradox," named after Richard Easterlin, who found that economic growth has little correlation with aggregate happiness. Poorer nations were often happier than richer nations, and even in countries like the US, which had enormous economic growth between 1946 and 1970, the average citizen was not happier as a result.[34] Easterlin's results have sparked some controversy, but even the most critical studies suggest that if increasing income in developed nations is correlated with happiness, the correlation is very small.[35] As researchers have pointed out, this calls into question the explicit or implicit assumption of governments that economic growth ought to be of paramount concern in policy consideration.[36]

Increasingly, social scientists have turned their attention from whether current policies are effective to the question of what policies would promote wellbeing. Some researchers are quite circumspect in policy recommendations, other than proposing more funding for research on wellbeing,[37] while others have made proposals for large-scale policy changes. For instance, Richard Layard has suggested that governments should look to policies that reduce the number of hours people work, and promote more egalitarian distribution of income.[38] Derek Bok makes the following recommendations:

> With such a change of emphasis [from the assumption that economic growth ought to be the overriding policy goal] in mind, government officials could draw upon the new research to rethink their priorities and make a more balanced effort to promote well-being. For example, happiness research reinforces the importance of programs to strengthen marriage and family; encourage active forms of leisure; cushion the shock of unemployment; guarantee universal health care and a more secure retirement; improve child care and preschool education; treat mental illness, sleep disorders, and chronic pain more effectively; and focus education policy on a broader set of goals. Progress on these fronts could well do more for well-being than such familiar proposals as redistributing income, putting more people in prison, subsidizing even further the retirement savings of the well-to-do, or promoting the kind of suburbanization that brings longer commutes and added traffic.[39]

There are three points that ought to be made. First, implementing each of these programs in the US, for instance, would require an enormous investment of public money. In total these programs would require public investment orders of magnitude greater than happy-people-pills.[40] The second point is that even if governments took all the advice and implemented such programs, their cumulative effect would probably be much smaller than what happy-people-pills could do. For, as we have seen, genetics is the single greatest contributor to individual differences in happiness, and happiness promotes other aspects of wellbeing. Third, it is clear that there is no need to accept the choice between trying to make policy reforms to promote wellbeing and altering the biological basis of wellbeing. As we have said before, the best results will no doubt be had if we get the oars of nature and nurture pulling in the same direction. The point here of drawing these comparisons with alternate policy recommendations is simply to show that happy-people-pills give enormous bang for the buck, not that these other policies are not worthy of pursuit. If I were made king, I would implement them all.

It may be protested that even if this is a good way for welfare state liberals to spend money in the developed world, still it does not show that it is a good use all considered. Surely it would do more for the collective wellbeing of humanity to help the impoverished of the two-thirds world.

The objection may be answered from a theoretical and a practical perspective. Let us concede that from a theoretical perspective utilitarians and egalitarians would direct a billion a year to the two-thirds world rather than develop happy-people-pills. What this shows is that given the choice, we should feed the two-thirds world. The trouble is connecting this choice with any question we are likely to face.

If we are addressing resource allocation from a theoretical perspective, we should be asking how to spend the entire wealth of the world, or of a nation, as opposed to worrying about the ten billion as if it were the only money that is of relevance. With reference to the US, it may be advisable from an egalitarian or utilitarian policy standpoint to strip most of the wealth from the top 10 percent of the people in the US, who own two thirds of all the wealth, and redistribute it across the globe. There is a superabundance of wealth in the US, so there is not a single reason to feel forced to choose between happy-people-pills and feeding the two-thirds world. From a theoretical perspective it should strike us as bizarre to hear an objection to spending ten billion on something that could potentially bring so much good to so many people in a world where individuals own personal yachts the length of football fields with helicopter landing pads. The problem is not that there are not enough resources to go around; the problem is how to get the wealthier to equitably share resources. Consider an analogous question: Should the fire department save the four adults upstairs or the three children downstairs? There is no moral dilemma here. The right answer is to reject the question. The fire department should save the children and the adults. Of course we can stipulate that the fire department can only save the adults or the children, just as we can stipulate that we can only support the two-thirds world or the development of happy-people-pills. Although such stipulations may make for interesting discussion in the philosophy classroom, there is no reason to think that this dilemma will be relevant next time the fire department gets a call or when adjudicating national budgets. In both cases, do both.

Turning to practice, consider that NASA's budget has often been criticized along the lines that exploring space is misspent money when there are so many problems here on earth. Even if we agree that this sounds good in theory, in practice there is little causal relation between reducing research budgets and giving more to foreign aid. Similarly, there is little reason to suppose that not investing in happy-people-pills will result in more aid to the two-thirds world. Certainly it would be incumbent on our opponent to show that there is in fact such a connection when history indicates the opposite. So, there is little reason to suppose that those who think the richer nations' priorities should be on helping the two-thirds world should oppose the development of happy-people-pills in particular.

We can in fact draw a stronger conclusion: there is some reason to think that developing happy-people-pills will result in greater social justice. The problem of social justice, for the most part, as we have noted, is one not of resources but of will. Sufficient food is produced on this planet to feed everyone; we simply lack the will to distribute it in a manner that ensures adequate food for everyone. But it might be wise for those concerned primarily about the two-thirds world to endorse the development of happy-people-pills as a side bet. Making the world happier through the development of happy-people-pills may increase the chances of turning the tide against starvation. The bet is not capricious: we have seen evidence that happy people tend to exhibit more prosocial behavior. Happy-people-pills may at least partially address the root problem here: a lack of good will. This is not to suggest that happy-people-pills are a silver bullet for all such concerns. The fight for greater social justice is, and no doubt will continue to be, a multi-pronged offensive. The side bet is that altering our biology with happy-people-pills will have some positive effect in the fight for justice.

Research on antidepressants as a short-term stopgap measure can be carried out relatively inexpensively. As noted in Chapter 7, volunteer-run trials could be conducted for next to nothing. Physicians prescribing antidepressants for enhancement "off label" can run less formal trials. Even full-scale Phase III clinical trials run in the US can be done for less than 100 million dollars, so there is no significant *financial* obstacle to testing antidepressants for enhancement. Just distribution of antidepressants for enhancement may also not be a serious issue, since so many of the major antidepressants are off patent, e.g. Zoloft, Prozac, Effexor, Wellbutrin, and Lexapro. Of course it would be a shame if the only antidepressants that worked for enhancement were under patent, but this seems increasingly unlikely.

10.7   Release the Hounds of Corporate Greed

Libertarians, the arch-foes of welfare state liberalism, who reject as unjust public money spent on anything but absolutely essential public services such as a military and a police force, will reject the argument of the previous section. For no doubt happy-people-pills would be seen by libertarians of this stripe as not an absolutely essential public good, so the use of public money would be unjust. As is perhaps obvious, this form of libertarianism has little traction in current Western politics, for the overwhelming majority subscribes to some version of welfare state liberalism. Most political parties in the West, for example, endorse at least some public support for higher education and scientific research.

It is also true that at least some versions of welfare state liberalism may consistently reject the claim that there is an obligation by the state to support the development of happy-people-pills. After all, there is much debate within welfare state liberalism as to what activities the state should support, and to what extent; for instance, should the state support access to health care, and if so, to what extent? One possibility, then, is for a welfare state liberal to say that although the state has an obligation to support such basic goods as higher education and health care, happy-people-pills are a luxury. The state has no duty to support their development, especially when the market will do so without public money. We will address the viability of this view below, but for the moment we want to see what follows if we accept it.

Even if we accept market forces as the mechanism to support the development and distribution of happy-people-pills, not all hope is lost. After all, there may be some reason to think that the profit motive may be sufficient inducement for privately held pharmaceutical companies to research happy-people-pills. Recall that the US pharmaceutical industries claim to spend about 30 billion dollars annually on research. Individual research projects typically target a small segment of the population; for example, high blood pressure affects a minority of the population, as do depression and insomnia. The fact that the target market for happy-people-pills is the majority of the population would surely be alluring to investors as a potential source of profit. For if there is profit to be made in selling antidepressants to people with clinical depression, say about 5 to

10 percent of the population, then imagine how pharmaceutical executives might salivate at the prospect of potentially selling a pharmaceutical to the majority of the population.

The potential for success would be increased if governments sent a strong signal to investors that it would be legal to sell happy-people-pills. Part of the problem here for investors is the high level of uncertainty. It is not clear, in many jurisdictions, what would happen if tomorrow it were announced that happy-people-pills had been successfully developed in some secret lab. Would governments allow them to be sold over the counter, much as vitamins are now? Would the pills be available through medical prescription only? Would governments ban them as they have marijuana? Investors hate uncertainty. The fact that there is so much uncertainty about the legal status of happy-people-pills would no doubt make investors very wary. Governments that want to encourage the free market to develop happy-people-pills should send a strong signal that it would be legal to sell such a product.

Indeed, the previous arguments indicate a stronger conclusion: states have a duty to send a clear signal that happy-people-pills could be sold on the open market. The reason is that it would cost the state nothing to make manifest the legality of happy-people-pills, and would encourage the market to pursue their development. More generally, the conclusion can be derived from the general argument that the development of happy-people-pills will benefit many people, and from the premise that the state has an obligation to benefit its citizenry when it costs the state nothing. In this case, the total cost to the state would be the cost of putting pen to paper to indicate that selling happy-people-pills, should they be developed, is lawful.

It might be thought that all welfare state liberals should be enticed by the market option. If the free market will develop happy-people-pills, why waste precious public dollars? One worry is that this course might mean that happy-people-pills were available only to the wealthy. It is not hard to imagine that a company that develops and patents happy-people-pills will charge exorbitant prices for them. We have ample evidence of this from current practices: the pharmaceutical industry has profit levels that make even pirates blush. The fact that only the wealthy could afford greater happiness and achievement would surely rub many welfare state liberals the wrong way.

As noted in the previous chapter, the problem of access for the impoverished classes would be mitigated by the fact that patents eventually run out. Once the patent runs out, the price will drop to a small fraction (typically in the case of therapeutics to about 20 percent of the original price) once generic formulations of the product come to market. The fact that the problem of inequality will have a shelf life – its biggest impact would be felt for 20 years – would be of some comfort. Still, welfare state liberals have some complaint: happiness delayed is happiness denied.

Moreover, again as noted at the end of the last chapter, even if big pharmaceutical companies develop happy-people-pills, all is not lost, since other measures are available to close the inequality gap. There are comparatively mild remedies, such as state subsidies or tax deductions for happy-people-pills, to help minimize the effects of income disparity, to more appropriate measures like nationalizing big pharmaceutical companies and putting their corporate heads on pikes.

The larger problem with the free market alternative is that the big pharmaceutical companies have proven time and time again that they are not interested in basic research, and they are lousy innovators. Anyone who thinks otherwise should read Marcia Angell's *The Truth About the Drug Companies*. She argues convincingly that big pharmaceutical companies have found it more profitable to invest in "me too" products and marketing rather than in basic research. Most basic research of the type that would be required to reverse-engineer the hyperthymic is done by public institutions like university labs, and to a lesser extent smaller biotech labs. The research divisions of big pharmaceutical companies perform an almost imperceptible amount of basic research. Still, the argument is mostly a historical induction: this is the way big pharmaceutical companies have operated in the past. Perhaps tomorrow some company will emerge that looks toward the long term and is highly innovative. Just don't hold your breath.

Still, pessimism about the private model for financing happy-people-pills should be tempered by the fact that the cost of the research should drop over time as the prices of the associated technologies drop in price. For instance, the first human genome was sequenced for a price of about three billion dollars in 2000. The price has dropped precipitously since then: soon it will cost less than $1000 to have your genome sequenced. Accordingly, the price for examining the genetics of the hyperthymic will also fall. So although the price tag for doing the basic research today may be too much for any private company to gamble, in ten years the investment may look more attractive. Of course this would mean a delay in the development of happy-people-pills, and happiness delayed is happiness denied.

Obviously the public and the private alternatives are not mutually exclusive: there are possibilities for public and private cooperation at all stages, including investment in research, testing, manufacturing, and distribution. Another possibility is for something like an "X-prize" for bio-happiness research. The X-Prize (or the Ansari X-Prize as it was renamed) offered ten million dollars for the first private reusable spacecraft to reach space twice in two weeks. The prize was claimed in 2004 by a team financed by Paul Allen. The idea behind the X-Prize was of course to spur private development of space technology. Using this model, the H-Prize could be privately financed by donations and offered to those who can achieve certain milestones along the developmental path to creating happy-people-pills.

In terms of efficiency and justice, I believe the public model of development is best. However, making this case in detail would resolve some more fundamental questions about distributive justice that are beyond the scope of this work. We have seen that in either distributive system there is hope that happy-people-pills might be developed, and that they would be justly distributed *according to the percepts of each distributive model*. Residual complaints about the just distribution of happy-people-pills are about the economic theories themselves, not against the distribution of happy-people-pills in particular.

10.8   Liberty and the Duty to Take Happy-People-Pills?

Thus far we have assumed that people ought to be at liberty to take happy-people-pills, but it may be wondered at this point whether this position is too weak. If mood boosters promise so much for so many, perhaps it may be thought that we have a duty to take them. I believe there is something to this view. To see what is valuable in it, we should first consider the distinction between enforceable and non-enforceable duties.

Suppose I have promised my mother a Mother's Day card. Do I have a duty to send one? Most would say yes. Is this an enforceable duty? Probably not. It would hardly seem appropriate for the state to put me in leg irons if I fail to keep my promise, even though I have a duty to send my mother a card. Certainly it may be appropriate to morally criticize me: if I fail in my duty I may be justly criticized for not sending a card to my dear mother. So, while I have a duty to send my mother a Mother's Day card, the duty is not an enforceable duty. On the other hand, I have a duty not to kill my neighbor when he starts mowing his lawn at 5 o'clock on a Sunday morning, and this is an enforceable duty. The state would be right to restrain me if I were to act on this impulse. A similar point applies to receiving health care and a higher education. We might think that you should agree to physician-recommended surgery, despite your fears, so that you can continue to look after your family, or that you have a duty to yourself to finish your postgraduate degree. Still this is entirely consistent with rejecting the idea that the state has a right or a duty to enforce these duties.

To the extent that we think we have self-regarding and other-regarding duties, we should take the same attitude to the question of the duty to take happy-people-pills. Most people's lives would be improved by taking happy-people-pills and so most people might be rightly criticized by family and friends for failing to take the opportunity to makes their lives better. From the point of view of the state, taking happy-people-pills ought to be viewed as a liberty: a decision up to the discretion of the individual. The justification for this is simply the usual apology for non-enforceable duties: even those in favor of very strong forms of paternalism must admit that it is extremely difficult for the state to force people to do certain things like get an advanced degree, exercise or take their medications.

10.9 Concluding Unscientific Postscript

When I talk about happy-people-pills a criticism I often hear in the question period has to do with the utopian nature of the proposal: the FDA and other government officials would never allow happy-people-pills, so why should we waste our energies thinking and talking about them?

Such remarks always strike me as extremely parochial. Few read Hegel's *Philosophy of History* today, and even fewer read it with more than a historical interest. For how could we take seriously pronouncements such as: "The History of the World travels from East to West, for Europe is absolutely the end of History, Asia the beginning"?[41] Why should we believe something so preposterous? Hegel offers the following "enlightenment":

> The History of the World is the discipline of the uncontrolled natural will, bringing it into obedience to a Universal principle and conferring subjective freedom. The East knew and to the present day knows only that *One* is Free; the Greek and Roman world, that *some* are free; the German World knows that *All* are free.[42]

Of course we can only smile at the Eurocentrism and the grand teleology that Hegel offers. I suggest that we let the same smile shine upon those who raise this triumphant objection: the FDA would never approve of the use of happy-people-pills. The US is only one country in a world where capital, monetary and social, is very fluid. Consider what happened when the US government tried to reign in stem cell research. Social capital, for example research scientists, and monetary capital fled the country to places like the UK, Singapore, and Australia. World history did not end in Germany, nor does it end at Silver Spring, Maryland, USA, headquarters of the FDA. It takes only a single country to provide a regulatory framework conducive to happy-people-pills research. Any country willing to do so will no doubt add to its material prosperity and ultimately be a benefactor of humanity at large. For once happy-people-pills show their promise in one place, it seems likely people everywhere will demand them.

Nor do we have to wait for some country to boldly step forward to make an "Apollo Project"-type announcement about happy-people-pills. As noted, researchers in universities still have some limited discretion over their research activities. Some may choose to study the genetics, psychology, and physiology of the hyperthymic – all on the public dime. A few people with good will towards happy-people-pills at least would be a start.

So, in the end, we need only convince some – perhaps even just a few initially – of the promise of happy-people-pills for the revolution to have a good chance to succeed. The situation is not so happy for bioconservatives: they must convince every country to unite against it. The possibility of all countries agreeing to renounce happiness enhancement seems exceedingly unlikely, although bioconservatives like George Annas, Francis Fukuyama, and Leon Kass have not given up hope, calling for a global ban on certain types of technologies.[43] And this is what makes their task so difficult: it takes only one country – the country that aspires to be to happy-people-pills what Singapore is to stem cell research – to thwart their bioconservatism.

The moral arguments in favor of happy-people-pills are compelling. We have every reason to suspect that if we were to increase the average happiness, people would achieve more in the workplace, have better relations with others, and have better health outcomes. This is why we have an obligation to see happy-people-pills realized. So, while there is no historical inevitability, solace may be had in the fact that the numbers and the moral arguments are in our favor.

Notes

1. Locke, *Two Treatises of Government*, Section 21.
2. Mill, *On Liberty*, Ch. 1.
3. Ibid., Ch. 4.
4. Cohen and Neumann, "What's More Dangerous, Your Aspirin or Your Car?"
5. Ibid.
6. Repantis et al., "Antidepressants for Neuroenhancement in Healthy Individuals."
7. Although, as Angell argues (*The Truth About the Drug Companies*), this tendency is not nearly as strong as it should be. Too many "me too" drugs are put on the market by big pharmaceutical companies that have little or no clinical advantages over their competitors' earlier efforts.
8. Uhr et al., "Polymorphisms in the Drug Transporter Gene ABCB1 Predict Antidepressant Treatment Response in Depression."
9. Pearce, "Amineptine."
10. Haddad, "Do Antidepressants Have Any Potential to Cause Addiction?"; Bertschy et al., "Amineptin Dependence"; Perera and Lim, "Amineptine and Midazolam Dependence."
11. Quaglio, Schifano, and Lugoboni, "Venlafaxine Dependence in a Patient with a History of Alcohol and Amineptine Misuse."
12. Crenshaw, Goldberg, and Stern, "Pharmacologic Modification of Psychosexual Dysfunction."
13. Castleman, "Wonderful Wellbutrin?"
14. Gibbons et al., "Relationship Between Antidepressants and Suicide Attempts"; Isacsson et al., "Decrease in Suicide Among the Individuals Treated with Antidepressants."
15. Davidson, Mostofsky, and Whang, "Don't Worry, Be Happy"; Pitt and Deldin, "Depression and Cardiovascular Disease."
16. Two other previously mentioned technologies for increasing positive affect, preimplantation genetic diagnosis and genetic engineering, would change our genotype, at least in terms of allele frequency in humanity's genetic pool.
17. We need not assume here that the mind can be reduced to or is identical with the brain. A weaker claim will suffice: differences in the mind, such as differences in levels of positive affect, will have correlated differences at the biochemical level.
18. Thanks to Glynis Baguley for this metaphor.
19. Fukuyama, *Our Posthuman Future*, 171.
20. Ibid., 172.

21. Ibid., 173.

22. Buchanan, *Beyond Humanity?*

23. Fukuyama, *Our Posthuman Future*, 51–2.

24. Rawls, *A Theory of Justice*.

25. Cohen, *If You're an Egalitarian, How Come You're So Rich?* There is a large debate too as to exactly what policies of equality should target, which we must pass over, e.g. Rawls's primary goods, Sen's capabilities, Arneson's equal opportunities for welfare, Dworkin's resources, and so on (Rawls, *A Theory of Justice*; Sen, *Choice, Welfare and Measurement*; Arneson, "Equality and Equal Opportunity for Welfare"; Dworkin, *Sovereign Virtue*).

26. I am taking certain liberties here in formulating the goal of welfare state liberalism in a manner that might sound excessively consequentialist given that the term 'welfare state liberalism' is intended to be a large umbrella. Thus, one might think that Rawls, for example, would object to this formulation. A Rawlsian might formulate the goal of welfare state liberalism as honoring the requirements of justice. However, the formulation here of promoting wellbeing is meant to describe the effect of policy decisions rather than to express a commitment to a certain view of normative ethics. Thus, honoring Rawls's conception of distributive justice will often have the effect of promoting the wellbeing of society as a whole. Furthermore, Rawls's understanding of justice is hardly disconnected entirely from the question of wellbeing; for instance, an important linkage is made in his conception of 'primary goods.'

27. Gagnon and Lexchin, "The Cost of Pushing Pills."

28. The lower figure comes from Angell, *The Truth About the Drug Companies*; the upper figure is cited in Adams and Brantner, "Estimating the Cost of New Drug Development."

29. The $800 million figure, for instance, builds in opportunity cost. If I ask you how much your new car costs and you say $20,000, this doesn't figure in opportunity cost. If you had taken the $20,000 and invested it in the stock market, then in ten years, when the car is scrapped, you would have had $40,000, so the car "really" costs $40,000. Half the cost of the commonly cited $800 billion figure that these economists estimate is opportunity cost. The sort of accounting that would make even pirates blush. Furthermore, this $800 billion figure is often cited as an average for all drugs, whereas in reality the figure is for a small subset of drugs that big pharmaceuticals develop, namely, drugs for which the research costs are significant because they are effectively new drugs.

30. Khachaturian and Khachaturian, "Prevent Alzheimer's Disease by 2020."

31. NASA, "NASA's FY 2010 Budget"; Stockholm International Peace Research Institute, *SIPRI Yearbook 2009*, 184.

32. Snyder and Dillow, *Digest of Education Statistics: 2008*.

33. Bentham, *The Principles of Morals and Legislation.*
34. Easterlin, "Does Economic Growth Improve the Human Lot?"
35. For recent support see Layard, *Happiness.* For criticism see Stevenson and Wolfers, "Economic Growth and Subjective Well-being." The correlation studies do not address the arrow of causality: if there is some correlation between happiness and wealth in the developed nations, this may be explained by happiness creating wealth, not wealth creating happiness.
36. Diener, Lucas, and Schimmack, *Well-being for Public Policy*; Layard, *Happiness.*
37. Diener, Lucas, and Schimmack, *Well-being for Public Policy.*
38. Layard, *Happiness.*
39. Bok, *The Politics of Happiness*, 208.
40. Consider, for instance, that the cost of adding a year of preschool is in the order of ten billion dollars a year in perpetuity (Barnett and Robin, "How Much Does Quality Preschool Cost?").
41. Hegel, *The Philosophy of History*, 103.
42. Ibid., 104.
43. Annas, "Why We Should Ban Human Cloning"; Fukuyama, *Our Posthuman Future*; Kass, "Wisdom of Repugnance"; Annas, Andrews, and Isasi, "Protecting the Endangered Human."

References

Adams, C. P. and V. V. Brantner. "Estimating the Cost of New Drug Development: Is It Really $802 Million?" *Health Affairs* 25, no. 2 (2006): 420–8.

Angell, M. *The Truth About the Drug Companies: How They Deceive Us and What to Do About It.* New York: Random House, 2004.

Annas, G. J. "Why We Should Ban Human Cloning." *New England Journal of Medicine* 339, no. 2 (1998): 122–5.

Annas, G. J., L. B. Andrews, and R. M. Isasi. "Protecting the Endangered Human: Toward an International Treaty Prohibiting Cloning and Inheritable Alterations." *American Journal of Law and Medicine* 28 (2002): 151–78.

Arneson, R. J. "Equality and Equal Opportunity for Welfare." *Philosophical Studies* 56, no. 1 (1989): 77–93.

Barnett, W. S. and K. B. Robin. "How Much Does Quality Preschool Cost?" National Institute for Early Education Research Working Paper, Rutgers, 2006.

Bentham, J. *The Principles of Morals and Legislation.* Buffalo, N.Y.: Prometheus Books, 1988.

Bertschy, G., I. Luxembourger, P. Bizouard, S. Vandel, G. Allers, and R. Volmat. "Amineptin Dependence. Detection of Patients at Risk. Report of 8 Cases." *L'Encéphale* 16, no. 5 (1990): 405–9.

Bok, D. *The Politics of Happiness: What Government Can Learn from the New Research on Well-Being.* Princeton, N.J.: Princeton University Press, 2010.

Buchanan, A. E. *Beyond Humanity? The Ethics of Biomedical Enhancement.* Oxford: Oxford University Press, 2011.

Castleman, M. "Wonderful Wellbutrin?" *Salon*, September 26, 2000. http://www.salon.com/sex/feature/2000/09/26/wellbutrin/index.html.

Cohen, G. *If You're an Egalitarian, How Come You're So Rich?* Cambridge, Mass.: Harvard University Press, 2000.

Cohen, J. T. and P. J. Neumann. "What's More Dangerous, Your Aspirin or Your Car? Thinking Rationally About Drug Risks (and Benefits)." *Health Affairs* 26, no. 3 (2007): 636–46.

Crenshaw, T. L., J. P. G. Goldberg, and W. C. S. Stern. "Pharmacologic Modification of Psychosexual Dysfunction." *Journal of Sex & Marital Therapy* 13, no. 4 (1987): 239–52.

Davidson, K. W., E. Mostofsky, and W. Whang. "Don't Worry, Be Happy: Positive Affect and Reduced 10-year Incident Coronary Heart Disease: The Canadian Nova Scotia Health Survey." *European Heart Journal* 31, no. 9 (2010): 1065–70.

Diener, E., R. Lucas, and U. Schimmack. *Well-being for Public Policy.* New York: Oxford University Press, 2009.

Dworkin, R. *Sovereign Virtue: The Theory and Practice of Equality.* Cambridge, Mass.: Harvard University Press, 2002.

Easterlin, R. A. "Does Economic Growth Improve the Human Lot?" In *Nations and Households in Economic Growth: Essays in Honor of Moses Abramovitz*, edited by P. A. David and M. W. Reder, 89–125. New York: Academic Press, 1974.

Fukuyama, F. *Our Posthuman Future: Consequences of the Biotechnology Revolution.* London: Profile, 2003.

Gagnon, M. A. and J. Lexchin. "The Cost of Pushing Pills: A New Estimate of Pharmaceutical Promotion Expenditures in the United States." *PLoS Medicine* 5, no. 1 (2008): e1.

Gibbons, R., C. Brown, K. Hur, S. Marcus, D. Bhaumik, and J. Mann. "Relationship Between Antidepressants and Suicide Attempts: An Analysis of the Veterans Health Administration Data Sets." *American Journal of Psychiatry* 164, no. 7 (2007): 1044–9.

Haddad, P. "Do Antidepressants Have Any Potential to Cause Addiction?" *Journal of Psychopharmacology* 13, no. 3 (1999): 300–7.

Hegel, G. W. F. *The Philosophy of History.* Translated by J. Sibree. New York: Dover, 1956.

Isacsson, G., A. Holmgren, U. Ösby, and J. Ahlner. "Decrease in Suicide Among the Individuals Treated with Antidepressants: A Controlled Study of Antidepressants in Suicide, Sweden 1995–2005." *Acta Psychiatrica Scandinavica* 120, no. 1 (2009): 37–44.

Kass, L. R. "The Wisdom of Repugnance: Why We Should Ban the Cloning of Humans." *Valparaiso University Law Review* 32, no. 2 (1998): 679–705.

Khachaturian, Z. S. and A. S. Khachaturian. "Prevent Alzheimer's Disease by 2020: A National Strategic Goal." *Alzheimer's & Dementia: The Journal of the Alzheimer's Association* 5, no. 2 (2009): 81–4.

Layard, R. *Happiness: Lessons From a New Science*. London: Penguin Books, 2005.

Locke, J. *Two Treatises of Government*. Cambridge: Cambridge University Press, 1988.

Mill, J. S. *On Liberty*. Indianapolis, Ind.: Hackett, 1978.

NASA. "NASA's FY 2010 Budget", 2010. http://www.nasa.gov/news/budget/FY2010.html.

Pearce, D. "Amineptine." From "The Good Drug Guide," n.d. http://amineptine.com/.

Perera, I. and L. Lim. "Amineptine and Midazolam Dependence." *Singapore Medical Journal* 39 (1998): 129–31.

Pitt, B. and P. J. Deldin. "Depression and Cardiovascular Disease: Have a Happy Day – Just Smile!" *European Heart Journal* 31, no. 9 (2010): 1065–70.

Quaglio, G., F. Schifano, and F. Lugoboni. "Venlafaxine Dependence in a Patient with a History of Alcohol and Amineptine Misuse." *Addiction* 103, no. 9 (2008): 1572–4.

Rawls, J. *A Theory of Justice*. Cambridge, Mass.: Harvard University Press, 1971.

Repantis, D., P. Schlattmann, O. Laisney, and I. Heuser. "Antidepressants for Neuroenhancement in Healthy Individuals: A Systematic Review." *Poiesis & Praxis: International Journal of Technology Assessment and Ethics of Science* 6, no. 3 (2009): 139–74.

Sen, A. K. *Choice, Welfare and Measurement*. Cambridge, Mass.: Harvard University Press, 1997.

Snyder, T. D. and S. A. Dillow. "Digest of Education Statistics: 2008." NCES 2009-020, National Center for Education Statistics, 2009.

Stevenson, B. and J. Wolfers. "Economic Growth and Subjective Well-being: Reassessing the Easterlin Paradox." NBER Working Paper no. 14282. National Bureau of Economic Research, 2008.

Stockholm International Peace Research Institute. *SIPRI Yearbook 2009: Armaments, Disarmament and International Security*. Oxford: Oxford University Press, 2009.

Uhr, M., A. Tontsch, C. Namendorf, S. Ripke, S. Lucae, M. Ising, T. Dose, M. Ebinger, M. Rosenhagen, M. Kohli, S. Kloiber, D. Salyakina, T. Bettecken, M. Specht, B. Pütz, E. B. Binder, B. Müller-Myhsok, and F. Holsboer. "Polymorphisms in the Drug Transporter Gene ABCB1 Predict Antidepressant Treatment Response in Depression." *Neuron* 57, no. 2 (2008): 203–9.

Index

Happy-People-Pills For All, First Edition. Mark Walker.
© 2013 John Wiley & Sons, Inc. Published 2013 by John Wiley & Sons, Inc.